REPRODUCTIVE ISSUES FOR PERSONS WITH PHYSICAL DISABILITIES

REPRODUCTIVE ISSUES FOR PERSONS WITH PHYSICAL DISABILITIES

edited by

Florence P. Haseltine, Ph.D., M.D.
Center for Population Research
National Institute of Child Health and Human Development
Bethesda, Maryland

Sandra S. Cole, Ph.D.
Department of Physical Medicine and Rehabilitation
University of Michigan Medical Center
Ann Arbor, Michigan

and

David B. Gray, Ph.D.
National Center for Medical Rehabilitation Research
National Institute of Child Health and Human Development
Rockville, Maryland

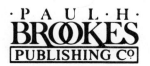

·P·A·U·L·H·
BROOKES
PUBLISHING CO

Baltimore · London · Toronto · Sydney

Paul H. Brookes Publishing Co.
P.O. Box 10624
Baltimore, Maryland 21285-0624

Support of the conference on which this work is based was provided by
the National Institute of Child Health and Human Development of the
United States Public Health Service. The National Association of
Rehabilitation Facilities was also a sponsor of the conference.

"A Guide to Pregnancy, Labor, and Delivery for Women with
Disabilities," by Judith Rogers is adapted from *Mother To Be: A Guide to
Pregnancy and Birth for Women with Disabilities*, by Judith G. Rogers
and Molleen Matsumura, copyright © 1991 by Demos Publications.

Photograph on page 331 by Brooke Hummer is courtesy of Chicago Women
in Philanthropy. Copyright © 1990.

Typeset by The Composing Room of Michigan, Inc., Grand Rapids,
Michigan.
Manufactured in the United States of America by
The Maple Press Company, York, Pennsylvania.

Library of Congress Cataloging-in-Publication Data
Reproductive issues for persons with physical disabilities / edited by
    Florence P. Haseltine, Sandra S. Cole, and David B. Gray.
      p.   cm.
    Includes bibliographical references and index.
    ISBN 1-55766-111-1
    1. Pregnancy in physically handicapped women—Congresses.
2. Physically handicapped—Sexual behavior. 3. Handicapped parents.
I. Haseltine, Florence. II. Cole, Sandra S., 1937–   . III. Gray,
David B.
    [DNLM: 1. Handicapped—congresses. 2. Pregnancy
Complications— congresses. 3. Reproduction—congresses.
WQ 100 R4253]
RG580.C48R47   1993
613.9'5'087—dc20
DNLM/DLC
for Library of Congress   92-48686
                                                        CIP

British Library Cataloguing-in-Publication data are available from the
British Library.

*To all the children
who have or will have
a parent with a disability*

Contents

Contributors

The Editors

Florence P. Haseltine, Ph.D., M.D., Director, Center for Population Research, National Institutes of Health, 9000 Rockville Pike, Bethesda, Maryland 20892. Dr. Haseltine is currently the Director of the Center for Population Research located within the National Institutes of Health. She is responsible for evaluating projects in order to set policy and encourage and highlight research areas in which promising advances are made in reproductive sciences. Her specialties are obstetrics and gynecology. She is a member of many population research-related committees and professional societies.

Sandra S. Cole, Ph.D., Professor, Department of Physical Medicine and Rehabilitation, University of Michigan Hospitals, 1500 East Medical Center Drive, Ann Arbor, Michigan 48109-0050. Dr. Cole is both Professor in the Department of Physical Medicine and Rehabilitation and Director of Human Sexuality Curriculum for medical students at the University of Michigan Medical Center. She is also the Director of the Sexuality Training Center and the Sexuality Evaluation Clinic at University of Michigan Hospitals. She is a Certified Sex Educator and Certified Sex Counselor through the American Association of Sex Educators, Counselors and Therapists (AASECT) and is currently serving on the National Board of Directors of AASECT as President. She has pioneered in the field of sexuality and disability for the past 25 years.

David B. Gray, Ph.D., Acting Deputy Director, National Center for Medical Rehabilitation Research, EPS 450W, 6120 Executive Boulevard, Rockville, Maryland 20852. Dr. Gray is currently the Acting Deputy Director of the recently established National Center for Medical Rehabilitation Research (NCMRR). He was also the Director of the National Institute on Disability and Rehabilitation Research (NIDRR). Dr. Gray is a member of the NIH Committee on

Employees with Disabilities and many professional organizations, including the American Psychological Association, the American Congress of Rehabilitation Medicine, the National Spinal Cord Injury Association, and the Spinal Cord Injury Washington Area.

The Chapter Authors

Marca Bristo, President and Chief Executive Officer, Access Living, 310 South Peoria, Suite 201, Chicago, Illinois 60607. As President and Chief Executive Officer of Access Living, Ms. Bristo is a nationally recognized leader in the disability rights movement. In 1979, she helped found Access Living as Chicago's only nonresidential independent living program for people with disabilities. Bristo directed the agency through its initial period of affiliation with the Rehabilitation Institute of Chicago and into full corporate autonomy in 1987. She is immediate past president of the National Council on Independent Living (NCIL), which she co-founded, and served on the congressionally appointed Task Force on Rights and Empowerment of Americans with Disabilities, which crafted the ADA.

Frances Marks Buck, Ph.D., Director, Women's and Children's Health Focus, Community Medical Center, 2827 Fort Missoula Road, Missoula, Montana 59801. Dr. Buck, a clinical psychologist, has specialized since 1978 in clinical care, program development, community advocacy, and research on persons with disabilities. She has served on the Scientific Advisory Board of the Paralyzed Veterans of America, the Board of Directors, and as 1991–1992 President of the American Association of SCI Psychologists and Social Workers, and the Board of Directors of Montana Mobility Impaired Housing. She conducted seminal research on children of parents with SCI and published and presented numerous papers on parents with disabilities.

Sandra Ann Carson, M.D., Associate Professor, Department of Obstetrics and Gynecology, University of Tennessee, Memphis, 956 Court Avenue, Room D324, Memphis, Tennessee 38163. Dr. Carson is Associate Professor of Obstetrics and Gynecology. A graduate of Northwestern University Medical School, she is board certified in obstetrics and gynecology and reproductive endocrinology. Dr. Carson is an NIH-funded investigator and directs the in-vitro fertilization program at the University of Tennessee, Memphis.

Richard V. Clark, M.D., Ph.D., Associate Professor of Medicine, Division of Endocrinology and Metabolism, Box 3027, Department of

Medicine, Duke University Medical Center, Durham, North Carolina 27710. Dr. Clark received his M.D. degree as well as a Ph.D. degree in cell biology from the University of Washington, Seattle, in 1977. He also completed his internship and residency training in internal medicine at the University of Washington and then did a fellowship in endocrinology and metabolism at the National Institutes of Health. He joined the faculty at Emory University School of Medicine in 1984. His research interests have been in male reproductive endocrinology, particularly evaluation and treatment of male infertility, and assessment of androgen action. He joined the faculty at Duke University Medical Center in endocrinology and metabolism in 1992.

Theodore M. Cole, M.D., Professor and Chairman, Department of Physical Medicine and Rehabilitation, University of Michigan Hospitals, 1500 East Medical Center Drive, Ann Arbor, Michigan 48109-0042. Dr. Cole is Professor and Chairman of the Department of Physical Medicine and Rehabilitation at the University of Michigan. He is a pioneer in the field of sexuality and disability and over the years has published more than 50 publications in medical journals, books, and texts on sexuality, disability, and other aspects of medical rehabilitation. In addition to many other professional activities, he is President-elect of the American Congress of Rehabilitation Medicine and is a member of the Advisory Board of the National Center for Medical Rehabilitation Research of the National Institutes of Health.

Alan B. Copperman, M.D., Department of Obstetrics and Gynecology, Yale University School of Medicine, Box 3333, 333 Cedar Street, New Haven, Connecticut 06510. Dr. Copperman is the Chief Resident of Obstetrics and Gynecology at Yale University School of Medicine. He has written extensively in the area of infertility treatments, hysteroscopy, and adhesions. He is also a Junior Fellow of the American Fertility Society and the American College of Obstetrics and Gynecology.

Nancy M. Crewe, Ph.D., Professor, Michigan State University, College of Education, Erickson Hall, East Lansing, Michigan 48824. Dr. Crewe coordinates the Rehabilitation Counselor Education Program at Michigan State University and is also on faculty in the Department of Physical Medicine and Rehabilitation of the university's College of Osteopathic Medicine. Prior to moving to Michigan in 1987, she was an Associate Professor in the Department of Physical Medicine and Rehabilitation at the University of Minnesota.

Alan H. DeCherney, M.D., Louis E. Phaneuf Professor and Chairman, Department of Obstetrics and Gynecology, New England Medical Center Hospital, Box 324, 750 Washington Street, Boston, Massachusetts 02111. Dr. DeCherney graduated from Temple Medical School in 1967 and completed his residency at University of Pennsylvania Hospital in 1972. This was followed by a tour in the Army in Tokyo, Japan. He then went to Yale University where he rose to become the John Slade Ely Professor of Obstetrics and Gynecology and the Director of the Division of Reproductive Endocrinology. He left Yale in September of 1991 to assume the Professorship and Chairman of Obstetrics and Gynecology at Tufts University School of Medicine.

Craig F. Donatucci, M.D., Fitzsimmons Army Medical Center, Aurora, Colorado 80045-5001. During fellowship under the tutelage of Dr. Tom F. Lue, Dr. Donatucci pursued research interest in both clinical diagnosis and therapy of erectile dysfunction and basic laboratory research into the pathophysiology of impotence. Specific research interests included the role of nerve growth factor in maintenance of erection and the role of the non-adrenergic non-cholinergic neurotransmission in erectile function.

Anne Finger, M.A., Senior Lecturer, Department of English, Wayne State University, Detroit, Michigan 48202. Ms. Finger is the author of a collection of short stories, *Basic Skills,* and an autobiographical essay, "Past Due: A Story of Disability, Pregnancy and Birth." She has won several literary awards and fellowships, most recently the D.H. Lawrence Fellowship.

Jean L. Fourcroy, M.D., Ph.D., Medical Officer, Division of Endocrinology and Metabolic Drug Products, 5600 Fishers Lane, HFD 510, Rockville, Maryland 20857, and Assistant Professor, Department of Surgery Unified Services, University of Health Sciences, Bethesda, Maryland 20814. Dr. Fourcroy is a urologist with primary interest in male reproductive endocrinology and toxicology. She has an appointment at the Walter Reed Army Hospital. As a medical officer at the Food and Drug Administration, she reviews applications for a variety of drugs affecting the male reproductive system.

William H. Graves, Ed.D., C.R.C., Head, Department of Counselor Education and Educational Psychology, Mississippi State University, Mississippi State, Mississippi 39762-5740. Prior to his appointment as Head of the Department of Counselor Education and Educational Psychology, Dr. Graves was the Director of the National Institute on Disability and Rehabilitation Research.

Lauro S. Halstead, M.D., Director, Male SCI Fertility Program, National Rehabilitation Hospital, Clinical Professor, Department of Medicine, Georgetown University School of Medicine, 102 Irving Street, NW, Washington, D.C. 20010. Dr. Halstead is an attending physician on the spinal cord injury service at the National Rehabilitation Hospital and is the Director of the NRH Spinal Cord Injury Male Fertility Program. Together with Dr. S.W.J. Seager, Dr. Halstead helped establish one of the first SCI male fertility programs in the country in 1984 in Houston, Texas.

Denise Sherer Jacobson, M.A., 423 Clifton Street, Oakland, California 94618. Ms. Jacobson is a trained sex and disability peer counselor/educator. She gives presentations to professional, parent, and disability-related groups across the United States on various aspects of disability including independent living, sexuality, and parenting. Her autobiographic articles have appeared in newspapers and literary magazines. She is currently finishing a book on the Jacobsons' adoption of their son, David.

Neil Jacobson, M.B.A., Vice President, Wells Fargo Bank, 423 Clifton Street, Oakland, California 94618. Mr. Jacobson is a Vice President of Wells Fargo Bank responsible for corporate systems architecture. He received his M.B.A. from Golden Gate University in 1984. Mr. Jacobson is the Board President and Co-Founder of the Computer Technologies Program in Berkeley. He also lectures on disability-related topics, such as independent living, parenting, and employment. Above all, he is the proud father of his son, David.

Barry R. Komisaruk, Ph.D., Professor II, Psychobiology, Rutgers, The State University of New Jersey, 101 Warren Street, Newark, New Jersey 07102. Professor Komisaruk discovered the pain-blocking effect of vaginal stimulation in laboratory animals and humans with his colleagues and is currently analyzing the possible applications of this phenomenon to women with spinal cord injury. This research utilizes an interdisciplinary approach, incorporating neuro-physiology, -endocrinology, -pharmacology, -anatomy, and psychophysiology, toward an understanding of the neurotransmitters that mediate the pain and motor inhibitory effects of vaginal stimulation, with the objective of developing novel means of controlling pain and spasticity.

Tom F. Lue, M.D., U-575, Department of Urology, UCSF, University of California—San Francisco, San Francisco, California 94143-0738. Dr. Lue has been involved in the research of neuroanatomy, physiology, pharmacology, and hemodynamics of penile erection

and impotence since the 1980s. He has developed several new diagnostic tests and treatments for patients with erectile impotence and
has helped many patients with physical disabilities to resume sexual intercourse.

John Money, Ph.D., Professor of Medical Psychology, The Johns Hopkins University School of Medicine, LL20 Old Town Office Center,
1235 East Monument Street, Baltimore, Maryland 21202. Dr. Money
has remained at The Johns Hopkins Hospital and School of Medicine where he is Emeritus Professor of Medical Psychology in the
Department of Psychiatry and Behavioral Sciences and Professor of
Pediatrics. He has maintained a full-time career in research, supported by grants from both the public and private sector. His current
research awards are from the National Institute of Child Health and
Human Development (30th year) and from the William T. Grant
Foundation. He has become internationally known for his work in
psychoendocrinology and the new and growing science of developmental sexology.

Mary Ellen Pischke, A.A., Southeastern Minnesota Center for Independent Living, 1306 7th Street, NW, Rochester, Minnesota 55901.
Ms. Mary Ellen Pischke has an Associate of Arts Degree and an
equivalency to a B.A. She is employed at the Southeastern Minnesota Center for Independent Living (SEMCIL). Her neck was broken as
the result of domestic violence in 1977. At the time, she had a
4-year-old daughter and was 2½ months pregnant. After she gave
birth to her second daughter, she had her tubes tied and was divorced. In 1983 she remarried. She had a tubal reversal and had two
sons and two miscarriages. She works full-time for SEMCIL as the
Independent Living Skills Program Coordinator.

Tara Reisner Pischke. Ms. Tara Pischke is 18 years old. She is a
sophomore at Rochester Community College. She intends to work
toward a master's degree in education. Other than going to college,
she works part time for a 19-year-old woman with quadriplegia.

Samuel A. Rhine, M.A., Genetics Consultant, Noble Centers—
Marion County ARC, 2400 North Tibbs Avenue, Indianapolis, Indi-
ana 46222. Mr. Rhine is an educator in the area of prevention of
disabilities and AIDS. He has presented more than 5,500 programs
on the causes and prevention of mental retardation, birth defects,
infant mortality, and AIDS. More than 3,200 of those programs have
been for high school, junior high, and elementary audiences for
more than 2,500,000 students. He has spoken to audiences all over
the United States, Canada, and Europe.

Carol Ann Roberson, M.S.W., Assistant Commissioner, Office of Equal Employment Opportunity, New York City Police Department, One Police Plaza, Room 1204, New York, New York 10038. Ms. Roberson is the former Director of the New York City Mayor's Office for People with Disabilities. She is actively involved in activities regarding issues of women and persons with disabilities. She lives in New York City with her husband and two teenage daughters.

Judith G. Rogers, B.A., OTR, A.C.C.E., Occupational Therapist, 1107 Shevlin Drive, El Cerrito, California 94530. Ms. Rogers has been working with a national nonprofit group, Through the Looking Glass, which has recently received a 3-year grant from NIDRR. Ms. Rogers is currently devising adaptive equipment to facilitate parenting by women with physical disabilities. She is a member of the American Occupational Therapy Association (AOTA), ASPO/Lamaze Association, Association for Pediatric Therapy of California, and the California Occupational Therapy Association.

Aimée B. Schimmel, B.A., Special Assistant to the Acting Deputy Director of the National Center for Medical Rehabilitation Research, 6120 Executive Boulevard, EPS 450W, Bethesda, Maryland 20852. Ms. Schimmel is responsible for evaluating and analyzing information regarding pending and active grants as they relate to the National Center for Medical Rehabilitation Research, National Institute of Child Health and Human Development, and other agencies funding medical rehabilitation and related research. Ms. Schimmel is also a graduate student of The George Washington University in the field of Public Administration.

S.W.J. Seager, M.D., Director of Research, Male SCI Fertility Program, National Rehabilitation Hospital, 102 Irving Street, NW, Washington, DC 20010-2949. Dr. Seager has spent his career studying reproduction in man and animals. He is considered to be a premier authority on obtaining semen by electroejaculation from men with spinal cord injuries and other neurologic impairments. He is continuing research in this field as well as training physicians worldwide in the utility of this technique.

Joe Leigh Simpson, M.D., Faculty Professor and Chairman, Department of Obstetrics and Gynecology, University of Tennessee, Memphis, 853 Jefferson Avenue, Room E102, Memphis, Tennessee 38103. Since 1986, Dr. Simpson has been Faculty Professor and Chairman, Department of Obstetrics and Gynecology, University of Tennessee, Memphis. Prior to that he served as Head, Section of Human Genetics, Northwestern University Medical School (1975–1986). As a reproductive geneticist, he has written extensively on disorders of sexual differentiation and pregnancy genetics diagnosis. He has written six major books, several edited volumes, and nearly 400 chapters and articles.

Marca L. Sipski, M.D., Assistant Professor of Clinical Physical Medicine and Rehabilitation, UMDNJ–New Jersey Medical School, Project Co-Director, Northern New Jersey Spinal Cord Injury System, Associate Medical Director, Kessler Institute for Rehabilitation, 1199 Pleasant Valley Way, West Orange, New Jersey 07052. Dr. Sipski is the Director of SCI Services at Kessler Institute for Rehabilitation and Project Co-Director of the Northern New Jersey Spinal Cord Injury System. Dr. Sipski lectures extensively and is an active researcher in the area of sexuality and spinal cord injury. Her major interest is the impact of the varying degrees and levels of SCI on sexual response.

Colleen Starkloff, B.S.P.T., Coordinator of Education and Training, Paraquad, Inc., (Independent Living Center), 4475 Castleman Avenue, St. Louis, Missouri 63110. Ms. Starkloff was Chief Physical Therapist at St. Joseph Hill Infirmary, Eureka, Missouri, for 2½ years and changed the department's emphasis from maintenance therapy to rehabilitation therapy. In 1976, she joined Paraquad, Inc., the Independent Living Center in St. Louis, Missouri. She has taught courses on independent living as a faculty member of the Washington University School of Occupational Therapy. She has co-authored articles on sexuality and disability and the impact of independent living on family members. Colleen Starkloff and her husband, Max, are the proud parents of three children, all of whom they adopted as infants.

Walter H. Verduyn, M.D., Medical Director, Physical Medicine and Rehabilitation, Covenant Medical Center, 2051 Kimball Avenue, Waterloo, Iowa 50702. Dr. Verduyn is currently the Medical Director of the Covenant Medical Center and a clinical instructor in the family practice department at the University of Iowa Medical School. Dr. Verduyn was also the recipient of a fellowship for spinal cord injuries and brain injuries at the Rocky Mountain Spinal Cord Injury Center, Craig Hospital from 1976 to 1977.

Sandra L. Welner, M.D., Clinical Director, Primary Care Programs for the Disabled, Washington Hospital Center, Washington, D.C. Dr. Welner is Clinical Director, Primary Care Programs for the Disabled for the Washington Hospital Center. Previously, she was an attending physician at Yale University School of Medicine. She is the author of a number of articles in the area of obstetrics and gynecology.

Beverly Whipple, Ph.D., R.N., F.A.A.N., Associate Professor, College of Nursing, Rutgers, The State University of New Jersey, 180 University Avenue, Newark, New Jersey 07102. Dr. Whipple's research focuses mainly on women's health issues and the sexual physiology of women. Additionally, she has quantified noninvasive methods of pain control. She has received a number of research awards and has been elected a Fellow in the American Academy of Nursing and the Society for Scientific Study of Sex.

Glen W. White, Ph.D., Schiefelbusch Institute for Lifespan Studies, 4099 Dole Building, Lawrence, Kansas 66045. Dr. White is currently an Assistant Professor in the HDFL Department at the University of Kansas and is interested in secondary conditions that affect people with physical disabilities.

Nancy L. White, B.S.N., St. Francis Hospital, Department of Rehabilitation Nursing, Topeka, Kansas 66606. Ms. White is currently a staff R.N. working with rehabilitation patients. She is interested in quality assurance in patient care delivery and in the area of self-esteem for newly injured patients. Adoptive issues as related to people with disabilities also is an area of deep interest.

Nathan D. Zasler, M.D., Director, Concussion Care Center of Virginia; Director, Brain Injury Rehabilitation Services, Sheltering Arms Hospital; Co-Director, Richmond Rehabilitation Physicians, Richmond, Virginia 23298. Dr. Zasler, a physiatrist with subspecialty training in brain injury, has served as Chairperson of the National Task Force on Sexuality and Disability with the American Congress of Rehabilitation Medicine for the last 4 years. He has published and spoken extensively on topics relating to sexuality and disability. His area of clinical specialization is in the neuromedical and rehabilitative care of persons with brain injury. Dr. Zasler also serves as Editor-in-Chief of *NeuroRehabilitation: An Interdisciplinary Journal* and is on the editorial boards of several major brain injury rehabilitation journals. He is nationally and internationally known for clinical and research work in his field.

Irving Kenneth Zola, Ph.D., Mortimer Gryzmish Professor of Human Relations, Department of Sociology, Brandeis University, P.O. Box 9110, Waltham, Massachusetts 02254-9110. Professor Zola is the Mortimer Gryzmish Professor of Human Relations at Brandeis University and currently Chair of the Sociology Department. He is a founding member of Greenhouse, a mental health clinic; of the Boston Self-Help center, an advocacy and counseling center for people with disabilities; of the Society for Disability Studies, an academic and professional society; and of Community Works, a greater

Boston progressive alternative to the United Way. Since 1981, he has been publisher, editor, and regular contributor of the *Disability Studies Quarterly* and the author of a dozen books and nearly 200 other publications. In addition, he writes out of his personal experience—polio at 16, an auto accident at 20 (multiple braces), the physical accompaniments of aging (arthritis), post-polio (carpal tunnel), and his genetic heritage (adult-onset diabetes).

Acknowledgments

This volume is a collection of some of the presentations made at a conference on reproductive issues for people with physical disabilities that was sponsored by the National Institute of Child Health and Human Development (NICHD) of the National Institutes of Health (NIH), National Institute on Disability and Rehabilitation Research (NIDRR) of the U.S. Department of Education, and the National Association of Rehabilitation Facilities (NARF). The Center for Population Research (CPR), the Center for Mothers and Children (CRMC), and the new National Center for Medical Rehabilitation Research (NCMRR), which are all components of the NICHD, support the scientific study of the issues presented at the conference and described in this book. The NIDRR has a history of sponsoring applied research and disseminating information on topics related to sexuality and disability. A 1979 conference held by the NIDRR was one of the first efforts to collect information on the topic. NARF is a major source of health service provision for people with disabilities.

Representatives of the agencies listed above worked together in developing the conference topics and selecting speakers. The conference was held in Herndon, Virginia, on March 25–28, 1991. We are extremely grateful for the support of the NARF staff. The conference and the book would not have been possible without the dedication of Ms. Aimée Schimmel of the NCMRR and Marge Perickles of the CPR. Their contributions are much appreciated.

We all wish to recognize and express our appreciation to Carol R. Hollander of Brookes Publishing for her outstanding technical editing, manuscript preparation, and guidance for the book's structure and coherence.

Preface

On a hot Saturday afternoon in August as I sat in my study, the telephone rang. A close friend whose son is a quadriplegic was on the other end asking me to visit a recently injured young man, his parents, and grandparents at a local hospital. As I rolled out the door and was getting into my adapted van, I remembered my own experiences in adapting to a life as an individual with only limited control over my arms and no control below my upper chest (quadriplegic).

When I arrived, the parents and grandparents wanted to speak to me privately. They asked if he would be able to walk again, move his arms and hands, finish school, earn a living, and become independent. Each question was difficult to answer. His parents wanted to know if he should go to a special school or return to his own high school. I encouraged the latter option to promote his adjustment to larger vistas than those available to individuals who are sheltered or shelter themselves from society. They seemed to appreciate that someone with a similar disability had survived and was able to support himself and a family. Yet, something seemed to be on their minds that they could not bring themselves to ask.

Finally, the mother asked me to speak to her son without anyone else in the room. I knew that one of his first questions would be, "Can I have sex and father my own children?" In 1981 the answer was that his chances were very small but that research was being conducted that might make fatherhood possible. He wanted more than fatherhood. He wanted to know if he would be able to feel sexual pleasure. How does one say to a 16-year-boy that not only is the current answer no, but that no one in the research community is asking the questions that might, someday, provide the opportunity for him to have, if not an orgasm in the traditionally defined sense, then an experience of intense sensual and emotional pleasure shared with another human being? "Do you think I'll be able to get a date with a woman without her going out because she pities me?" You will have to develop many personal characteristics, intellectual abilities, and emotional strengths that give you a uniqueness that overshadows your obvious physical differences.

Did I know of any research on adjustment to the sexual aspects of physical disabilities? Once again, the answer had to be that little work was being done, but that there were several books that described the experiences of people with disabilities.

His next question was "What about adopting children?" I thought to myself that this is a determined person. The problems associated with adoption for couples with no disabilities were and continue to be almost insurmountable. He was getting pretty discouraged. "Well, if there is a miracle and I can have my own kids or adopt them, do you think I can be a good father?" I finally had an answer, albeit personal. "Yes," I said. I have three children, each of whom I love and who love me. They have, in some ways, had their lives enriched by having a father who relies on them for assistance but who can give love, time, intellectual stimulation, and even financial assistance to make their lives happy and their dreams realities. He liked that answer. But answers based on the personal experiences do not contribute to a scientific body of knowledge that can determine factors of most importance for the many skills that people with disabilities need to develop if they are to have the opportunity to be parents. I left the hospital with the hope that the next decade would provide a scientific basis for answers to these important questions.

What has happened since 1980 to stimulate the National Institutes of Health to sponsor a conference and a book on the topics so important to this young man and many others with physical disabilities?

"My Left Foot," "Born on the Fourth of July," "Children of a Lesser God," and other movies have brought the sexual needs and desires of people with disabilities to the attention of the American public. Recent books such as *Enabling Romance: A Guide to Love, Sex, and Relationships for the Disabled (and the People Who Care About Them)* and *Sexual Concerns When Illness or Disability Strikes* provide excellent insights into how people with varying disabilities have developed intimate relationships, experienced motherhood, and raised families. On July 26, 1990 the Americans with Disabilities Act was passed by Congress and signed by President Bush. This law provides for the civil rights of people with disabilities in many important aspects of life, including equal employment opportunities, access to buildings and transportation, and protection from discrimination. This legislation has recently been interpreted to apply to the rights of people with disabilities to have equal access to health care (*Sullivan v. Oregon*).

Yet, even with the changes in media portrayals of people with disabilities and positive legislation, the opportunities for people with disabilities to enjoy the pleasures of intimate personal relationships, including sexual activity, pregnancy, and parenting, continue to be restricted both by negative societal attitudes and little scientific knowledge upon which to counter myths, stereotypes, fears, and prejudice. In their book, *Enabling Romance*, Ken Kroll and Erica Levy Klein express the current status as follows:

> There are millions of people with disabilities who eventually discover they can enjoy sexual satisfaction despite their physical limitations. Unfortunately, they often receive little support or information from parents or rehab professionals who may be too uncomfortable to attempt a discussion of this issue. Even in an era of sexual enlightenment, a code of silence seems to envelop the issue of disabilities and sexuality." (p. 20)

Can the problems that are in some ways unique to people with physical disabilities but in many ways shared by people without disabilities be subjected to scientific analysis? Despite some progress by scientists and clinicians in addressing these questions during the 1980s, a chasm remains between the descriptions of personal experiences and the scientific study of the variables that affect people with disabilities in satisfying sexual relationships and raising families. The research paradigms, models, and hypotheses used by most scientists continue to make assumptions that physical disability is an important causal factor in producing emotional, behavioral, and intellectual deficits for the person with the disability and his or her family.

At least a part of the reason for holding a conference on this topic was to bring scientists, clinicians, and service providers face-to-face with people with disabilities who have successfully managed to develop sexual identities, marry, have children, and contribute to their communities in a positive manner. The conference began with a panel of people with disabilities discussing how they struggled with developing the sexual identity and establishing intimate relationships. The comments made by members of this panel provided the conference attendees with a context for their presentations and a vision for future research. Their experiences underscored the need for better understanding the opportunities that allow people with physical disabilities to develop successful coping strategies for general life challenges and for the particular challenges of their physical impairments. For researchers and clinicians who have studied normal human development, the conference and this book open new vistas for applying their expertise and experiences to health and behavior issues of significance to people with physical disabilities. For people with physical disabilities, this book provides basic information on reproductive anatomy and physiology, sexually transmitted diseases, options for prevention of pregnancy, and the probabilities of having children with genetically transmitted conditions. Complications and solutions to problems associated with sexual activity, ejaculation, pregnancy, labor, delivery, and parenthood are also included.

D.B.G.

REFERENCES

Kroll, K., & Klein, E.L (1992). *Enabling romance: A guide to love, sex and relationships for the disabled (and the people who care about them).* New York: Crown Publishers.

Sandowski, C.L. (1989). *Sexual concerns when illness or disability strikes.* Springfield, IL: Charles C Thomas.

Introduction

This book is unusual because it contains personal perspectives and scientific analyses of issues of great importance to people with disabilities, which have rarely been addressed. The biologic capacity for reproduction can be altered with the onset of disability early in life or after maturation. Learning about sexuality and sexual relationships may be different and difficult for people with disabilities for a variety of reasons. Early onset disability may result in isolation that limits access to peers and reduces the chance for spontaneous learning of gender roles, facts about sex, and interactive skills such as communication with the opposite sex through language and touch. Changing from dependency to independence and developing interdependent relationships are all made more difficult by the physical, economic, and societal limitations that accompany disability.

Disabilities that occur after maturation can result in changes in body control, body image, established sexual behaviors, intimate relationships, gender identity, and family roles. Moving from sudden or progressive dependency to independent actions requires an enormous amount of relearning of old skills and the development of a significant number of new skills. Establishing an interdependent life with another and, together or alone, raising a family requires special skills, self-confidence, motivation, resistance to criticism, acceptance of assistance, persistence, and a bit of good luck.

The first section of the book provides an overview of the topics and perspectives contained in this volume. The first chapter, "Sexuality, Disability, and Reproductive Issues Through the Lifespan," is written by two of the pioneers in the field of sexuality and disabilities, Sandra and Theodore Cole. This couple has led efforts to improve the education of professional care providers in the sensitive domain of sexuality and reproduction of individuals with disabilities.

Chapter 2, "Contraceptive Choices: Male and Female," by Florence Haseltine is a summary of available options and their development, as well as a look at what is *not* available, by the Director of the Center of Population Research, National Institutes of Health.

The second section of this book presents issues associated with gender identity, sexuality, pregnancy, and parenting from the vantage point of people with disabilities. Interspersed in the first two sections are vignettes by Irving Kenneth Zola that provide poignant portrayals of what it means to live with disability in a society where concepts of beauty, sexuality, and reproductive worthiness are often based on television advertisements, movies, novels, and even textbooks that emphasize the importance of physical attractiveness.

"I Can Do Anything," by Carol Roberson, is a strong statement by a woman determined to live the full and meaningful life that she chose, committed to husband, family, and career, despite enormous prejudice and disapproval from society at large. This chapter is complemented by Chapter 4, "Rethinking Expectations," by Denise Jacobson, which provides a unique insight into the decision by people with disabilities to have a child by birth or through adoption. Chapter 5, "Parenting with a Disability," by Mary Ellen Pischke, provides another woman's perspective as she describes how she met the challenge of raising four children as a quadriplegic, both as a single parent and with her husband. The transformative power of children is the theme of Chapter 6 by Neil Jacobson, "Learning About Disability from Children," which gives a touching illustration of how the perception of disability can be altered by the love between father and child.

Two detailed accounts of pregnancy and birth by women with physical disabilities, Chapters 7 and 8, are concerned with how physical impairments may complicate pregnancy and delivery. Marca Bristo, a registered nurse who is a paraplegic, provides important insights in her chapter, "Pregnancy and Delivery: A Personal View." Judith Rogers interviewed 36 women with physical disabilities about their pregnancies and deliveries. In Chapter 8, "A Guide to Pregnancy, Labor and Delivery for Women with Disabilities," she reviews their experiences and offers their solutions to the wide range of difficulties that they faced in giving birth.

Two perspectives on the realities of the adoptive process are presented in Chapters 9 and 10. Colleen Starkloff discusses many of the problems associated with adoption that she and her husband experienced—unavailability of infants, high costs, lack of medical insurance coverage, and lack of counseling for both biologic and adoptive parents. Glenn and Nancy White provide an overview of the adoptive process for people with physical disabilities who want to adopt children in their chapter, "The Adoptive Process: Challenges and Opportunities for People with Disabilities." The authors take prospective adoptive parents through the social service and legal review processes and discuss several types of adoption.

The section "Personal Issues" closes with Anne Finger writing on "Mothers with Disabilities." This teacher and writer takes us through the halls of the university where she teaches to illustrate the social roles and expectations associated with women, motherhood, and disability. She raises the question of whether the traditional idea of mothers as providers of care can be reconciled with the almost instinctual response to persons with disabilities as requiring care. This chapter opens our eyes to possibilities through examples of current attitudinal gaps between capabilities and perceived inabilities.

Section III covers the medical research and clinical implications of the range of issues addressed in Section I. Joe Leigh Simpson clearly and comprehensively describes the causal factors associated with disabilities that appear during pregnancy or birth in Chapter 12, "Reproductive Disabilities: An Overview of Congenital Factors." The next three chapters provide clinical research on issues of particular importance to couples and families. In Chapter 13, Nancy Crewe presents her research and that of others on "Spousal Relationships and Disability." The scope of genetic counseling is addressed by Samuel Rhine in Chapter 14, "Genetic Counseling and Evaluation of Recurrence for People with Physical Disabilities." This chapter reviews conditions that can be inherited, the possibilities of transmission of a physical disability, the difference between acquired and genetic risks, the complexity of determining risk, and the variability of expression on genetic disorders. Chapter 15 by Frances Marks Buck, "Parenting by Fathers with Physical Disabilities," counters long-held assumptions about the parenting skills of fathers with research that has been conducted on parenting by men with spinal cord injuries. Here we have a research basis, albeit limited, for the positive parenting experiences described in Section II.

The complex and controversial issues of sexuality and eroticism of people with physical disabilities are introduced by John Money in Chapter 16, "Orgasmology: Relevance for Persons with Physical Disabilities." Thirty years after Dr. Money's research on the phantom orgasms of men with spinal cord injuries, researchers have begun to address some of the fundamental issues in the sexual experiences of men and women with spinal cord injuries. In Chapter 17, "Current Research Trends in Spinal Cord Injuries," Drs. Whipple and Komisaruk challenge the commonly held view that orgasm is not possible for people with spinal cord injury. They have used physiologic measures found to correlate orgasm in women without injury to serve as markers for sexual arousal and orgasm in women with injury. Differences and similarities in female sexual response are detailed in Chapter 18, "The Impact of Spinal Cord Trauma on Female Sexual Response." Marca Sipski provides a scientific framework for studying sexual arousal in women with spinal cord injuries, which includes both physiologic changes and self-reports of sexual pleasure. In Chapter 19, "A Summary of Normal Female Reproductive Physiology," Sandra Ann Carson provides a review of the complex interactions of the central nervous system and the hormonal system in controlling the activities of female reproductive organs.

Chapters 20 and 21 cover nearly neglected areas of clinical services and research. Nathan D. Zasler's investigations, reported in "Sexuality Issues after Traumatic Brain Injury: Clinical and Research Perspectives," describe portions of the neural anatomy that, if damaged, have serious consequences on both sexual relations and sexual performance. He reviews important clinical treatment and counseling considerations. In Chapter 21, Dr. Walter H. Verduyn shares his experience as a practicing obstetrician and the very limited clinical reports of pregnancy, labor, and delivery for women with spinal cord injuries. Despite the limited reports, Dr. Verduyn gives an encouraging picture to women with spinal cord injury who are considering pregnancy as well as helpful management advice to health care professionals.

Fertility, infertility, sexually transmitted diseases, and disability are addressed in Chapters 22–25. Richard V. Clark, in Chapter 22, "Male Reproduction: Fertility," reviews the process of sperm production in males without impairments in the hormonal system or urogenital tract. He further describes three broad categories of male reproductive failures and provides examples of specific syndromes associated with each category. Determination and treatment of male and female infertility are the subject of Chapter 23 authored by Drs. Copperman and DeCherney. Although this chapter focuses on the evaluation and treatment of infertility in people without disabilities, the procedures are applicable to assist couples with disabilities in their efforts to have children. Jean L. Fourcroy in Chapter 24, "Effects of Medications on Fertility in Males with Physical Disabilities with Sexually Transmitted Disease," describes the different types of drugs, indications for use, and possible complications in this population. Sandra L. Welner discusses the causes and effects of several common sexually transmitted diseases (STDs), and the particular problems of treatment, in women with sexually transmitted disease in Chapter 25, "Management Approaches to Sexually Transmitted Disease in Women with Disabilities."

Sexual dysfunction in males with disabilities and treatment options are sensitively detailed in Chapter 26, "Pathophysiology of Sexual Dysfunction in Males with Physical Disabilities," by Drs. Craig F. Donatucci and Tom F. Lue. Chapter 27, "Electroejaculation and its Techniques in Males with Neurologic Impairments," by Lauro S. Halstead and S.W.J. Seager recounts the pioneering efforts of these two clinicians to allow men with neurologic impairment to reverse ejaculatory failure in order to father children. The substantial progress in this process is described in terms of improved techniques, increased number of facilities, and number of successful pregnancies.

The fourth and final section of this book addresses future directions and needs that have been raised by the authors and issues of the preceding chapters. Dr. William Graves, former director of the National Institute on Disability and Rehabilitation Research (NIDRR) of the U.S. Department of Education, reviews the research accomplishments, and he outlines the need for further research in three areas: sexuality, reproduction, and parenting and schooling in Chapter 28, "Future Directions in Research and Training in Reproductive Issues for Persons with Physical Disabilities." Chapter 29, "Future Directions for Research on Reproductive Issues for People with Physical Disabilities," by David B. Gray and Aimée B. Schimmel, sets forth research issues and directions in this field.

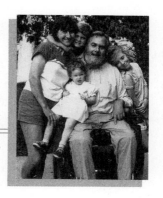

I

OVERVIEW

1

Sexuality, Disability, and Reproductive Issues Through the Lifespan

Sandra S. Cole
and Theodore M. Cole

The decade of the 1990s presents an opportunity for America to reflect on the progress that has been made in services, attitudes, and opportunities for people with disabilities. In her book, *Sex, Society and the Disabled*, Robinault (1978) reminds us that Margaret Mead said, "The character of a culture is judged by the way it treats its disabled." In the United States we are now implementing the Americans with Disabilities Act (ADA), and Margaret Mead would be pleased to judge our culture by our commitment to the ADA.

Biology is the determinant of anatomic sex. It is not the determinant of behavioral sex, and the primate learns sexual behavior. More is needed than biology alone—education influences the final product of sexual health. However, in animals, sexual behavior is determined neurochemically. It is related to reproduction, which is its final intent. In humans, reproduction and sexual behavior are not synonymous. Men and women must learn not only about sexuality, but they must also learn about sexual relationships. Add to this the need to learn about love, and it becomes apparent that both the tasks and the rewards become complex. Beyond sexual love is the more generic love for humankind, a noncoital love involving personal interaction and charm.

Historically, disability in the Western world has a grisly past. In early cultures, an imperfect child was usually killed. In the Middle Ages, such a child was tolerated but was the object of ridicule or fear. Court jesters were sometimes the adult products of birth defects. By the time of the Renaissance, many people with disabilities could look forward to living out their adult lives in asylums.

It was not until the 18th century that the first "modern care" for people with disabilities was begun, in Switzerland. In the 19th century, the first glimmers of education and scientific inquiry into physical disabilities and mental retardation were seen.

By the middle of the 20th century, what has come to be known as modern rehabilitation first appeared. It was the by-product of a society sympathetic toward survivors of military encounters. Now at the close of the 20th century, we are just beginning to demonstrate our concerns for personhood, body image, and human sexuality as a part of rehabilitation (Robinault, 1978).

AN OVERVIEW

Sexuality and reproductive issues encountered by people with physical disabilities during early childhood, adolescence, and early reproductive years are likely to be different from those that people without disabilities experience. Earlier years (infancy) and later years (adult reproductive years) have many similarities for both groups.

It is most convenient to think about these issues from four points of view: 1) sexuality and developmental disabilities, 2) sexuality and acquired disabilities, 3) reproductive issues, and 4) issues pertaining to the aging process.

Early onset disabilities are likely to affect sexual development in terms of gender roles, the language of sex, privacy, self-exploration, sex education, and personal learning. Socialization experiences in early childhood give direction and meaning to adult sexuality. Examples of medical correlates include musculoskeletal disabilities and neurogenic impairments that can affect fertility and sexual options (Hanks & Poplin, 1981).

Disabilities that are acquired after sexual maturity may affect these same areas, but in different ways. Gender roles may become blurred, past sexual patterns of activity may impede creativity needed after disability, and medical experiences may have a desexualizing effect upon self-esteem and libido. Birth control, sexually transmitted diseases, pregnancy, reproduction, and parenting present similar concerns for early onset and adult onset disabilities.

Individuals with and without disabilities have the same rights to information, services, and to health service providers with adequate knowledge, sensitivity, and experience in areas of sexual development. Self-empowerment, life skills, parenting, and medical concerns are common to everyone, but these are issues that may need special attention in individuals with physical disabilities. As individuals mature, new problems may be added to underlying disability issues: for example, further confusion of gender role, stigma, need for more adaptive equipment, societal expectations of the aging adult, and the anticipated transition from health to illness (Frank, 1988; Goffman, 1963).

DEVELOPMENTAL ISSUES

Gender

As children grow, a tremendous focus of energy and instruction, both from the individual and society, is on the careful preparation and development of the gender role of female or male. Much of the childhood experience lays the foundation for the masculinity and femininity of personalities and relationships with others. It must be recognized that the presence of a physical disability influences and in some ways may limit the development of psychosexual/social maturity.

It is reasonable to assume that parents, in anticipation of the birth of a child, have fantasies and dreams of what their "perfect little child" will be as a man or a woman. Needless to say, parents are generally not prepared for the birth of a child with a disability, and, although they can learn to understand and work with the presence of a disability, many of their dreams, plans, and preparations for the child and for the family will be altered (Darling, 1988; Shapiro, 1983).

Privacy

In the early years when children first demonstrate independence and curiosity, including curiosity about themselves and their sexual bodies, the child with a disability probably experiences some alteration in natural opportunities for privacy. He or she may be more closely observed or supervised by family or caregivers and therefore less able to be spontaneous and private with sexual curiosity than a typically developing child. This lack of privacy can affect a child's perception of his or her body, its function, and personal boundaries regarding appropriate or inappropriate touch. Most learning in children is

done spontaneously and includes a great deal of physical involvement with other children, adults, and with the environment—
physical involvement being a catalyst to learning. Spontaneity is
dramatically affected and can be severely limited by the presence of
a disability (e.g., affecting vision, mobility, speech and/or hearing)
(Cole & Cole, 1990).

Language and Communication Skills

During these years, children are simultaneously gaining language
skills: first, recognizing language; second, gaining cognition; and
third, developing individual skills to communicate with parents,
family, and the environment. During these early years, children are
also obtaining the "language of sex," learning terms and phrases for
body parts and behaviors, and striving to gain an understanding of
word usage in expressing thoughts and feelings about sex and sexuality. Their efforts sometimes range from embarrassing and silly to
dramatic. This phase is a time for adults and parents to provide
children with accurate language for body parts and their functions,
appropriate and accurate sex education, in addition to the usual
private and personal words, names, and sexual expressions used
within the family.

It is helpful for all children, including the child with a disability,
to know correct words, their usage, and to be able to express him- or
herself appropriately regarding sexual matters. This knowledge and
ability increases the child's self-confidence and self-esteem and can
be a contributing factor in prevention of sexual abuse, molestation,
or exploitation. Increased knowledge, awareness, and language confidence can help the child to recognize inappropriate behavior,
abuse, or violence that may be imposed on him or her, since persons
with disabilities are particularly vulnerable to sexual perpetrators
(Cole, 1986; Sobsey & Varnhagen, 1988).

Many common expletives in adult language make reference to
sexual activities. A child very likely will have heard such "swearing"
and, most naturally, tries to repeat those words to emulate adult
behavior, even if the words are not understood. This spontaneous
behavior of children frequently generates a startled reaction from
adults and can sometimes result in an immediate opportunity to
provide sex education, helping the child to distinguish appropriate
and inappropriate language and social situations. (Unfortunately,
occasionally the response from an adult is to admonish and punish
the child.) A child with a disability may be quite insulated from
having these spontaneous experiences. For children with disabilities, particularly those who have limited mobility, it is entirely

possible that a part of their development may be influenced by isolation or limited access to peers, and that they may not have had many opportunities to explore and learn about life and its events with their peers. As children with disabilities get older, these life experience omissions become more evident and they may experience social handicaps because of their lack of awareness or understanding of society and the behaviors of the adult world. Since most information about sex is learned quietly, covertly, and is greatly and dramatically influenced by peers and the media, children with disabilities may experience distinct limitations in knowledge and communication about sex education and sexual behavior (Robinault, 1978).

Touch

Touch is a major element in human development and has a powerful effect on all individuals. Infants and children first learn feelings of security, intimacy, and bonding through touch. Love and affection are expressed through touch and language. Children with physical disabilities have additional touch experiences that relate to medical care procedures or to assistance with activities of daily living (ADL).

Children with physical disabilities may require specific assistance with movement or positioning and may require apparatus or equipment to facilitate ambulation and mobility. As a result, they may experience a profound difference between being handled for management and health care purposes and being touched and held for tender and loving purposes. Many children with disabilities experience far more "handling" then tender loving caresses. Similarly, having a disability that requires medical attention presents the possibility of more public nudity than that experienced by a typical child. Having one's body examined and impersonally handled by health care providers often involves this type of physical exposure, and this type of touch most often is not negotiated with the child by health care providers. It is a common experience for individuals with disabilities to have medical procedures, examinations, and inquiries made by health care providers who touch their bodies for purposes of examination but who neglect to be sensitive to this intrusion. Any effort to acknowledge and negotiate personal boundaries of touch is generally overlooked, and the implications of being touched by strangers usually are left unresolved. Obviously, vulnerability to exploitation, misinterpretation, or misinformation is increased with these situations.

Such behavior is common, although inappropriate, in the health care professions. For example, a child with an orthopedic condition may have experienced many examinations that take place with five or more members of a health care team in attendance. In addition, the procedures may be videotaped and the child may be wearing only underpants during the examination. Vulnerability during pubescent years when children are naturally modest, particularly as they experience genital development, is heightened. Perhaps one of the most important lessons for professionals in health care to learn is to respect the individuality, personal dignity, and privacy of patients, something that is not often demonstrated in public examinations in amphitheaters or lecture halls.

When boundaries of appropriate touch are not clear, a child with a disability may not learn to distinguish between appropriate and inappropriate touch and may not have a healthy understanding of the subtleties between public and private nudity and public and private sexual behavior. For some children, especially in institutions, inappropriate touch may have been the only form of affection they have received, and, therefore, their ability to distinguish appropriateness has been impaired. It is well known that health care providers are not infrequently the abusers of persons with disabilities (Griffith, Cole, & Cole, 1990; Sobsey & Varnhagen, 1988).

These issues add to the well-established societal fact that adults handle and interact differently with male and female children (Allgeier & Allgeier, 1991). Adults tend to be more aggressive and physically firm in the way boys are handled in daily activities. Girls are more frequently stroked and caressed, spoken to softly, and handled gently. With all children, society begins to shape the gender roles of masculine and feminine from infancy. A child with a disability may experience additional limitations by being unable to participate fully in his or her expected and implied gender role (Gordon, 1975).

Self-Exploration

In early childhood, self-exploration of genitals is a natural activity. Male genitals are exposed, available, conspicuous, and of great interest to the little boy. Female genitals are hidden, less conspicuous, and much more mysterious and difficult to access for the little girl. For boys who are easily able to handle their own genitals, there is a direct opportunity to touch and stimulate their penises. Girls experience a more diffuse and sensual kind of touch in sexual expression, through caressing and stroking, as their genitals are hidden and more obscure. These distinguishing sexual aspects of masculinity and femininity are carried into adult sexual roles, each role having been developed and refined through puberty and adolescence. Some children with disabilities may have difficulty reaching and touching their own genitals. They also may lack the ability to experience touch sensation in their genitals. They may not directly experience their whole bodies, particularly if there is sensory loss and no feeling in some parts of their bodies. The spontaneous, curious, and innocent ways in which children learn about their bodies through touch may be less prevalent in the child with a disability than in typical peers, either through personal sensory limitations or through limitations such as lack of privacy, the need for assistance, and being discouraged in these activities by adults or by an environment controlled by adults (i.e., an institution).

The situations that have been described indicate the specific need for accurate and comprehensive sex education and gender role preparation for children with disabilities. Society must be more diligent in providing opportunities for children with early onset disabilities to acquire knowledge about themselves as sexual individuals, about sexual mores in the culture, and about the informal world of sex that their nondisabled peers more easily access. Toward that end, parents and educational systems are encouraged to provide structured sex education and to help children with disabilities to obtain accurate information about sexual health and to form positive role models for themselves.

Adolescence

During adolescence, the most common means of learning about sex is through private, informal, and perhaps secret opportunities alone or with others to rehearse the roles of a sexual man or woman. The need for opportunities for sexual rehearsal cannot be overemphasized, as it is during these occasions that adolescents begin to sort out the many mixed messages they have learned about sex and sexuality (Money, 1986). There are dramatic changes in their bodies as secondary sex characteristics begin to develop. It is a time for practicing and refining one's masculinity or femininity, and, similarly, it is during this time that the young adolescent boy and girl will begin to talk openly with peers about matters of sexual development, behavior, and desires. They will practice relating to peers and to the opposite gender in sexual ways and will enter into the dramatic, sensuous, and momentous experiences of rehearsing their adult roles (Gordon & Gordon, 1983).

As many adults recall, some of the most significant memories of adolescent sexual development were of those events that occurred privately and unobserved. These opportunities of spontaneous learning may not be available to adolescents with disabilities, who often lack easy accessibility to other adolescents. Dynamics change considerably if, as a teen, one has to be catheterized, transferred into an electric wheelchair, assisted into a van, and delivered to a friend's home or public event where further assistance is needed to get into the building. At the end of the event, all of the maintenance activities are repeated in reverse. Spontaneity and social experiences and risk-taking are inhibited in these circumstances. Women who experience a disability before adolescence report their first social and sexual experiences later than their peers for these reasons (Rousso, 1988).

Society has a tendency to reinforce the dependency of children and young adults with disabilities. They are frequently infantilized in their relationships and communications with adults. A child may quickly learn that he or she is perceived and treated as helpless or less able, and this may actually facilitate the development of a "helpless individual" or "learned helplessness" (Romeis, 1983).

The pubescent child with a disability can be at risk for stigmatization by an insensitive, uncaring, and ignorant able-bodied society. At a time when conspicuousness and vulnerability is at its peak in boys and girls, the presence of a disability can further compound the difficulty of natural sexual and social development. The young person may have had so little opportunity to spontaneously interact with peers that he or she may not have the ability to develop the social skills of adolescence so necessary to carry out the culturally expected roles of male and female.

Perfection/Body Image

Society places enormous positive value and emphasis on having a perfect body. This message is taught and reinforced in the early years by the presence of role models with perfect bodies and by the lack of role models with disabilities. Advertising and media rarely show a person with a disability. By the time a child acquires language, he or she has already learned that to be disabled is to be different, imperfect, and perhaps unacceptable (Fine & Asch, 1985). To be imperfect is to be asexual and anonymous or overlooked in the sexual spectrum of adult life. The continuing emphasis on the healthy and physically fit adult (who must also achieve a perfect body) is a concrete message learned repeatedly from early childhood through media and advertising. This is often a further assault on the vulnerability of self-esteem for all people without perfect bodies, increasingly reinforced for persons with disabilities (Bogdan, Biklen, Shapiro, & Spelkoman, 1982; Brolley & Anderson, 1986; Ruffner, 1984).

Social Opportunities

Social opportunities for adolescents to interact with peers assist young adults to gain self-esteem. Clothing and fashion, music and the media, community activities, social events, and school experiences are major contributors to gender development at this age. The technical aspects of having physical access to settings where social events occur are often taken for granted by the nondisabled population. These years are times for intense peer interaction, communication, and learning by watching, doing, and rehearsing. Parental influence and values are challenged during these years and often are replaced by peer and media influences. Each adolescent matures at a different rate, but, all in all, these years are extremely full of sexual and sensual overtones, messages, and activities for those who can access them.

The sexual messages in the media about perfection and the artificiality of adult life as presented on television and in magazines tend to be one-dimensional and value-laden and provide few opportunities for the adolescent to discuss and clarify such values and their implications. These aspects of sexual socialization strongly shape and influence the emerging adult (Blackwell-Stratton, Breslin, Mayerson, & Bailey, 1988). It is entirely possible that the adolescent with a disability may have to be a spectator on the sidelines rather than a participant in exciting and demanding experiences of social-sexual development.

Socialization opportunities are essential to growth and development. If the process is healthy, essential self-esteem is achieved through daily activities, social events, and by wearing particular clothing and observing contemporary fashions. It is assumed that the child has access to settings in which these events occur. For most children, the setting does not limit them to the role of spectator but allows active participation and peer interaction. The child with a physical disability may have a more passive than active role, and learning may result more from reading and watching than from doing and experiencing.

Medical Issues

More and more, medical care includes educating the individual and the family about physical, emotional, and behavioral aspects of the disability. Even so, education is frequently presented from the perspective of the health practitioner and may be more technical than useful to the individual and family (Biklen, 1988).

Issues that should be included in patient education are mobility limitations, weakness and fatigue, management of spasticity, and adaptation to somatosensory and perceptual dysfunctions (e.g., loss of vision, hearing, smell, or touch). This material is always best presented in a nonjudgmental fashion, while the educator helps to broaden the individual's and family's concept of human diversity (Cole & Cole, 1990).

In terms of sexuality, it is advisable to avoid a narrowly defined concept of sexuality (e.g., coitus and reproductive physiology). It is useful to include information that helps the adolescent or adult prepare for sexual fantasies and activities. Avoiding unwanted pregnancy and sexually transmitted diseases would be high on the list of desirable topics to be taught. It is all too possible that an individual with a physical disability may have alterations of body functions that interfere with the timely and accurate recognition of symptoms of sexually transmitted diseases.

Inherent in this more modern approach to health care is the assumption that the physician and other health professionals are educated and knowledgeable, both about human sexuality and the individual and the specific disability (Sandowski, 1989). It is pleasing to see that some medical examination rooms incorporate examining techniques and equipment that are user-friendly to the "disabled customer." The paraplegic woman will readily attest to the awkward, if not embarrassing, experience of being subjected to a pelvic examination that is carried out on a traditional and inaccessible examining table—too high for transfers, too narrow for safety, and with stirrups that require leg positions that may be impossible (Ferreyra & Hughes, 1982).

ISSUES CONCERNING ACQUIRED DISABILITIES

Disabilities acquired in early adulthood after maturation may most specifically affect the established and well-developed sense of masculine or feminine identity of the individual. In fact, the elaborate preparations for masculine and feminine roles of individuals are interrupted by the onset of the disability. Life plans, goals, dreams, and ideals are significantly challenged and perhaps changed by the onset of disability. The individual will most likely experience grieving, not only for specific body changes and losses, but also regarding the trauma of having one's private dreams altered, including one's sexual identification as a man or woman.

Stable and Progressive Disabilities

A disability acquired as an adult may be characterized as stable (e.g., a spinal cord injury) or progressive (e.g., multiple sclerosis). There are differences between these types of disabilities. Although the trauma of an acquired disability is undeniable, once the disability is stabilized, an individual can proceed with organizing his or her life and achieving some semblance of control, with adaptation.

It is more complicated, however, to experience a progressive disability, because it is hard to predict the course medically and physically. It is therefore difficult to be confident about being in charge or in control of daily living, spontaneity, and planning for the future. When individuals are in the stages of dating or planning a family, these uncertainties may complicate the usual challenges of relationships and family living.

Through the rich use of memory and the creative use of fantasy, much pleasure can be retained from previous sexual experiences of individuals who have acquired disabilities in adult life. Sensuality can be enhanced through memory and retained throughout various sexual pleasures and activities, even with physical changes or limitations. With some disabilities, intimate behaviors and preferred sexual positions may have to be changed or adapted. However, severe physical losses (e.g., for a male with spinal cord injury) often cause distinct and serious concerns about fertility and the ability to be a parent, in addition to general and obvious concerns about erectile dysfunction and being accepted by society as a "real" man or woman (Mooney, Cole, & Chilgren, 1975; Neistadt & Freda, 1987; Rabin, 1980; Sha'ked, 1981).

Partners of persons with disabilities may experience the dual roles of personal care assistants and of intimate partners. These challenges can create feelings of conflict for both the partner and the person with the disability and may contribute to stress in the relationship. Efforts must be taken by the health care worker to be sensitive to these situational dilemmas and to assist in creative problem-solving recommendations (Griffith et al., 1990).

Persons socialized in contemporary American culture are surrounded by traditional societal messages about parenting and disability (Hahn, 1981). It is imperative that health care practitioners avoid falling into the trap of stereotypical responses of pity, avoidance, infantilization, and excessive attention to persons with disabilities. Independence, personal esteem, positive body image, and positive sex messages should be emphasized. Silence from the medical community concerning disability, sexuality, and reproductive issues relays the stronger message of rejection and repression and gives the impression that parenting is not to be considered. This approach is not helpful.

GENERAL MEDICAL CARE

Men and women with acquired disabilities frequently avoid general medical care. The reason commonly given is that they believe that physicians providing general health care are not sensitive to the specific urologic and gynecologic needs and conditions of a person with a disability. Women who have disabilities often find that their gynecologist is not trained in alternative methods of conducting a pelvic examination on women with a variety of physical limitations. Many health care facilities and offices are not even accessible for the individual with a disability.

Among the general population, it is well established that sexual exploitation occurs in one out of three females and one out of seven males before they reach adulthood (Finklehor, 1979). The statistics are even more grave among those with disabilities (Mullan & Cole, 1991; Sobsey & Varnhagen, 1988). Early research has indicated that men and women with disabilities are more frequently sexually exploited than nondisabled persons and that it is almost always done by someone known to the individual. As is the case with all sexual exploitation, the psychological effect can be traumatic, and, when the trauma experienced is compounded by a disability and a lack of sex education or healthy sexual experiences, we can only assume that understanding and concerns about sexuality and confidence about one's sexual self-esteem are dramatically affected.

Certainly, there is great recognition that particular medical attention should be paid to persons with disabilities, not only to be observant to clues or indications of sexual abuse, but also for opportunities to provide information about birth control and the prevention of sexually transmitted diseases.

Consistent with the general lack of sex education available to people with disabilities, there is also an equal lack of knowledge regarding specific reproductive technology and birth control options. The sensitive clinician provides pertinent and accurate education and information (Neistadt & Freda, 1987). Such a clinician increases sexual knowledge, personal skills, and self-confidence regarding sexual health.

Sexually Transmitted Diseases

An important consideration in adolescent and adult sexual experiences is the threat to health and fertility from acquiring sexually transmitted diseases (STDs). Accurate and explicit information regarding the prevention of STDs, including AIDS, must be available to all children and adults in our society.

Of particular concern are persons with disabilities, who may lack basic sex information and education that make them more vulnerable for acquiring these diseases. Specific recommendations for STDs and pregnancy prevention must include the use of latex dental dams and of condoms that contain nonoxynol-9. Information about the identification of symptoms and management of various STDs should be as available to individuals with disabilities as it is to others. This requires deliberate efforts by health practitioners.

Options

Just as artificiality and awkwardness are recognized by nondisabled individuals as an occasional accompaniment to sexual activities, they are also recognized by persons with disabilities. The difference is more one of quantity than quality. However, technology can be helpful for all people. A sizable portion of the nondisabled population has found that sexual diversity and adaptation can be welcome in the bedroom. So, too, people with disabilities can find that technology can be of assistance in sexual activities as it is with other activities of daily living. Surgery has contributed to the advances in technology affecting sexuality (e.g., breast enhancement, penile prosthesis). The rehabilitation practitioner or other professional should supplement the technology with information to facilitate its use. Insights into sexual kinesiology or "the athletics of sex" can be as helpful as the technology itself. Thus, the practitioner assists the person with a disability in coping with pain, fatigue, or spasticity as they affect sexual activity.

Ten percent of the population in the United States has a homosexual orientation (Kinsey, Pomeroy, & Martin, 1948; Reinisch, 1990). This should be kept in mind, so that the information and technology provided does not burden the recipient with the need for "gender translation." All medical care should be extended nonjudgmentally (Moses & Hawkins, 1982).

Physical disabilities that produce sexual dysfunctions or concerns are seen in everyday medical practice. Most practitioners encounter a patient every day with neurotrauma, skeletal disease, cardiopulmonary disabilities, metabolic diseases, dermatologic disorders, pain, malignancy, or sensory disturbances, any one of which can and usually does affect sexuality in major or minor ways.

SPECIFIC REPRODUCTIVE ISSUES AND OPTIONS

Basic reproductive concerns for men and women in the general population are also of concern for the person with a disability and, in
addition, specific topics require particular attention.

Family Planning

Medical advice may facilitate pregnancy and the activities of preparing for pregnancy. Spontaneity of intimacy must also be considered.
A woman who is beginning intimacy with a disabled man may wish
to consider the gender role into which she has been socialized. She
may be well advised to be assertive and playful and to take greater
initiative. If her partner is paralyzed and cannot initiate physical
activities, it may no longer be sufficient for her simply to "not say
no."

In the area of family planning, there must be more linkages
between those who provide these services and the rehabilitation
professionals who understand and work with the problems imposed
by physical disabilities. So, too, medical information needs to be
tailored to a more diverse population that includes people with
physical disabilities. Research in this area is not abundant. Information for the public is not generally available, and many practitioners
are unprepared to think about issues of fertility, conception, pregnancy, delivery, or even the monthly occurrence of menstruation for
women with physical disabilities (Miller & Morgan, 1980; Neistadt
& Freda, 1987).

In discussing reproductive options and potentials with an individual with a disability, one must assess whether the disability influences fertility and fertility options (Neistadt & Freda, 1987). Evaluation must include whether genital sensation and genital function
are affected. An example would be a male with a spinal cord injury
who is unable to ejaculate. This is a case in which a urologist,
specially trained in electroejaculation procedures, would be instrumental in assisting with the evacuation and obtaining of sperm for
insemination.

Some birth control methods may be contraindicated for women
with specific disabilities. For example, a woman with spinal cord
injury who is unable to feel sensation in her genital area and has
diminished hand function from quadriplegia would not be a candi-
date to insert and use a diaphragm. There may also be unrecognized
and ongoing medical conditions that affect fertility, such as irregular
menses and chronic infection. What reproductive choices might be
available for a woman with a disability? She would need to be evalu-

ated to determine if she could physically carry a fetus to full term once she conceived. If this is contraindicated, it may be important to consider other alternatives for reproduction, perhaps using a female surrogate. Evaluating and recommending the type of delivery suited for a woman with a disability is extremely important for the safety of both mother and child. Many obstetricians are not trained to specialize in pregnancies of women with physical disabilities and should consult physiatrists who can assist in consultation and health care of the patient. The presence of sexually transmitted diseases would need to be identified, as would be necessary for any pregnancy.

Additional Considerations

There are several other considerations related to the ability to reproduce that are not routinely considered but potentially could have a tremendous impact on an individual with a disability and his or her partner.

People with disabilities frequently live on fixed incomes or are medically subsidized in some way. Therefore, money and finances may be limited or strained, which creates limitations on one's ability to socialize, establish relationships, and find partners (Hanks & Poplin, 1981). Does the individual with a disability have life skills that include the ability to parent? Does the possibility exist of someone assisting with parenting tasks? In addition, does the individual with the disability require a personal care assistant or someone to assist with general daily living tasks? What is the person's level of independence? What kinds of reasonable accommodations can be provided?

Social skills, body image, self-esteem, and personal integrity are central to one's ability to enjoy life and to participate in the development of relationships, intimate behavior, and preparation for pregnancy, birthing, and parenting (DeLoach & Greer, 1981).

When medically evaluating individuals for fertility, the potential for substance abuse, the use or abuse of medications and, as mentioned earlier, a routine evaluation for determination of sexually transmitted diseases or other genital disorders must also be assessed. What previous investigation has been done in the form of tests, procedures, and assessment of sexual activities regarding reproduction? Does the individual understand his or her exact situation and options from a medical perspective? If so, then the individual deserves commendation for determination to learn and challenge a rather passive medical system until there are more answers and solutions.

AGING

As we age as sexual individuals, we continue to function in our male and female roles, which have been established since adolescence. We experience normal changes of aging, which can include physical disabilities. These changes affect the flexibility and ease with which we are able to conduct our daily lives. Additions such as wheelchairs, new and unfamiliar devices, apparatus, or equipment, which support the body, increase mobility, or enhance and make safe daily living tasks, can be cumbersome and awkward. Changes such as these can be overwhelming to the individual and his or her sense of self-confidence, dignity, and self-esteem.

We are sexual until our death. However, the gender roles we have carefully created for ourselves can be eroded during the aging process by the realization and personal experience of being slow, being viewed as less important, feeling incapable from time to time, and experiencing a general loss of personal value. These experiences can seriously affect one's confidence and the maintenance of femininity or masculinity. Negative or hesitant reactions from life partners or family members who have become caregivers for the aging individual, health care professionals who do not understand geriatrics, and society in general can increase the vulnerability of one's self-esteem.

The transition from being a healthy adult to one who experiences traumatic or chronic illness or disability can be difficult for many (Trieschmann, 1987). Elderly individuals become keenly aware of their frailties. Inaccurately and inappropriately, society may increase the potential for guilt and shame, which it associates with aspects of aging. This can be directly experienced, for example, by a woman who is incontinent and vulnerable to conspicuous embarrassment in social situations, or by the man who experiences erectile difficulties due to aging or the presence of disease.

It is time that new horizons be recognized and that we cease to add further societal burdens on individuals experiencing natural aging difficulties. Medical and societal recognition of sexual health, sexual development, gender socialization, and fertility issues pertaining to persons with disabilities will serve to pave the way for all individuals to age with sexual dignity.

There has been progressive recognition of the need to liberate people with disabilities who are oppressed. The Rehabilitation Act of 1973 that has been updated and amended is an example of the recognition of the rights of individuals with disabilities. The community of people with disabilities is working together to better state what needs to be addressed by federal legislation. The Americans with Disabilities Act of 1990 (ADA) (PL 101-336) is a civil rights act and an advance for people with disabilities. The ADA does not deal specifically with sexuality, but it does empower the individual.

Sexuality and fertility concerns are natural experiences for persons with disabilities. We cannot artificially separate sexuality from the spectrum of life for anyone.

Civil rights, which are the rallying points of those who are oppressed, include the *right to reproductive information* that is comprehensive and accurate.

REFERENCES

Allgeier, E.R., & Allgeier, A.R. (1991). *Sexual interactions.* Lexington, MA: D.C. Heath.

Biklen, D. (1988). The myth of clinical judgment. *Journal of Social Issues, 44*(1), 127–140.

Blackwell-Stratton, M., Breslin, M.L., Mayerson, A.B., & Bailey, S. (1988). Smashing icons: Disabled women and the disability and women's movements. In M. Fine & A. Asch (Eds.), *Women with disabilities: Essays in psychology, culture, and politics* (pp. 306–333). Philadelphia: Temple University Press.

Bogdan, R., Biklen, D., Shapiro, A., & Spelkoman, D. (1990). The disabled: Media's monster. In M. Nagler (Ed.), *Perspectives in disability* (pp. 138–143). Palo Alto, CA: Health Markets Research.

Brolley, D.Y., & Anderson, S.C. (1990). Advertising and attitudes. In M. Nagler (Ed.), *Perspectives on disability* (pp. 147–151). Palo Alto, CA: Health Markets Research.

Cole, S.S. (1986). Facing the challenges of sexual abuse in persons with disabilities. *Sexuality and Disability, 7*(3/4), 71–89.

Cole, T.M., & Cole, S.S. (1990). Rehabilitation of problems of sexuality in physical disability. In F.J. Kottke, G.K. Stillwell, & J.F. Lehmann (Eds.), *Krusen's handbook of physical medicine and rehabilitation* (pp. 988–1008). Philadelphia: W.B. Saunders.

Darling, R.B. (1988). Parental entrepreneurship: A consumerist response to professional dominance. *Journal of Social Issues, 44*(1), 141–158.

Deloach, C., & Greer, B.G. (1981). The third disabling myth: The asexuality of the disabled. In *Adjustment to severe physical disability: A metamorphosis* (pp. 65–99). New York: McGraw-Hill.

Ferreyra, S., & Hughes, K. (1982). *Table manners: A guide to the pelvic examination for disabled women and health care providers.* Oakland, CA: Sex Education for Disabled People.

Fine, M., & Asch, A. (1985). Disabled women: Sexism without the pedestal. In M.J. Deegan, & N.A. Brooks (Eds.), *Women and disability: The double handicap* (pp. 6–23). New Brunswick, NJ: Transaction Books.

Finklehor, D. (1979). *Sexually victimized children.* New York: Free Press.

Frank, G. (1988). Beyond stigma: Visibility and self-empowerment of persons with congenital limb deficiencies. *Journal of Social Issues, 44*(1), 95–117.

Goffman, E. (1963). *Stigma: Notes on the management of spoiled identity.* Englewood Cliffs, NJ: Prentice-Hall.

Gordon, S. (1975). *Living fully: A guide for young people with a handicap, their parents, their teachers, and professionals.* New York: John Day.

Gordon, S., & Gordon, J. (1983). *Raising a child conservatively in a sexually permissive world.* New York: Simon and Schuster.

Griffith, E.R., Cole, S.S., & Cole, T.M. (1990). Sexuality and sexual dysfunction. In M. Rosenthal, E.R. Griffith, M.R. Bond, & J.D. Miller (Eds.), *Rehabilitation of the adult and child with traumatic brain injury* (pp. 206–225). Philadelphia: F.A. Davis.

Hahn, H. (1981). The social component of sexuality and disability: Some problems and proposals. *Sexuality and Disability, 4*(4), 220–234.

Hanks, M., & Poplin, D. (1981). The sociology of physical disability: A review of literature and some conceptual perspectives. *Deviant Behavior: An Interdisciplinary Journal, 2,* 309–328.

Kinsey, A.C., Pomeroy, W.B., & Martin, C.E. (1948). *Sexual behavior in the human male.* Philadelphia: W.B. Saunders.

Miller, S., & Morgan, M. (1980). Marriage matters: For people with disabilities too. *Sexuality and Disability, 3*(3), 203–212.

Money, J. (1986). *Lovemaps: Clinical concepts of sexual/erotic health and pathology, paraphilia, and gender transposition in childhood, adolescence, and maturity.* New York: Irvington Publishers.

Mooney, T.O., Cole, T.M., & Chilgren, R.A. (1975). *Sexual options for paraplegics and quadriplegics.* Boston: Little, Brown.

Moses, A.E., & Hawkins, R.O., Jr. (1982). *Counseling lesbian women and gay men: A life-issues approach.* St. Louis: C.V. Mosby.

Mullan, P.B., & Cole, S.S. (1991). Health care providers' perceptions of the vulnerability of persons with disabilities: Sociological frameworks and empirical analyses. *Sexuality and Disability, 9*(3), 221–243.

Neistadt, M.E., & Freda, M. (1987). *Choices: A guide to sex counseling with physically disabled adults.* Malabar, FL: Robert E. Krieger Publishing Co.

Rabin, B.J. (1980). *The sensuous wheeler: Sexual adjustment for the spinal cord injured.* San Francisco: Multi Media Resource Center.

Reinisch, J.M. (1990). *The Kinsey Institute new report on sex: What you must know to be sexually literate.* New York: St. Martin's Report.

Robinault, I.P. (1978). *Sex, society, and the disabled.* New York: Harper & Row.

Romeis, J.C. (1990). Alienation as a consequence of disability: Contradictory evidence and its interpretations. In M.Nagler (Ed.), *Perspectives on disability* (pp. 47–57). Palo Alto, CA: Health Markets Research.

Rousso, H. (1988). Daughters with disabilities: Defective women or minority women? In M. Fine & A. Asch (Eds.), *Women with disabilities: Essays in psychology, culture, and politics* (pp. 139–172). Philadelphia: Temple University Press.

Ruffner, R.H. (1984). The invisible issue: Disability in the media. *Rehabilitation Digest, 15*(4).

Sandowski, C.L. (1989). *Sexual concerns when illness or disability strikes.* Springfield, IL: Charles C Thomas.

Sha'ked, A. (Ed.). (1981). *Human sexuality and rehabilitation medicine: Sexual functioning following spinal cord injury.* Baltimore: Williams & Wilkins.

Shapiro, J. (1983). Family reactions and coping strategies in response to the physically ill or handicapped child: A review. *Social Science Medicine, 17*(14), 913–931.

Sobsey, D., & Varnhagen, C. (1988). *Sexual abuse, assault, and exploitation of people with disabilities.* Ottawa: Health and Welfare Canada.

Trieschmann, R.B. (1987). *Aging with a disability.* New York: Demos Publications.

~~~~~~

The Last Goodbye

Irving Kenneth Zola

Your given name was Frances, but I don't remember many people using it. To everyone I knew, you were Fagie. You were my aunt, my mother's younger sister. But no such simple description captures what you mean to me. You were my friend, my confidante, my ally and soon I was going to lose you.

We were being warmed by the late afternoon sun as we sat on the deck. You looked worn out as you lay there in the chaise lounge. To a stranger you might have seemed sunburned, but I knew it was the side effects of the radiation treatment.

I had made you a gin and tonic and sat nearby with a chilled club soda in my hand. We were alone. Lee, my wife, and Paul, your husband, had taken the kids to the beach. Tomorrow you were leaving to go back to the Mainland.

Your breaking of the silence was typical. "Well, smart-ass, it looks as if you've done OK."

"You mean the house . . . yes it's quite . . . ."

"No," you interrupted, "I mean your life."

"Well," I said, "I had lots of help . . . especially from you."

You let this pass and looked into your glass for a few moments. As you raised it to your lips, you added as if in a toast, "Well . . . it's been a long time."

"So it has," I answered, raising my glass in turn. And then I laughed, "Do you remember the time when . . . ?" And so we drifted in and out of memories all afternoon.

Innocence Claimed

Your favorite childhood story had to do with how I always got away with murder. As my mother's younger sister and only 16 years my senior, you were my first and favorite babysitter. While I loved your attention I was not so generous when you bestowed it on others. And one day, in the throes of the "terrible 2s," I showed it. Left alone in the

---

livingroom of your then boyfriend, Doobie, I completely destroyed his portable radio. When the loud crash brought you both in, you gasped, "What happened?" Undaunted, I said, "Doobie did it," pointing my finger directly at the culprit, your boyfriend.

Sleepless Nights

The age of 8 found me temporarily quartered in your apartment. It was June and my family had just moved to Mattapan, a streetcar suburb of Boston. It was too late to transfer to another school and, since we had no car, too far to commute daily. So everyone agreed that I should stay with you for the remaining few weeks of school. With Uncle Paul away in the service, we shared the same bed. I don't know what this did to my incipient sexual fantasies, but it *did* disturb my rest. Some people talk in their sleep; others snore; you back up. In fact, you were so vigorous that I found it necessary to wrap myself around the bedposts lest I fall off. But I never complained, for fear you'd exile me to another room or worse yet send me home. But one night it was no use—with a mighty heave you did it. And there *I* was on the floor, awake and tearful, trying to respond to *your* queries of why *I* was so restless a sleeper.

Sidetracked on the Road to Manhood

As the first grandson to reach Jewish manhood, my Bar Mitzvah was an eagerly awaited and much fussed-over event. You, while proud, were nevertheless determined to bring me down to earth. There I stood on the platform that cold January morning addressing the congregation in very solemn tones about taking my rightful place among Jewish men. Specifically, I was in the process of claiming that I was about to become "a brick in the wall of Judea." For emphasis, I looked down and spoke directly to my mother. You, sitting beside her, promptly crossed your eyes and stuck out your tongue. For your efforts you received a jab in the ribs. I, in turn, delivered the rest of my speech to the clock in the second balcony.

No More Interruptions

After I had polio, the climb up four flights of stairs to my home seemed to take forever. So we devised a system of stops and rests. The first was at your place, reached after traversing the first two outside flights. And there I sat, coffeed, and chatted, till my strength returned. But long after this stopover was necessary, we continued the practice much to the annoyance of my mother. Maybe she was jealous of our closeness. Whatever the reason, she would inevitably yell down the stairs, "Irving! Irving! Are you there? When are you coming up?" One day she reached her limit and yelled down, "Irving! Irving! What's taking you so long? What are you *doing* down there?" You, too, must have reached your limit, for you answered back, "Screwing!" She never interrupted us again.

Lessons Learned

It was clearly in the area of sex that you opened the most taboo areas. While my mother played the role of a classic hysteric, often claiming that she never understood a dirty joke or even the location of erotic zones, you were by contrast quite vivid and charmingly obscene. It was from you I learned about sexuality in general and women's sexuality in particular. And while the terms and framework might be Victorian— as you referred to "the curse," "your monthly friend," and "men's needs"—whatever else you did, you led me into a mysterious world long before the women's movement made that world more public.

The Overacceptance of Irving

Though always my ally and defender, there were some ways in which your acceptance went too far. I know you remember my accident well. Polio at 16 was bad enough, but having to be confined for a year in a cast at the age of 20 was even worse. By now, though I was getting along pretty well on crutches, I made a private decision. Consulting with my orthopedist, we decided that I could get rid of the crutches and use just a cane if I was willing to wear a long leg brace. For months I practiced at school until I finally had it right . . . until I could walk without the crutches and with just the cane. On that Friday, I showed up at your doorstep, walked into your house, and said proudly, "Well, what do you think?"

"About what?" you asked.

"About how I look?" I answered.

"Oh!" you said stepping back so you could survey me more care-fully. "You know how I am about not noticing things," and then added with obvious satisfaction . . . "You've cut your hair differently."

We'll See Who's Not Good Enough!

And then there was the time when I took you aside to tell you that Lee and I had decided to marry several months earlier than planned and that her father seemed quite concerned. You asked but one question, "Is she pregnant?"

"No," I laughed with some embarrassment.

You went on, "It doesn't matter to me . . . I just wanted to know all the facts."

It turned out that "the facts" that upset you the most was my prospective father-in-law's concern about my adequacy as a husband . . . monetarily, emotionally, and physically.

"Don't worry," you said, "I'll take care of him."

But even I was not prepared for the scene that followed. After a serious man-to-man chat at his hotel room, I brought my future father-in-law to meet my aunt.

As we came in the door, I looked at him. He was impeccably suited in a somber gray coat, a trimmed fur collar, and a newly blocked hat upon his head. We rang the bell. And there you were, my Aunt Fagie, in an outfit that would have put Carol Burnett's charwoman to shame. With a towel wrapped around your head, you stood there poker-faced, wearing a moth-eaten terrycloth robe, tied over a set of rolled-up flannel pajamas, with mismatched socks flopping over your slippers, a broom in your hand, and a lit cigarette dangling precariously from your lips.

Clearly taken aback, he stammered, "I'm sorry . . . . I didn't know . . . if we're . . . ."

"Oh, of course not, Felix," you said with a smile and extended your hand, "Please come in," and added in measured tones, "We were expecting you."

The sound of children's voices brought this time to a natural close. Our eyes were filled with tears—of joy, sadness, love, and loss all mixed together. With your hand in mine I tried to speak but the words remained in my head. I think of your leaving in quite selfish terms. Who will I call first to tell my good . . . or bad news? Who will I turn to when there is no place else to go? You are my closest friend, my kindest critic, my strongest support, my longest love. No one will ever replace you. Maybe no one should.

My throat ached from the held-back anguish. "I'll miss you" was all I could croak out.

"I know" was all you said in reply.

The next day you and Uncle Paul left. You stood on the railing of the ferry and waved to all of us on the pier. I heard later that when we were out of view you collapsed. I never saw you again. You died a week later.

2

Contraceptive Choices
Male and Female

Florence P. Haseltine

The ability of people to regulate their fertility is an important factor in their physical and mental well-being. Indeed, many social and health problems are associated with unintended or accidental conception. Studies have shown that children who are wanted are better cared for and have fewer psychological and health problems as they develop than do children whose conceptions are unintended and unwanted. Yet, according to studies from the National Survey of Family Growth (NSFG), over half (53%) of pregnancies are unplanned. This means that pregnancies occurred before the women felt they were ready to have a child or when they did not want any children at all. The NSFG survey found that about 20% of all pregnancies occur while a contraceptive method is being used. (The data cited above are based on unpublished tabulations from the NSFG [1988].) Of the unintended pregnancies, 42% generally end in abortion. For teenagers (women under the age of 20), 40% of pregnancies end in abortion. The survey demonstrates that inadequate contraceptive methods play a role in a large number of induced abortions and that more and better contraceptive methods could greatly reduce the use of abortion as a method of family planning.

CONTRACEPTIVE OPTIONS

Even in this highly sophisticated Western culture, very few contraceptive methods are available to couples. Not only is there a high rate of unplanned pregnancies among people having intercourse, but the contraceptives that are available are unreliable for the population as a whole. Very often, a woman who becomes pregnant even after using a contraceptive thinks that she used the method incorrectly or that she did not understand her cycle very well. It is important for women to understand that they can be absolutely correct in their use of a contraceptive method and still experience a failure.

The difficulties of providing contraceptives for the national population also include physical considerations. At the moment, we are very limited in our selection of contraceptives and in the ability to adapt them to the needs of each person. Contraceptives have not been designed for the unique needs of a person who has a physical disability, and persons with physical disabilities must select a contraceptive method that was not developed with their needs in mind. For example, some methods, such as the diaphragm or cervical cap, require mechanical dexterity and may be impossible for people with certain types of disabilities to handle. The fact that some individuals need an assistant to insert and remove a vaginal mechanical device needs consideration. Furthermore, other methods, such as the birth control pill, may be inappropriate for certain people, such as those subject to thrombophlebitis.

Controlling fertility is a social issue and one that appears to have many anxieties attached to it. These anxieties are often fueled by fears generated by articles and accounts that sensationalize the pitfalls involved in contraception. The ability to control fertility so that people can have—or not have—children when they so choose requires an understanding of the way sex leads to conception. It is important to understand how the contraceptive methods interfere with the ability of the sperm and the egg to fuse.

Barrier Methods

Contraception works by interfering with fertilization, by preventing sperm from coming into contact with an egg. This can be done mechanically by putting a barrier in the vagina that prevents the sperm from entering the uterus. When a sperm barrier method is used by a woman, the device inserted in the vagina is called a diaphragm. The diaphragm is placed over the cervix so that sperm in semen ejaculated from the penis into the vagina cannot penetrate the rubber barrier and enter the uterus. Different forms of diaphragms are available; one variety, the cervical cap, covers only the cervix and does not spread out to cover the entire upper vagina.

To be effective, a diaphragm and similar barrier methods should be used in conjunction with spermicidal creams or jellies, and, if intercourse occurs more than once in 6 hours, the vaginal jelly should be reapplied. The jellies are considered safe and the use of contraceptives has not been shown to be teratogenic. Also, the diaphragm should remain in place for at least 6 hours following intercourse. One of the advantages of using the diaphragm is that spermicidal jellies not only kill sperm but also are effective in killing other microorganisms, thus reducing the likelihood of contracting a sexually transmitted disease such as gonorrhea or chlamydia. A diaphragm does not totally prevent the transmission of disease, but it does help.

Problems that can occur with the diaphragm include the timing of insertion into the vagina so that it does not interfere with intercourse, the difficulty some women have in inserting or removing it (although a partner can help in this process if the woman feels comfortable enough to allow her partner to help), and the skin irritation that it can cause. Sometimes, the skin irritation can become severe enough to cause bladder infections. Cervical caps alleviate some of these problems, although the difficulty with insertion and removal may still be a problem. Allergies to contraceptive jellies used in conjunction with the diaphragm may also occur. Another drawback is that the devices need to be fitted by a medical practitioner, which is costly and time consuming, and contraceptive jellies are expensive. These are the reasons why women may stop using the diaphragm after they have chosen it as a contraceptive method. The most common reasons given for not choosing the diaphragm as a contraceptive method in the first place is because of its inconvenience and because women believe that it may not be available when they need it.

Although the side effects and contraindications to using the diaphragm and jellies are few, their effectiveness is variable. Effectiveness is not only user-dependent but fit-dependent, and, in addition, the size of the vagina changes so much during intercourse that it is difficult to determine an accurate size that accommodates to a vagina that is one size when not aroused and larger during intercourse. The efficacy of this method ranges from 65% to 95%.

Other devices similar to the diaphragm are the cervical cap and the vaginal sponge. The cervical cap is also a barrier method but has the advantage of being smaller and therefore not as apt to press against the vaginal wall and cause discomfort. It is also less likely to cause skin irritation. It is recommended that the cervical cap be removed within 24 hours of insertion. The vaginal sponge, as the name implies, is a polyurethane sponge that is impregnated with the spermicidal agent, nonoxynol-9. The sponge should be well-moistened with water and placed inside the vagina no more than 24 hours before intercourse. It should be left in place for 6 hours following intercourse and can be removed by the string attached to it. The sponge should not remain in the vagina longer than 24 hours because the risk of toxic shock syndrome (TSS) increases after that time. It should also not be used when a woman is menstruating because that increases the incidence of TSS. One problem with the cervical sponge is not a medical side effect, but is a problem with dryness of the vagina. The dryness is caused by the sponge's absorption of water from the vagina immediately after insertion, which can become a practical problem if the couple wants to engage in immediate intercourse.

All of the vaginal devices must be used with care if a woman has had TSS, repeated urinary tract infections, is being treated for a cervical lesion, has recently had cervical surgery, or has just had a pregnancy. Both the diaphragm and the cap have to be individually fitted. Fitting the cervical cap requires more care and attention to exact fit. The sponge can be purchased over the counter of a drug store. Mechanical dexterity is important in being able to use both devices.

The diaphragm and the sponge reduce the risk of common infections, but increase the risk of TSS. Again, the risk of TSS to a single individual is very small, while the lowered risk for infection is great. This is a case of the risk–benefit ratio being dramatically in favor of use.

ORAL CONTRACEPTIVES

The introduction of the "pill," as the birth control pill became known in the early 1960s, changed our thinking about contraceptives and their acceptability. The birth control pill works by interfering with the reproductive cycle in at least three phases needed to promote ovulation, implantation, and fertilization of an oocyte. The pill changes the pituitary pattern of gonadotropin release so that the ovary does not regularly ovulate; it acts on the lining of the uterus so that, even if an oocyte is released and fertilized, there is not a receptive endometrium on which to implant; and it makes the mucus of the cervix inhospitable to the sperm that travel through it into the uterus. The pill is the single most popular method of contraceptive used by nonsterile couples and has been tried by 80% of women in their reproductive years. Ten million women are using the pill at this time in the United States (Mosher & Pratt, 1990).

The first birth control pills have been labeled high-dose pills because the active compounds were administered in doses higher than are needed for contraception. Studies showed that women were at greater risk for cardiovascular side effects. Lowering the dosage has resulted in decreasing thromboemboli, but it is unclear whether the very low-dose pills on the market today do not have some other long-range problem.

There are some absolute contraindications to using the pill; these are thrombophlebitis or thromboembolic disorders, cerebrovascular disorders, heart disease, pregnancy, carcinoma of the breast, and liver tumors. There is no way to know in advance which pill will cause minimal side effects for an individual woman. The only real criterion for the caregiver and the woman is to evaluate the side effects of a specific drug and then to change the medication if it seems to be appropriate.

The pill is administered so that the woman takes the active hormone 21 consecutive days and then takes a placebo, iron, or nothing for the next 7 days. Originally, it was reasoned that women wanted a 28-day cycle so that they would feel "normal" and be reassured that pregnancy had not occurred. Clearly, several assumptions are made. One is that women consider it normal to bleed every month; another is that perpetuating this assumption is desirable. The drug companies even went so far as to develop pills called triphasics. These pills have three different types of combinations in a month in order to mimic the normal hormonal changes. There is no rationale for this type of thinking except as a marketing stunt. Medications are given to change the cycle, not to replicate it.

Chemically, the pill is made up of one or two of the steroidal compounds that are related to hormones that the body produces normally during the menstrual cycle. The hormones are estrogen and progesterone. The natural estrogen molecule is modified to be a more active form of estrogen and, therefore, a smaller dose of the medication is needed. The two compounds currently in use in the U.S. are ethinyl estradiol (EE) and mestranol. EE is the most active estrogen in use in this country, and mestranol is inactive until it is converted by the liver to become EE. Thus, the two forms of estrogen are basically the same. However, the dosage can be confusing, since the mestranol is converted to EE. One of the problems with the medication containing the lower estrogen dose is that the pill is no longer 100% effective. The overall efficacy for the birth control pill is 95%–99%.

The amounts and kinds of estrogen in the pills are really quite straightforward compared to the types of progesterones that pills contain. There are six different types of progestational agents in pills: norethindrone, norethindrone acetate, ethynodiol diacetate, norgestrel, levonorgestrel and norethynodrel. The effectiveness of different progesterones is determined by the ability to prevent the onset of endometrial bleeding. The activities are so different between the medications that they cannot be evaluated simply on the basis of dosage. Dosage of a pill with an estrogen and a progesterone component refers to the strength of the estrogen, not the progestin. Also, progestins vary in the amount of estrogenic activity that they have and in their androgenic or anti-estrogenic effects. The noticeable estrogenic effects are increased breast swelling and some fluid retention. Androgenic effects include acne and hirsutism, as well as changes in the blood lipid patterns to a lower HDL/LDL pattern that is more characteristic of men than women. Estrogenic or androgenic effects are mediated not only by the drug but also by the extent of suppression of the woman's ovaries, adipose tissue, and adrenal glands and the interaction with the pill steroids. The progesterone with a high level of estrogenic component but no androgenic component is norethynodrel. The other extreme is the compound norethindrone acetate, which has little estrogenic activity but is very androgenic.

Birth control pills include inserts that list the many possible side effects, but they do not provide any indication of how common or rare any one of these side effects might be. The estrogenic effects attributed to use of the pill are classically nausea, breast tenderness with increase in size, fluid retention, headaches, thromboembolic complications, pulmonary emboli, cerebrovascular accidents, hepatocellular adenomas, hepatocellular cancer, telangiectasias, and growth of fibroids. The complications that are associated with the progesterone side effects are increased appetite and weight gain, depression, fatigue, decreased libido, acne, oily skin, increased breast size, decreased carbohydrate tolerance, diabetes-related symptoms, headaches, pruritus, increased low-density lipoproteins (LDL), and decreased high-density lipoproteins (HDL). Other complications may be headaches, hypertension, myocardial infarction, and cervical dysplasia. The reduction in the amount of estrogen has reduced the risk of heart attacks, but not the risk of strokes. Smoking, of course, increases the side effects of cardiovascular disease and many physicians will not prescribe the pill to any woman over 35 who smokes. The use of the birth control pill continues to menopause if a woman has had no difficulties. There is no information that long-range side-effects of taking the pill are a problem; that is, women who took the pill at a young age and have now gone through menopause do not appear to be at risk for other diseases. But we must be cautious because it is not possible to extrapolate the data from 20-year follow-ups to a 50-year follow-up. Information on this first group of users is minimal because these women are only now in their first decade of menopause.

THE INTRAUTERINE DEVICE (IUD)

The intrauterine device (IUD) is inserted into the uterus where it causes an inflammatory reaction. Its efficacy is 94%–99%. Studies have shown that, although ovulation occurs, the oocyte does not get fertilized. This may be because the sperm have a poor chance of getting past the cervical mucus that is hostile because of the secondary inflammation in the uterus, or because the uterine environment is responding to the IUD, causing spermicidal toxins to be produced by the endometrium. Thus, the oocyte, even if fertilized, might be unable to implant because the lining of the uterus is inhospitable.

The two IUDs now on the market contain medication. One contains progesterone in small quantities and needs to be replaced every year. The other is an IUD containing copper that lasts for 3–5 years. The additional agents make the IUD more effective than the previous, nonmedicated type, and they reduce the increased menstrual bleeding that was frequently associated with IUDs.

The advantage of an IUD is that it does not have to be inserted before intercourse. The disadvantages are that menstrual periods tend to be heavier and irregular bleeding can occur. An IUD should be removed if a pregnancy is suspected. An IUD should be checked if a woman has an unexplained fever and if she complains of flu-like symptoms. It is important to check the uterus if a woman feels pain on intercourse or has a foul-smelling discharge. The woman should check to make sure the string that is attached to the IUD is intact, and if she cannot find it she should have her health care provider see if the IUD is still in place. The most common problems associated with the IUD are expulsion from the uterus, a low-grade inflammation in the uterus, and perforation of the uterus and migration into the abdominal cavity. IUDs are not recommended for women who have never had a pregnancy. Perforation of the uterus with migration of the IUD into the abdominal cavity happens most often during insertion but can also occur at other times. Frequently, the IUD can be removed through the laparoscope. If an infection is suspected, the IUD should be removed at once, and antibiotics administered to clear the infection. To reduce the chance of infection at time of the insertion, antibiotics can be taken just before doing the procedure. However, antibiotics that are taken at other times for therapy can reduce the effectiveness of an IUD because if the antibiotic causes the low-grade uterine infection to subside the effectiveness of the IUD will be compromised.

The litigation against IUDs because of infection and pelvic damage has made the pharmaceutical industry very cautious. It is not possible to obtain an IUD without signing a detailed consent form that details the risks of infection and bleeding and their sequelae. The informed consent form places the responsibility for correct use of the IUD in the hands of the patients, and the list of contraindications is very long. The problem with these forms, as well as the package inserts, is that there is so much information, and specific applicability to a specific individual is difficult to appreciate, so that the inserts are not very helpful.

OTHER CONTRACEPTIVE METHODS

Norplant is an implantable form of the progesterone levonorgestral and can last as long as 5 years. It must be surgically inserted and removed and it is usually placed into the anterior arm. Uterine bleeding becomes irregular and this is the principal reason for having the implant removed. The unpredictability of the bleeding might make this method difficult for women who have major physical disabilities. However, the total blood loss from vaginal bleeding is less than normal so that, on the whole, this method may be acceptable for that reason.

Other contraceptive methods for women include vaginal rings, RU-486, and natural family planning. Vaginal rings that release contraceptive drugs have recently been approved for marketing. RU-486, an antiprogestin developed in France, is not a contraceptive specifically but it is used to produce an abortion. The utilization of this compound for pregnancy termination was the direct result of knowledge that the establishment and maintenance of pregnancy are dependent on progesterone. This compound terminates an early pregnancy if used in combination with various prostaglandins and does so with high efficacy (95%) and minimal side effects, the principal one being bleeding. The drug is currently marketed only in France and the prospects for marketing it in other countries is uncertain. In this country, it has been the subject of very heated debates. Natural family planning, which is promoted in this country as a method of birth control, involves identifying the periods in a woman's cycle when it is safe or unsafe to have intercourse if pregnancy is to be avoided. The method requires a great deal of under-

standing about the menstrual cycle and is based on periodic abstinence, which is linked to high user motivation. The efficacy is in
the same range as the barrier methods, that is, 65%–90%.

Condoms are the only form of completely reversible contraception that a male can use, and 10%–15% of couples use them. Condom use has apparently doubled since the awareness of autoimmune
deficiency disease (AIDS). The most effective condom is latex that
has been stored in a rolled form. Although the condom provides the
best method to prevent the spread of sexually transmitted diseases,
it is not a very effective method of birth control. There are several
reasons for this. The condom must be put on at the time of intercourse and must be removed from the penis as soon as intercourse is
over. It must be rolled correctly onto the penis. It must be held on
the penis during withdrawal so that it remains in place and will slip
off if the penis becomes flaccid within the vagina. It can break during intercourse and, in that case, there is no protection against sexually transmitted venereal disease for the woman or man. The failure
rate for condoms is a little greater than 12% among typical users.
Natural membrane condoms are made from the caecum of lamb
intestine, but these do not survive the rigors of intercourse as well,
nor are they as effective in preventing the spread of viral infections.
Since many people find using a condom uncomfortable because of
the sensation of dryness, it is recommended that vaginal contraceptive jellies be used as a lubricant, which add additional spermicidal
and antimicrobial protection. The biggest advantage of condoms is
that they are readily available and inexpensive, although a single one
can cost $1 or $2, and that both women and men can feel comfortable buying them. Condoms do need improvements, and some major improvements would include condoms that could be placed on a
flaccid penis, stay on throughout intercourse, and that would remain
on the penis when the erection subsided.

Sterilization, a major contraceptive method in this country, is
available for both women and men. Almost 30% of couples rely on
either ligation of the fallopian tubes in the female or ligation of the
vas deferens in the male. The reason that such a high percentage of
women choose tubal ligation is that methods of contraceptive are so
limited and the failure rate is so high. Sterilization methods used in
the U.S. are very effective, and are considered permanent. In women,
a surgical procedure of closing off the fallopian tubes is performed
through the abdomen. In men, the scrotum is incised to reach and to
ligate the tubes.

Except for the condom and sterilization, there are no male contraceptives on the market today. That is not to say that attempts

have not been made to develop injectable forms of medicine that would prevent sperm formation. A primary concern, however, is that the method not interfere with a man's libido. Reversibility and the long-range effects on health are important to both men and women, but specific concerns are assigned different priorities for men and women. The effects of contraceptives on women's libidos have never been of equal concern.

There is no evidence that men, if provided with safe and convenient contraceptives, would not use them. Certainly, as child support laws are more effectively enforced in many states, men will find themselves at greater risk for financial commitment for child support, which, in turn, should eventually lead to stronger feelings among men that they, as well as women, should have control over their fertility.

IMPLICATIONS AND COMPLICATIONS OF CONTRACEPTIVE USE

The United States has fewer contraceptive options available than western European countries. Why are so few contraceptive choices available? The reasons vary according to how the question is asked and who is answering. Reasons range from concerns about public safety and liability issues, to the inability of pharmaceutical companies to develop or introduce new methods. Only one major pharmaceutical company in the U.S. does any contraceptive research. Explanations of why research is not being conducted have ranged from the lack of need to introduce new contraceptive agents to the concern that new products will incur major liabilities for the pharmaceutical companies. Frequently, the media highlight the risks of adverse side effects and the problems related to using a particular contraceptive method; these may exacerbate fears because the accounts do not fully explain what is meant by the term "risk." Furthermore, busy medical practitioners may not take the time necessary to acquaint women and men with the risks and benefits of each method. Fear is as real a part of making contraceptive choices as any of the side effects. It is almost as though people make contraceptive choices by weighing their fears rather than weighing the positive and negative aspects of one method over another. To deal with contraceptives from another point of view is not to acknowledge a major reality.

It is clear that many contraceptives have not been studied in people with physical disabilities, so that published health risks relate to women who have no medical or physical disabilities. It is important that people understand the meaning of the term risk and the difference between risk to an individual and risk to an entire population. For example, if there are two large groups of women, and one group is taking an oral contraceptive and the other is not, there is an increased risk of liver tumors for the entire population taking the pill. However, the risk to each woman is small. For the women not using the pill, the risk of a liver tumor (hepatic angiosarcoma) would be approximately 1 in 1,000,000, which is a very low risk for any one woman. For the women who were taking the pill, the risk is 5 in 100,000, which is still low for an individual. This risk is a high *relative* risk, because the possibility of developing a liver tumor is 500 times greater for the woman taking the pill, but the *absolute* risk is low, because the disease is so rare to begin with. In situations with a very high relative risk but a low absolute risk, most cases are due to the exposure. Whether it is absolute or relative risk, however, makes very little difference in public health terms, because so few people develop the disease. However, that may not be how an individual person *perceives* the risk.

A public health risk *would* include women who develop thrombophlebitis as a result of oral contraceptives. In this situation, the relative risk is low but the absolute risk is higher, because the disease is more common than liver tumors (normally the risk is around 1 in 1,000). Diseases that are prevalent, such as breast cancer, are studied because even a very low relative risk might be a high absolute risk.

At the present time, no increase in breast cancer has been seen among women who have ever used oral contraceptives. There may be a risk for some women, while others may be protected from breast cancer because of their use. The data simply indicate that the population of women using oral contraceptives are not at greater risk because of that use. After 30 years of studying the epidemiology of breast cancer, a host of risk factors have been identified, but they account for only a small portion of the cases. These include reproductive risk factors, such as age of menarche and parity, family history of breast cancer, and various dietary risk factors.

It is very difficult to describe the risks of complications in terms of their lives. The particular areas that can terrify women are the risks mentioned, such as relative risk versus actual risk, and the risk of using a contraceptive versus the risk of having an unwanted pregnancy. Cost and convenience are important factors in choosing a contraceptive method and can determine if the contraceptive will continue to be used.

In clinics and medical offices throughout the country, people repeatedly express their frustration about contraceptive choices and realize that there is no currently available method with which they will be completely happy. The questions usually asked and the anxieties generally expressed are hard to list in any priority, but the ones that make the headlines and that medical practitioners get the most calls about generally are related to questions regarding safety and health. People are concerned that their chosen method will not harm them. Women often have questions about whether using the birth control pill may increase their chances of getting cancer. Others are concerned that using an IUD will cause them to become sterile, or that using a diaphragm will be too messy, or that their partners will refuse to use a condom. More often than not, contraceptives are viewed as a negative decision rather than as a means of gaining greater control.

In the context of persons who have physical disabilities, the type of disability and how it may affect their use of a particular type of contraceptive are important considerations. One of the most important issues that people must face when deciding upon a contraceptive method is acknowledging to themselves and to those who are advising them as to what their sexual practices really are and when they need contraception. Another consideration is the phase of life they are in and whether they should have more than one contraceptive method available. There is no reason that a person should always use the same method, because needs may be different at different times in their lives. For example, there may be times when an individual is regularly having intercourse and there may be other times when he or she is not. The woman who is breast feeding has to think about whether her contraceptive method will affect her breast milk. For example, oral contraceptives are not recommended for nursing mothers because some hormones can get through to the milk.

As mentioned, other countries offer a wider range of products and more available methods of sterilization than those offered in the U.S. Oral contraceptives are available that offer a wider range of progestational and estrogenic agents. Contraceptive hormones are widely used elsewhere, and injectable forms of contraceptive steroids are available. Intrauterine devices come in many more forms than those available in the U.S. and incorporate a greater variety of spermicidal agents. Other countries use advanced nonsurgical methods of occluding the fallopian tubes and the vas deferens, and these methods have a higher potential for reversibility than the surgical methods currently available in the U.S.

In sum, how does one choose a method of contraception? It depends. It is up to the individual or couple to consider all factors involved, including how the contraceptive method will be used in their daily lives, and to make a choice based on personal needs and priorities.

BIBLIOGRAPHY

David, H.P., Dytrych, Z., Matejcek, Z., & Schuller, V. (1988). *Born unwanted: Developmental effects of denied abortion.* Prague: Czechoslovak Medical Press.

Forrest, J.D., & Singh, S. (1990). The sexual and reproductive behavior of American women, 1982–1988. *Family Planning Perspectives, 22,* 206–214.

Gray, M.J., Haseltine, F., Love, S., Mayzel, K., Simopoulos, A., with Jacobson, B. & the editors of Consumer Reports Books. (1991). *The woman's guide to good health.* Yonkers, NY: Consumer Reports Books.

Hook, K. The unwanted child: Effects on mothers and children of refused applications for abortion. In *Society, stress and disease* (Vol. 2, 1987–1992). Oxford: Oxford Medical Publications.

Institute of Medicine Committee on the Relationship Between Oral Contraceptives and Cancer. (1991). *Oral contraceptives and breast cancer.* Washington, DC: National Academy Press.

Jones, E.F., & Forrest, J.D. (1989). Contraceptive failure in the United States: Revised estimates for the 1982 National Survey of Family Growth. *Family Planning Perspectives, 21,* 103.

Judkins, D.R., Mosher, W.D., & Botman, S. (1991, September). *National Survey of Family Growth: Design, estimation, and inference.* DHHS publication No (PHS) 91-1376, Series 2, No. 109.

Kelsey, J.L., & Gammon, M.D. (1991). The epidemiology of breast cancer. *CA: Cancer Journal for Clinicians, 41*(3), 146–65.

Maine, D. (1981). *Family planning: Its impact on the health of women and children.* New York: Center for Population and Family Health, Columbia University.

Mastroianni, L., Jr., Donaldson, P.J., & Kane, T.T. (Eds.). (1990). *Developing new contraceptives: Obstacles and opportunities.* Washington, DC: National Academy Press.

Mosher, W.D., & Pratt, W.F. (1990). Contraceptive use in the United States, 1973–1988. Advance data from Vital and Health Statistics, No. 182.

Potts, M., & Diggory, P. (1983). *Textbook of contraceptive practice* (2nd ed.). New York: Cambridge University Press.

Rantakallio, P. (1985). *Unwanted children: A longitudinal study.* Paper presented at the first International Workshop on Longitudinal Studies of Unwanted Children, Oulu, Finland.

Schlesselman, J.J. (1990). Oral contraceptives and breast cancer. *American Journal of Obstetrics and Gynecology, 163,* 1379–1387.

Weller, R.H., Eberstein, I.W., & Bailey, M. Pregnancy wantedness and maternal behavior during pregnancy. *Demography, 24*(3), 407–412.

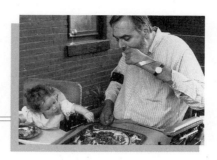

II

PERSONAL ISSUES

3

I Can Do Anything

Carol Ann Roberson

When Carl and I decided to marry 19 years ago, we had several major stumbling blocks to making our marriage work: Carl is black and I am white, and I have a significant disability. More than strong cultural differences, however, my physical disability brought us face to face with attitudes that could have destroyed our relationship. As in any marriage, compromise and adjustment to new responsibility are important ingredients. Negative expectations, prejudice, and spurious ideas regarding disability have been present throughout our marriage, but in those first few years, serious damage to our relationship could easily have been done.

At age 5 I was paralyzed by poliomyelitis in one of the last major epidemics just prior to development of the Salk vaccine. I was placed in an iron lung for breathing and was otherwise given no therapy, so polio destroyed much of my physical ability. Today, I am considered quadriplegic and have the use of only one arm for steering my motorized wheelchair. Early on I became quite proficient in using a pen held between my teeth and a mouthstick for activities such as turning pages and writing. Carl knew when he married me that there were many things that I physically could not do on my own. This includes all of my personal care, dressing, feeding, and positioning me correctly in my wheelchair. He was willing to do all of these things for me, even though his motives were questioned from the very start of our relationship. On some level, his life would certainly have been easier if he did not have both the physical work as well as the emotionally charged questioning that comes with marrying someone "different."

Friends, relatives, and especially strangers view ours as a very strange relationship. They find it difficult to understand what Carl gets from it. They have a view of disability from a medical model and see only a "damaged partner," who could not possibly contribute to the relationship, but rather only take. What could I possibly give that would make an able-bodied man want to spend his life with me?

When we were married for 1 year, I got pregnant. Even before marriage I had been cautioned, by "friends" and relatives, to remain single until after my childbearing years. The thought of my having a child and rearing it in the context of my disability was unthinkable. Carl, of course, was as delighted as I. This was part of the purpose of our union. We were not afraid of the difficulties that would arise because of my disability. We knew that together we could find solutions; however, attitudes of those around us proved to be outrageous. In the seventh month of my pregnancy, a lady I hardly knew approached me on the street to tell me that my crooked spine would certainly damage my unborn child.

These unrequested, unwanted, offensive statements were often made during my two pregnancies as well as while my two daughters were growing up. People with disabilities are not supposed to be sexual, not supposed to be partners, and certainly in no way should we assume the role of parents.

Eighteen years ago, when my daughter Nicole was born, there was little information and no encouragement to have a family if one had a disability. I was told by several physicians that I should not get pregnant. When I asked for the medical reasons I was instead questioned, "How will you be able to care for a child?" or, "Do you realize what you are asking of your husband?" There was also an unspoken question that was very clear: "What will you do when he leaves you?" The assumption was that Carl and I had not discussed these issues. I was 27 when my daughter was born, held a master's degree in social work, and had an excellent work record with increasingly greater responsibility. Yet, there was an assumption that I had not thought this through, and that Carl, also an intelligent, hard-working, and extremely thoughtful man, had gotten into something that was beyond his control.

We searched for quite some time and finally, through a nondisabled woman friend, found an obstetrician willing to accept me as his patient. He was very clear in answering all of our questions based on his medical expertise, which was what we wanted. He did not question our motives for having a child, and, frankly, if he had begun that line of questioning we would have continued our search.

Of course, as we began to get to know him, we did discuss concerns and solutions to problems that might come up, but these were the conversations of any couple about to introduce a baby into their relationship.

One of my earliest concerns was that of normal childbirth or c-section. Dr. W. stated that he was reasonably sure that I would need a c-section and explained that because I did not move and stretch, he was concerned that the vaginal opening was not pliable enough for the baby to be born without possible damage. He assured us that he would keep us informed of all of the medical facts, and he did so to our satisfaction. My first child was born by c-section after I went into labor. Because of my immobility, he suggested that I get up in my wheelchair as quickly as possible. I did so the following day, and my baby and I were home in 8 days. My stay in the hospital was uncomplicated. Carl was allowed to arrive prior to visiting hours and to stay as late as he could so that he could assist me with my personal care and learn with me the care and routine that we would follow at home. I was able to see what I could do physically, such as how to hold my baby comfortably both for me and so that she would feel secure, as well as feeding and directing others in her care. We had arranged for help with the baby at home during the day, and in the evening Carl and I cared for her ourselves.

On outings we often carried Nicole in a baby carrier rather than have a carriage and my wheelchair. Often Carl would strap her onto me so that she could feel my warmth and be held close to me. The carrier was excellent for this because it allowed me to hold her without the use of my arms, which were not strong enough. People are not used to seeing a woman in a wheelchair with a baby and we were often stared at or whispered about. One instance that I can recall was on the way home after doing some grocery shopping. Nicole, who was approximately 2 months old, had been asleep in the carrier and resting comfortably. About 2 blocks from home she woke up and began to cry. As we waited for a light to change, two women who were also waiting for the light began to talk to each other in whispers just loud enough for Carl and me to hear. They were concerned about the "poor baby" and wondered, "How could someone do that?" They clearly were expressing their concern that I was not fit to care for my child. My initial response was to wonder if they had never before heard a baby cry, but by the time we arrived at home I was devastated. I cried and told Carl that I would no longer carry the baby outside. Their words cut deeply and only too clearly restated what I knew most people felt. The negative attitudes toward my parenthood, as well as my own feelings of inadequacy as a new mother, might have stopped me from enjoying some of my most precious memories; however, my husband replaced the negatives with positives. Did I really intend never to hold my child in full view of others? Was I going to allow ignorance to stop me from doing what I knew was right? The answer, of course, was and is, "No!"

Stereotypical ideas have abounded as Carl and I have raised our children. Our decision, 14 years ago, to have Carl stay home and care for the girls while I work, was not easy for people to comprehend. Today, fathers are expected to participate in childrearing, but then we were trend-setters. Our reasoning made sense to us because I was unable to do all of the things that are necessary physically, but certainly able to work and pull in a good salary. The rationale was not always as apparent to family and friends.

In all of our activities my disability became a central theme because of the prejudice about people with disabilities. I have been told that I was fortunate to have had girls because they will help me; that my participation at graduation ceremonies, or parent–teacher conferences was not necessary, and that the teachers would understand my inability to participate, rather than to simply change the site from an inaccessible site to one that is accessible; that I needed an "adult" to get into a movie theater with my 5- and 7-year-old—obviously my disability kept me from participating as a parent. We have been stared at, prayed over, "tsk, tsked" at, and all because I have a visible disability, and people with disabilities should not have children.

Our children have grown to young adulthood, despite my disability. One daughter is presently attending college while the other is a sophomore in high school. We have, clearly, not done things in the traditional manner; we haven't been able to. Our girls are fun-loving, intelligent, athletic, musical, and independent. They have developed as wonderful young women even though society believed that their chances were slim. If my disability has inhibited them, it is only in the way that others perceived me; my daughters think I can do anything.

~~~~~~

But It Hurts Too Much

Irving Kenneth Zola

*I*t was after 1 and she still wasn't home. I should be used to it now but I'm not. It didn't seem to matter whether I was out with someone else, though it did help.

So I lie here festering—that's what it feels like. A car goes by. Is it her? No, it doesn't have the familiar rumble.

I wonder where she went tonight. I know she's with him again though I pretend to her I don't. What a stupid-ass game I'm playing.

Lights are reflecting off the window but somehow I know she won't be coming from that direction.

She loves to dance. Maybe that's what they did. If I could really dance, would it make a difference? There's a part of me that would like to think so. Then I could blame all this—what she needs, what I need—on my physical limitations. Strange that that would make me feel better. Maybe it's because I then wouldn't have to examine the us, or the me that's making me feel so lousy.

I think I heard a door slam. So I push myself out of bed and limp slowly to the window and wait . . . and wait . . . and wait. Maybe the fifth car will be her. Let's see if the first one is black and the second green then . . . now I'm into magical thinking. I feel like a child. I want her home now . . . now. I laugh to myself. I think of my mother. When I used to trek in at 3 A.M. she would ask, "What could you be doing till 3 A.M.?" I don't have to ask that here. I know what she was doing. Funny I can't, really won't, picture it. I won't let myself think of her in bed with someone else. Sometimes I think that if I could just purge myself I'd feel better. But I won't. I feel like crying but I won't. I just moan inwardly.

Another car door. I think this is it.

I hear a click, the back door is being unlatched.

I climb back in bed.

I hug my pillow tighter. I'll pretend I'm asleep. Now I hear her on the stairs. But she's stopped. She's going to the bathroom. Why does she take so long? What is she doing in there?

She's in the room. I hear her but my own breathing comes evenly. The message to her is that I'm sleeping restfully, unbothered by her new freedom.

The closet door creaks as she hangs up her dress. She's beside the bed almost immediately. Why didn't it take that long? Does that mean that some of her clothes were already off? I've got to stop this obsessing.

She's getting into bed. I can feel her weight. If she reaches over and touches me then I'll know she still loves me.

Her lips brush my shoulder. And I, pretending to have wakened, roll over. Now we face each other. No words yet pass between us. We come closer and we kiss, gently but warmly . . . but I can smell him.

"I love you," she whispers.

"I know," I answer, but the words are a lie.

"I really do," she says again. And as she does I pull her tighter, repeating to myself her words like a mantra. I'm trying to hear it. I am. I am. But it just hurts too much.

4

Rethinking Expectations

Denise Sherer Jacobson

I have had cerebral palsy since birth, and from the time I was a child I was very much aware of the double standard that existed concerning my family's expectations in regard to my future and that of my nondisabled sister. For Shelley, they spoke of marriage and children. For me, well . . . since I was fairly bright, I'd go to college and have a successful career (a rare expectation for someone with significant CP even nowadays). In those days, of course, the two—family and career—were mutually exclusive.

CHILDHOOD EXPECTATIONS

I am grateful that they did have expectations, that they did encourage me to be as independent as they thought possible. Yet, dreams are so much a part of childhood existence—a very normal part—except for children who are significantly disabled. Perhaps professionals and parents feel that it's better not to talk about dreams since, in the end, those dreams are so "unattainable" that it would lead to only heartbreak and despair. In reality, even children with cerebral palsy have dreams about love, partners, babies, and yes, even sex.

It wasn't often that I'd talk about my desire to get married and have children because I knew that society did not expect it of me. Ironically, however, I am a product of my society; I very much wanted to get married, to become pregnant (perhaps, in part, to prove that, even with my disability, I was a woman), and to have a baby. Perhaps if I had been encouraged to talk openly, I could have

49

explored the possibility of motherhood so that I would have been more confident and prepared for it.

OPTING TO ADOPT

Neil, my husband, had always wanted to adopt a disabled child. I was wary. I felt that adopting an older disabled child (3 or 4 years old) might be more than we could handle—both physically and emotionally. For over 30 years I had struggled to become independent, to dress, groom, and feed myself. Neil and I used an attendant only for cleaning house and meal preparation—activities which were both too time- and energy-consuming for us to do on a daily basis. Having a disabled child could mean that we would most likely need more help for an extended, and perhaps unlimited, period of time. In addition to that adjustment, I felt that it would be easier to bond with an infant, whereas an older child might have already built up some anxiety about being parented by two people with disabilities. The reality was, however, that babies were, and still are, in such demand by nondisabled couples. We had, I thought, no chance of adopting one.

Then one day I received a desperate call from a stranger (Colleen Starkloff) 2,000 miles away. She was offering me a baby—a baby whose adoption had been arranged through a private agency before he was born, but whose placement 5 weeks after his birth had fallen through because inconclusive medical tests showed that he might have cerebral palsy. Suddenly this blonde-haired, blue-eyed, beautiful (according to Colleen) infant was less desirable. WHY? The reasons are, indeed, too complex to examine here, for the issues range from social stereotypes of disability, to inadequate medical prognosis, to economic considerations (in his first 6 weeks, this infant's medical bill rose to $8,000), to one's personal assessment (given limited and often inaccurate knowledge) of his or her capability to raise a disabled child.

Fortunately, our decision to adopt David had very little to do with those issues. Neil, who's otherwise very logical about everything (to my frustration during heated arguments), would have brought David home the very same day of Colleen's phone call, if that had been possible. I was the stick-in-the-mud, and decided that I would have to see this baby to "assess" whether adopting him would be "right" for us. This time I had to be the logical one, and I, of course, was very "realistic" when it came to my disability. But, sometimes a decision can't be made with your head; it's made with your heart. I've heard it said that babies are the most powerful creatures on earth, and it's certainly true! When that 2-month-old baby was placed in my arms and looked at me with his magnetic blue eyes, I knew that my belief that it would be my choice was a fallacy. David gazed up at me with such an intense assuredness that seemed to demand, "Hey Mom, what took you so long?"

PHYSICAL CARE

Because our needs as a disabled couple with a baby were unique, we debated about hiring an au pair. After a brief experience with one, we concluded that an attendant would fit in better with our lifestyle and prove more economical. An attendant came for 2½ hours in the morning to bathe David, dress him, feed him breakfast, and prepare his bottles. Another came in the late afternoon to make dinner and help with David's evening routine. Attendant management presented many difficulties. The people we employed had other jobs and also had to be educated in baby care. Being an anxious new mother, I found it stressful at times to coordinate and supervise everything that needed to done within those hours. On the average, 4 months was about the length of time an attendant would stay in our employment. So just when things began settling down, we had to start trusting and getting used to someone new again.

David helped Neil and I explore and discover our physical capabilities. We were able to diaper him using disposable diapers—I apologized to the environment, but for us disposable diapers were safer, easier, and more sanitary than cloth diapers. At most, it took Neil 10 minutes to change David's diaper. It could take me up to 40 minutes, depending on what was in the diaper and how tired I was at that particular time of the day.

Babies have a greater instinct and intelligence than they're given credit for. As we adapted to David, he adapted to us. When Neil or I would diaper him, David stayed still; he'd squirm for others who weren't disabled. Whenever he'd bump into something, he'd crawl over to me and pull himself on my wheelchair up to a standing position so that I could lift him into my lap to comfort him. He started doing that at 6 months. He'd grasp my forefinger that I'd dip in oatmeal to steady it as I fed him, since I couldn't feed him with a spoon. All three of us were, and are, very comfortable with each other.

EMOTIONAL/PSYCHOLOGICAL CARE

Comfort extends beyond the physical. I'm often approached by mothers who wonder how I keep David from running away from me in stores or on the street. There have also been times when we've been among nondisabled people when David has fallen and has insisted that I'm the only one who can comfort him. And then there are times when David and I battle wills. Luckily, I'm just as stubborn as he is.

RETHINKING EXPECTATIONS

As a parent with a disability, I now find myself facing another double standard. A child is expected to learn responsibility, independence, consideration, cooperation, and caring within the family. Yet, I'm aware of those who voice concern about David's being too independent or David's being at risk for falling into the role of our attendant because Neil and I are disabled. Disability is an easy scapegoat, and although our disabilities do influence our lives as individuals and as a family, they are just like our other strengths and weaknesses; they just happen to be more visible. What others may not realize is that Neil, David, and I have our own expectations of each other based on love and knowledge of our needs as mother, father, and child.

Why Marcia Is
My Favorite Name

Irving Kenneth Zola

*T*here was no other word for it. My friends were just pushy. I knew
they meant well but the last thing I wanted to do was go to a dance,
especially in my condition. "In my condition." The words rankled. If I
just looked at myself in the mirror, I felt okay. Not bad looking. No
adolescent acne. Some people even said I had nice eyes. But I was most
pleased with my face—no peach fuzz. I stroked my cheeks. This 5
o'clock shadow felt like one of the few good inheritances from my
father's side of the family. Besides, the idea of having to shave every day
made me feel masculine, a virile 16½. But if I stepped back, the rest of
my image undid me. I didn't feel strong leaning on these two crutches
and dragging myself around at a snail's pace. And though I knew I'd
improve somewhat, my doctor had been brutally honest. "The 1951
Red Sox will have to do without you. . . . Contact sports are out. You'll
never run a race again nor will you ever walk unaided." Such was my
polio legacy.

The phone was ringing. Maybe I could tell Zummie and Hank
that I wasn't feeling well. Besides it was a long schlep down the stairs
and perhaps even harder to get into the community center. But as I
hopped to the phone, I knew they wouldn't buy it. They'd already
worked out how, if necessary, they'd carry me up the stairs. "But I'll be
embarrassed," I argued. "Bullshit," they eloquently countered.

The phone call set the time. They'd be by to pick me up at 8. For
the tenth time I went into the bathroom to comb my hair. I felt like an
ass. It was as if this was the only part of my body I could control. "How
do I look?" I asked as I made my final appearance in the hallway. My
mother stopped washing the dishes and smiled, "Very handsome." My
father shook his head in agreement and came over to give me a few
dollars spending money. My younger brother Michael just giggled.
When the bell rang and I turned to go, they all kissed me good-bye,

told me not to stay out too late but, thank God, didn't say 'Be careful."

My friends were at the door. A little too ready and eager, I thought to myself. It was easier to go downstairs if I didn't have two crutches under the same arm, so I asked Zummie if he'd take one. Then leaning on the railing for support, I began the slow descent down the three flights from our apartment.

Once in the car, I asked who was going to be there. "Oh the usual crowd" was the reply and we began to joke about the likelihood of any "action." The trip was quick—less than 15 minutes.

As I slowly climbed the stairs to the community center, I realized that no one was paying much attention. Perhaps with no visible scars, people just thought I'd had an athletic injury. The first few minutes were easy. As we settled in a corner, others came by to say "Hello!" "Good to see you again!" "How've you been?" The questions required little of me. "Okay." "Thanks." "Fine." I answered with a smile. But down deep I was wondering what the hell I was doing here.

I could hear the music playing but I certainly wasn't in a hurry to follow it. I would have been content to just sit on the staircase but the casual, "C'mon, let's see what's doing!" dashed that hope. Using the banister for support, I was back on my crutches. I wondered where in the dance hall I could hide. But when we got there a moment later, I realized it wasn't necessary. I was hardly the only guy not dancing. In fact, relatively few of my friends were. All of us milled to one side, looking over the girls, commenting on who was dancing with whom, who that new girl was, and wow did that one look great in a tight sweater.

Almost imperceptibly conversation turned to next week's big event—a weenie roast down Nantasket Beach. "Sounds like fun," I said.

"Who are you gonna take?" asked Zummie.

"My mother," I answered sardonically.

"C'mon, seriously," chimed in Hank.

"I hadn't thought about it." It was a lie. I'd been thinking about it for weeks but it had been a long time since I'd been out on a date. It didn't seem fair to call up a girl out of the blue. I wasn't so much afraid that she'd say no but that she'd accept out of pity or worse, ignorance of what she was getting into. I felt girls should at least see me face-to-face before going out. For these reasons I wouldn't let my friends fix me up.

"Why don't you take Marcia?" suggested Zummie with a not-so-believable innocent air.

"Who?" I asked.

"Marcia. You know, the one over there with the frizzy hair."

I looked over in the direction he was pointing. She was dancing with another girl. At least that meant she didn't have a steady. I looked at her very closely. She was cute—brown curly hair, freckles, nice Jewish nose, and figure which showed off quite well in a short-sleeve blouse.

"She doesn't even know me."

"Sure she does. She was even asking about you."

"Bull," I said. Part of me wanted to believe, but I let it go. So did my friends. In reality none of us did. We were merely biding our time.

After what seemed like a decent interval, I asked, "What did you say that girl's name in the green blouse was?"

"Marcia, you dumb asshole," answered Hank.

Subtlety was clearly going to get me nowhere. "How do you know that she's interested in me?"

"Contacts," he winked.

"What if she says 'No'?"

"She won't . . . you're too cute," said Gerry who'd been standing on the edge of our threesome. I tried to hit him with my crutch but I missed.

"What have you got to lose?" asked Zummie.

Everything, I thought to myself. But somehow the pressure was difficult to resist. I knew my friends really cared about me and wouldn't have set me up for a fall. So, ambivalently, I hopped over to where she stood talking with a girlfriend.

"Marcia?" I interrupted.

She turned to me smiling. Five minutes after we'd spoken I had *no* recollection what I'd said! All I knew was that she'd accepted my invitation and I'd agreed to call during the week to make final arrangements. I was so excited by her reply I didn't even think to spend the rest of the evening with her. Maybe I thought if she got to know me better, she'd change her mind.

During that week panic set in. Amongst the arrangements I thought of making was calling the whole thing off. The whole situation was crazy. She didn't know me. I didn't know her. Besides a weenie roast was a hell of a way to have a first date.

Somehow the 7 days passed and Saturday night was here. Again my parents were solicitous. But when my mother told me to bundle up, I got very upset.

"But it's nearly 80° out there!" I snapped.

Undeterred she went on, "Still you never can tell. . . . When it gets late, you might get cold."

Her remark sparked in me a minor anxiety attack. In it I saw a veiled reference to the fact that Marcia might possibly go off and leave me alone. It's happened to other guys before, I thought to myself. Only my 8-year-old brother's query, "Why can't I go along?" kept me from exploding. That weenie roasts were only a place for big boys sent him away in a huff but allowed all of us to laugh anxiously.

My friends soon arrived and off we went to pick up Marcia. Luckily it was the style of the time to announce one's arrival with a beep of a car horn. Thus I was spared having to climb the stairs to her house and meet her parents. I didn't know what they would or would not ask me. I just didn't want to have to deal with any questions. Marcia quickly bounced down the stairs and squeezed in beside me. The long ride to Nantasket passed quickly. We talked about previous jobs, friends, school, plans.

My sense of ease was broken when we encountered the beach. I'd forgotten how difficult it was in sand to keep my crutches from slipping and me with them. Marcia went first. With guiding remarks like, "This place looks solid enough to lean on," we finally made it to the bonfire. I didn't feel like moving so I suggested a nearby spot for the blanket. When she spread it out, anchoring the corners with rocks, I tried to ease myself down. It was no use. The trek from the car had exhausted me so I somewhat ungracefully plopped to the ground.

Only then did I realize how difficult it was going to be to play the manly role—coming back and forth with drinks and food. But Marcia spared me. "What would you like on yours?" she said, jumping to her feet. It was only then I let myself really look at her. She was wearing shorts and a halter with a pullover tied around her waist. She looked lovely but all I wittily could say was, "I'll take the works."

The early evening passed in talk, food, and songs but as the fire died down, couples began to take their blankets and drift away. A sea breeze wafted across the water. Awkwardly I put my arm around Marcia to fend off the cold. At least that would be my excuse if she pulled away. But she didn't. Someone turned on their portable radio. As romantic music filled the night, I whispered, "It's beautiful enough to dance to and you are beautiful enough to dance with but I . . . ."

She interrupted me with her lips, answering in that kiss far more questions about myself than I had ever imagined I was asking.

5

Parenting with a Disability

Mary Ellen Pischke

In September 1977, my neck was broken at the C7 level as the result of domestic violence. I was also 2½ months pregnant and the mother of a 4-year-old daughter. I was brought to St. Mary's Hospital in Rochester. I was asked if I wanted an abortion so it would make things easier for me, but I said no because I felt there had to be a purpose for that life inside of me. When I was 8 months pregnant I was moved to Methodist Hospital because St. Mary's didn't deliver babies, and the nurses on Rehab were afraid that I would go into labor and not know it. While I was waiting for my baby to come, I worked on daily living skills in therapy. I practiced changing diapers on a doll, cooking meals, and other skills. When I was 9 months along, a doctor who had an 8-month-old baby brought her baby in to see if I could handle him. I could hardly hold the child because he wiggled all over and, being 9 months pregnant, I didn't have much lap room. A few days later some doctors and other hospital staff sat down and asked me to consider putting my baby up for adoption, or having someone else raise my baby for the first years of its life, since I was going to be a single parent with a new disability to get used to. I told them to forget it, and I would manage.

The delivery of my child was induced as I was getting tired of being in the hospital and my baby was ready. My doctor thought it would be easier if we knew when my baby would come so we could plan for everyone to be there. Labor lasted for nearly a whole day. All of a sudden my blood pressure went sky high and I experienced the worst headaches of my life, so my doctor gave me medicine to bring my blood pressure down. This kept happening until my baby was ready to come out and the doctors were able to keep my blood pressure down by giving me oxygen and keeping me calm. I was able to deliver my baby as naturally as possible. My doctor used forceps and another doctor helped me push. My baby girl was perfect. My doctor thought it best to tie my tubes after my delivery, so I did that before going home. I was able to nurse my daughter, change her diapers, dress her, bathe her, and carry her in a carry bag that hooked on my wheelchair so she could snuggle on my chest.

I stayed with my brother until my body was ready to go back to Rehab so I could learn personal care, bladder training, and how to drive. When I left Rehab for good, I was able to live in an apartment with my girls and take care of myself and my family. It was a lot of work, and I needed help on occasion from my friends and relatives; however, I was quite capable of being independent in most of our care.

After a year of living in my hometown of Red Wing, I decided to go back to college to eventually earn a living for my family, so we moved to Rochester. I had no friends in Rochester, but I was able to get the help I needed to begin college within a month of moving. I was able to maintain my home and children, go to college full time, and have an active social life. A few years later I decided to accept a marriage proposal. After we were married for a year, we looked into the possibility of having a tubal reversal. It took much work and the surgery was painful, but it was worth it. I got pregnant about 10 months after the surgery.

During my pregnancy I worked part time for the Southeastern Minnesota Center for Independent Living (SEMCIL), teaching daily living skills to other people with disabilities. After several bladder infections, learning to cath myself, and doing transfers with a large stomach throwing me off-balance, I went into labor. The first time I went into labor my doctor had to stop the labor because it was too early. This happened a couple of times. Finally my doctor induced labor so everyone needed for delivery could be there. I had an epidural so my blood pressure would stay under control, and it worked. I was able to lie back with very little discomfort and watch my baby boy being delivered. After delivery, I was able to hold my baby and nurse him. He was perfect. Although I wanted my tubes tied right away, my doctor convinced me to wait for awhile. I did get pregnant again, and after 2½ months I had a miscarriage.

I got pregnant again 2 months later, and when I was 4 months along I miscarried again. I was devastated and wanted nothing more to do with babies. I was going to have my tubes tied again, but the day before I chickened out. I got pregnant a few months later. Again,

I had a rough pregnancy with cathing myself, more bladder infections, and lots of swelling. I was working full time until I was 7 months along, then I could only work half days. I went into labor when I was 8 months pregnant. After doing an amniocentesis, we discovered my baby's lungs were healthy, so labor was continued. An epidural was used again, and after a day of labor my baby popped out. In fact, literally, because of all the water I had retained, my baby came out with gallons of liquid. My baby boy was perfect and I nursed him for a month, then I had my tubes tied. When I nursed my babies I would usually lay a pillow under my arm on the side I was nursing because otherwise my arm would fall asleep. Since my last baby was a preemie I had to nurse every 2 hours, so I was pretty exhausted. My bladder training was back to normal within the first month after delivery.

I change my baby on any table I can wheel under. I just put a blanket down for my baby's comfort and get the job done. I'm much slower than everyone else, but I can do it. As my baby gets bigger, it gets harder because he tries to crawl away from me; however, after much struggling we complete the job.

I have a baby chair to sit him in for feeding that fastens on each side with Velcro, and it has been a lifesaver for holding my baby. Most of my babies' clothes have snaps or a lot of stretch. Sometimes I have friends put Velcro on the clothing. Now that my girls are older, they have been very helpful with our babies. I have been able to go back to work full time. My husband works second shift at IBM and I work days at SEMCIL. My girls fill in the afternoon until I get home, or if I have evening meetings. When I travel I need personal care assistance because of my bladder, so I usually bring my children with me as my daughters have learned to help me. As my babies get older, they learn to climb up on my lap by using my wheelchair as a ladder. I have a seat belt on my wheelchair that fastens with Velcro so they can sit securely on my lap. I'm able to get them in and out of their car seats so we can shop, go to church, and go other places together. I've used a power wheelchair since I had my boys, for ease and to save my strength.

Discipline can sometimes be difficult, but I try to instill respect for authority in my children while they are still young. It is important for me to look at what I can do for my children and not at what I can't do.

POSTSCRIPT

Being the child of a disabled person does not make me feel different than someone who isn't, unless someone tells me I am. Even then I don't know why. I, as a person, still am normal. My mother does not expect me to do anything unusual that a mother without a disability has her children do.

I think having a mother in a wheelchair has more good qualities than people realize. It gives me a chance to help out more around the house and learn responsibility. Also, we get great parking spots!

Tara Reisner Pischke

Is It All Right To Be Sad?

Irving Kenneth Zola

*I*t was a very hot night . . . not that I needed any excuse. But as soon as dinner was over, I mounted my stair-o-lator to the second floor and quickly stripped off all my braces. This brought up memories of my mother. Behind closed doors, of course, she would recite the litany of her day and sigh with relief as she stripped off every confining garment from high-heeled shoes to garter belt to girdle. As the sweat poured off me, I matched her item for item and probably sigh for sigh.

Letting my whole body breathe I stretched out on my high bed, watched the sunset, and grabbed for my latest paperback mystery. I didn't get very far because I could hear Kyra, my 7-year-old daughter, crying in the other room. Ordinarily, that in itself would have caused me to either leap (only figuratively) out of bed or at least call out, "What's the matter?" But I could hear Judy's soothing voice in the background so I sank back into my reading.

Soon Kyra appeared at the foot of the bed, carrying the ever-comforting panda bear in one hand with the thumb of her other firmly implanted in her mouth. With tears streaming down her face I could barely understand a word she was saying so I reached out and helped her climb up. Words were still not forthcoming, only racking sobs. So holding her close enough so that her tears now were staining my nightshirt, I waited.

"Daddy, I'm so sorry and I hope you won't think I'm being mean . . . ."

It was such a strange combination—her tears and the supposed meanness—that I didn't really know how to respond or even if I should. So I didn't.

"Daddy," she began very haltingly, repeating again her apology, "I know you do so much. I know you do puzzles with me and games and lots of things that Mommy won't do . . . ." The longer the list of my virtues got, the greater became my anxiety. But I had learned over the years with Kyra, that having such long-winded parents, the last thing

---

she wanted was to be interrupted—especially when she so obviously had a well-rehearsed or rather thought-through prologue.

"It's just," and out it came with tears still flowing, "that sometimes I want you to swim out to the dock with me and sometimes I want you to go bicycling with me and sometimes I want you to go on long walks with me and sometimes I want you to climb or go hiking with me . . . ."

As the list continued I knew that she knew all the things I could do, but that didn't matter. I started to formulate an answer that included a greater use of a motorized wheelchair, when she, far wiser than I, said what had to be said.

"You know Daddy, I asked Mommy if it was OK to talk about something sad even though you can't do anything about it. She said it was and even that it can be good to get it out. Is it really OK?"

As I whispered "Yes," she mumbled through her loud sucking, "I feel better now." "So do I," I said in return as we lay there cuddling.

6

Learning About Disability from Children

Neil Jacobson

It is important to stop and learn some of the lessons children have to teach us. I am convinced that I have learned as much, if not more, from my son than from anyone else about disability. I will give you a few examples.

When David was 3 or 4 months old, he used to wake up at 2 A.M. hungry. Do you know what he did when he was hungry? He cried! He didn't ask if I could please feed him. He didn't ask how difficult it was for me to drag myself out of bed. He cried! He insisted that I be there for him. How utterly marvelous it felt to have another human being not care about my disability but instead insist that I attend to *his* needs! The same thing happened at 4 A.M. when David needed to poop. Again, he didn't get into a big philosophical discussion about whether my disability would allow me to change him. He didn't spend much time or energy wondering how I might feel about having to get up again. He just pooped. He knew, indeed, he demanded that I be there for him and, by golly, there is always a way.

When David was a little older, perhaps about 2, I was surprised that he often demanded that I do things for him even when there were other, "more capable" people around. For instance, sometimes, when I'd come home from a rough day at work and find we had some nondisabled friends over for dinner, I'd figured that they could change him. After all, what I could do in 18 minutes, they could do

63

in 45 seconds. *Wrong!* If I were home, I had to do the honors. What causes this illogical behavior in children? The answer is quite simple. I'm Daddy and that's what Daddy does. This simplicity I find very refreshing.

So as not to have you think that all experiences with David were pleasant, I want to tell you that when David was about 3½ years old, his daycare teacher informed us that he had somewhat of a behavior problem. Oh no, my son had a behavior problem—there goes his Stanford scholarship! Furthermore, it had to be my fault. Being keenly aware of my own disability, it was natural for me to blame his problem on my disability. After all, I had a hard time catching him when he ran away from me. I couldn't get him down from climbing on furniture. I couldn't get him to sit in his car seat when I wanted him to. What kind of father was I? After several months of beating myself over my disability, it was pointed out to me that the problem had nothing to do with my disability—I was just being a wimp! I was letting this little guy get away with murder! While studying for my M.B.A., no one taught me how to manage a 3-year-old! Let me tell you, it's different than managing anyone else! Once I realized that it was my wimpiness and not my disability, I became somewhat more strict. David's behavior problem did indeed subside. The point here is to show how easy it is to blame something as blatant as a physical disability when often the problem has absolutely nothing to do with the disability.

Before ending, I do want to relate one last story that has to do with adopting David. As you know, in order to adopt, you need to get about 2,000 people to vouch on your behalf. We got 1,998 people—the two who felt we were wrong in our desire to adopt David were my mother and my ex-doctor. We don't have time to discuss my mother, but my ex-doctor offers a lesson to be learned. He wrote to the adoption agency that he felt that two parents with disabilities such as ours posed a "potentially problematic situation in rearing a child." After finding another doctor to vouch on our behalf, I asked my ex-doctor why he did that. He said that he had two major reservations. One was that the child would develop our speech patterns, and the other was that the other children might tease the child because of our disabilities. I informed him that we had indeed thought about both issues. As for the speech, I was convinced that the child would pick up normal speech patterns from radio, TV, school, friends, and neighbors, among others. My parents had pronounced Polish accents that my brother, sister, and I did not pick up. Furthermore, it's not "natural" to sound CP—you really have to work at it! As far as other children go, I had no doubt that there will be kids who will make fun of David's parents. My hope and my goal is that David will feel so good about who he is and so good about who his parents are, that he will be able to proudly face those kids and say, "So what?"

And the Children Shall Lead Us

Irving Kenneth Zola

*I*t was freezing cold. I sat huddled behind the wheel of my car waiting, as I do every Wednesday, for Amanda to get out of school. The radio was blaring, the heater was rumbling, and I was absorbed in a paperback novel, so I didn't hear the first knock. With the second, I saw Amanda pointing to the window. Anything that let the cold in seemed outrageous, so I only opened it a crack.

"Daddy, you're such a silly," she said with a certain exasperation. "I meant the door, not the window?"

To me that seemed silly and I told her so, "You know you can't climb over me that easily. Why don't you go in the back door . . . like always?"

With a patience that a 9-year-old develops to deal with the older generation, she gave me a benign smile. "I don't want to come in. I want you to come out." And then, acknowledging with her hand another snowsuited young girl, she explained, "I want you to show Kristin your leg."

"My what?" I stammered in surprise.

"Your leg, the one with the brace," she said offhandedly.

"My leg," I answered softly to no one in particular.

"Yes," she went on, "Kristin often asks me about it. So when she brought it up today, I thought now was a good time."

Her matter-of-factness was almost hypnotic. And so turning in my seat, I first placed my left foot outside and then with my hands lifted my right to join it. And there I sat . . . a grey-bearded 42-year-old clad in an olive-drab parka and his favorite blue jeans.

"Well there it is," said Amanda pointing triumphantly at my leg. We all looked at it. Amanda, Kristin, and another friend who stopped on his way home. The only "it" that was immediately visible was the bottom of my brace, two pieces of shining aluminum attached to the

---

Copyright © 1991 by Irving Kenneth Zola. Used by permission.

heel of my shoe. Kristin shook her head and when she falteringly asked, "How, umm, umm . . .?" I knew the question. "You mean how high does it go?" She nodded in response.

"It goes all the way up here," and I traced the brace from my ankle to my hip. Very young children want to touch it and say so, but this older audience said little and so I didn't offer.

"Why do you wear it?" asked the boy.

Amanda smiled, "I've told them about the polio but," and she pursed her lips knowingly, "you should tell."

And so I did, telling briefly about polio—a disease already to them a piece of history—something they knew about only indirectly, by "the sips they once had to take in school" to avoid having it. But they were more interested in how the brace worked. And so I began to explain, "Because of the weakness in my right leg . . . without the brace, my knee would keep bending and I'd fall. But this way," and I patted it, "the brace keeps my leg stiff and unbending."

"You know, Daddy. Your leg doesn't look weak. I mean," and she waved toward both of them, "they look the same to me."

"You're right," I laughed, a little nervously. This was something she'd never mentioned before, "They are almost the same. But if you look close—some day when I'm not wearing the brace, I'll show you— the right leg is a little thinner than the left. And if you look at me carefully in shorts you'll see that I'm pretty big all around here" and I let my hands fall across my rather thick chest, "but that I'm much thinner below the waist."

This clicked off a memory in Amanda and she turned to her two friends, "The other day my daddy and I were in a restaurant and we saw a waitress without a real leg." The two children gazed at her disbelievingly. "She had something else. I don't know what you call it. I think it was made of wood or plastic and looked sort of like a leg but not exactly. I know you're not supposed to stare but my Daddy said it was better to be curious than be uncomfortable and look away . . . ." And then with a conclusive sigh, "It was amazing. She did real well," and nodded her head approvingly.

Her friends agreed and looked toward me.

"Do you have any more questions?" Amanda said in her most teacherly fashion. No, they nodded, and smiling at both of us whispered, "Thank you," and trotted away in the snow.

Amanda with an air of satisfaction settled in the back seat. I turned around and asked what that was all about. "Well, Kristin often asks me questions about you and about your leg. And when she asked again today, I thought you could do it better."

"Better?"

"Yeah, there's only so much I could say. Some things you have to see."

"Oh," I answered rather speechlessly.

"And besides I knew you'd oblige."

"Yes," and she gave me a coy look, tilting her head downward. "I thought you'd be comfortable doing it. You were, weren't you?"

As I shifted the car to start, I nodded yes. But to myself I added . . . and everyday I get a little more comfortable.

7

Pregnancy and Delivery
A Personal View

Marca Bristo

I became disabled in 1977. I dived off a pier into Lake Michigan and broke my spine.

GETTING PREGNANT

Although I was reassured by my doctors early on that I was physically capable of having children, I had many concerns and fears about my safety and about my ability to care for the child. Almost all the medical information I had obtained said giving birth would be no problem. I understood this cognitively, but I had a lot of doubts on a personal level. Why hadn't I seen many parents with disabilities? Think about it as you go out into the community. Even though our visibility is increasing rapidly, it's still rare to see significant numbers of people with disabilities interacting. Seeing people with disabilities interacting with their own children is even more rare.

Becoming involved in the independent living movement brought me in contact with parents with disabilities who were inspiring role models for me. I knew if they could do it, I could too, if I went about everything in the right way. This exposure was invaluable in helping me decide to have a child.

THE PREGNANCY

Still, the overwhelming emotion during my pregnancy, labor, and delivery was fear of my own mortality. It was not unfounded. I had worked as a labor nurse and had read several articles on autonomic hyperreflexia. Some women had died or had strokes during labor. I didn't talk about it much, but I went through the majority of my pregnancy really wondering if I was going to make it.

So carefully selecting the right physician and medical team was of the utmost importance in putting my mind at ease as much as I could. I am fortunate to have adequate health insurance, which the great majority of women with disabilities do not. We have a 65% unemployment rate and because of this and the discrimination of insurance providers, most of us have little if any medical coverage. We more or less enter a medical lottery when we have to see a doctor and must take whom we get.

I knew I would need a high-risk medical team, so I selected a hospital renowned for its medical research. I brought to my first physician's appointment an annotated bibliography of hyperreflexia, pregnancy, labor, delivery, and spinal cord injury. I suppose I brought it because it gave me some psychological relief. As I expected, they had limited experience delivering women with spinal cord injuries and none with anyone with an injury as high as mine.

It was also important to me that my physicians respected the idea that, in many ways, I knew better than they what was best for me. The experience I gained from living with a disability for 13 years and managing my own care was not something I was willing to give up. My medical team cooperated well with me. They deferred to my expertise for things like controlling spasticity and transferring techniques.

It was also important that the members of my medical team communicated with each other. For example, I had more bladder infections than usual during pregnancy, so I wanted my obstetric and gynecology team to be in contact with my urologist. The team worked very well in this way too, which meant better care for my baby and me and reduced my own fear.

Having a game plan was also vital to me, so my obstetrician set up an appointment with me with the anesthesiologists early on. Doing this was the single greatest factor in controlling my anxiety. Although this team had not dealt with hyperreflexia during delivery, I learned they had done a lot of homework. We talked at great length about procedures, and they gave me confidence they could handle what could occur.

My body experienced other changes. As I got bigger, my balance was thrown off more than I expected, and toward the end of both pregnancies I used a transfer board more often than usual. Also, as my hips began to spread, I literally outgrew my wheelchair. Chairs like mine cost about $2,000, and I wasn't prepared to buy a new one just to make it through pregnancy. I borrowed a wider chair, but it wouldn't fit through my bathroom door at home. So I stayed in my original chair, even though the tight fit gave me tread marks on my hips that remain today. I was extra careful about watching out for dangerous skin abrasions.

My spasticity increased during pregnancy in frequency and intensity. The changes occurred toward the end of the first trimester. I experienced a new kind of spasm, which I call a trunk spasm. My upper body would tense rapidly, throwing me back in my wheelchair. One time my chair even tipped over backward in the bathroom, and I sustained a concussion from hitting my head on the floor. Wondering when this would happen again added a new level of fear, but knowing other people with disabilities provided the solution again. One of them told me about an anti-tip device I could add to my chair. It prevented me from tipping too far back without otherwise limiting my mobility.

My body sensations changed during pregnancy, too. I have irregular sensation because of my incomplete lesion, but basically I am without sensation from the breast line down. But while pregnant, my sensation increased, particularly in the genital area. That was a good side effect as I was able to feel intercourse more than usual.

My endurance and respiratory capacity were decreased. I wasn't able to push my chair far because I was too short of breath. I understand this shortness of breath is common even for women without disabilities. It was particularly troublesome for me at night. Often I would feel like I could not breathe at all and would have to prop myself up in bed with pillows. By the end of my pregnancy I was sleeping with seven pillows behind my back, practically upright.

I noticed changes in my body's ability to regulate its temperature. People with my type of injury have a very hard time adjusting to temperature extremes. We are very hot and uncomfortable in hot weather and when it is cold, we can shiver for hours. But when I was pregnant with my first child in winter, it was the first winter I slept without shivering, without needing a hot water bottle or anything else to warm me up. The majority of my second pregnancy was in the summer, and it was not beneficial this time around. I was extremely hot throughout the latter part of the pregnancy, so much so that it greatly reduced my mobility.

Because of my higher bladder infection rate, during the first pregnancy we decided to take a specimen during every visit, which the nurses assisted with in the latter part of the pregnancy. With the second pregnancy, the physicians chose to not treat the bladder infections unless I was running a high fever. Therefore, the team felt it was unnecessary to take samples at each visit, making my visits a great deal easier.

All this necessitated a flexible approach to my care. My medical team learned a lot from me. For instance, the medical facility didn't have an electric exam table that could be lowered so I could transfer onto it myself. At first the nurses lifted me onto a regular table, but two problems developed. First, bad spasms were triggered by the stirrups. Second, as I grew heavier, lifting became more difficult. So we agreed that most of my exams during the latter part of the pregnancy would be done on a regular bed. This made a big difference.

Of course, physical accessibility took on renewed importance. The medical facility I used during my first pregnancy had close parking, and I was able to park my car and transfer from it and get to the physician's office pretty much on my own. The parking wasn't nearly as good the second time, which increased my difficulty. I also found it harder and harder to transfer out of the car as I got bigger. I usually transfer myself, but as the pregnancy progressed, I preferred to have assistance. Physicians can help a lot by being aware of this and having the necessary assistance available or alternative suggestions.

My husband and I did a lot of the things most people do in preparation for the arrival of our new family member. Access and accommodation were again major variables. I searched quite a while to find a Lamaze instructor who was flexible about my needs since a lot of Lamaze exercises are not practical for me. I found an instructor who worked very well with us and made us feel very much a part of the class. The facility was accessible, and we were able to participate up to a point. This exposure was very, very important later in labor, especially having learned some nontraditional positions for pushing. It also involved my husband much more thoroughly in the whole process and eased our transition into parenthood.

I was recommended for genetic counseling during my second pregnancy, since this is standard for women over 35 and I was 36. I went, even though my counseling experience with my first pregnancy was not good at all. There was a clear bias. Obviously, they were accustomed to dealing with the nondisabled. The message I heard was, "If you, heaven forbid, should be carrying a deformed (i.e., disabled) fetus, there are many options including abortion." I've been pro-choice most of my life, but sitting there as a disabled adult, I was uncomfortable with the way it was being presented. There was no discussion of alternatives so I could make an informed decision. I raise this because it is loaded with attitudinal issues regarding disability. In addition to providing abortion as an option, they could have said to me, "If you happen to have a disabled child, there are many community organizations and techniques and treatments being developed, and that person can have a meaningful life." There is no way of predicting the severity of disability. This attitude reflects a lack of knowledge about societal, scientific, and technological changes regarding disability.

I was quite pleased that the genetic counselor I saw during my second pregnancy was, coincidentally, a woman with a disability. She was much more thorough. She was very quick to point out there were a number of options, and I was very pleased with that.

Our final step in preparation was establishing an accessible place in our home for child care. One of the biggest problems, strangely, was finding a crib I could operate. I never thought that most cribs operate with a toe release that frees the rail to slide up and down. That did not work for me, and it was difficult to find one with a hand release.

The only other modification I made was to use my desk as a changing table. Most changing tables have shelves or cabinets or something below them so I could not push underneath to get close enough. The desk with the changing pad on top of it was the simple solution.

LABOR AND DELIVERY

A dilemma my doctors and I faced as the due date drew nearer was whether or not I would be able to feel labor pains. Some women with spinal cord injuries can and others cannot. I could either be admitted to the hospital around my due date and wait, or I could hope to feel the pains. We opted for the latter. My physician spent a fair amount of time counseling me, holding my hand and assuring me that I would know when it was time to come. Having been a labor nurse, I knew how to manually detect labor pains by palpating the fundus, and I used that technique a great deal.

Let me share with you a funny anecdote about peer counseling gone awry. When I first learned I was pregnant, I wanted to speak to some other women with disabilities, and a nurse I knew gave me the name of someone she knew. I called the woman and asked if she had been able to feel her labor pains. She said, "I'm not sure I'm the person you want to speak to. I had just gotten over the flu and was having stomach cramps. I thought I needed to go to the bathroom and I transferred onto my commode chair. All of a sudden I heard this baby crying. I looked down and I had the baby in the commode chair!" Fortunately, she said, everything worked out. She had a portable telephone in her bathroom and she called 911. The 911 operators didn't believe her until they heard the baby crying.

I mention this for two reasons. First, it shows how a spinal cord-injured woman who is not well-counseled on what to expect might misinterpret symptoms or not feel labor pains the way she is expecting to. Also, it shows how using peer support, of which I am a strong advocate, needs to be done with discretion. Not everyone is the right match. It turned out I learned a lot from this woman so I don't regret having spoken to her, but her misadventure did add a lot to my anxiety.

I was able to detect my labor. I experienced Braxton-Hicks contractions for about 2 weeks before my due date. I could feel a tightening of my abdomen with my hand. I had small hyperreflexic rushes with mild goose bumps and mild sweating that would come and go with these infrequent contractions. I woke up one morning at dawn and the contractions were 20 minutes apart, and the hyperreflexia was much more severe. I went into the hospital more because of the hyperreflexia than the contractions.

My cervix was only dilated 1 centimeter, but my blood pressure was phenomenally high, something like 200/120 or higher, as I recall. The staff was very busy when I arrived, and it took some forceful urging on my part to get them to take my blood pressure right away. The nurses were not familiar with the specifics of my case so when I told them the contractions were not too regular they were not alarmed. But after they took my blood pressure, things started happening rapidly.

It was frightening. There were more people in the room than I could count. They inserted an epidural line but had some trouble determining whether the anesthetic was at the right level because I couldn't feel the pin pricks. They basically had to guess. The first dose of anesthetic made me so dizzy I nearly passed out. So they elevated my legs and finessed with the dosage until they got it right and were able to maintain my blood pressure at an acceptable level throughout labor and delivery.

In addition to the epidural line and catheter, there was also an arterial line to monitor my blood pressure. During my first pregnancy, they also put in a fetal monitor. My labor was very sluggish, but I didn't want to be induced, so I held out as long as I could. Eventually they convinced me I needed some assistance so they gave me some pitocin. They turned it off after about 5 minutes when there was some fetal deceleration. But apparently it was just enough to accelerate my labor because soon I gave birth to my beautiful 8-pound son, Sammy. It was a mid-forceps delivery with an episiotomy.

I had labored for 20 hours and pushed for 4. It was a little bit less in my second pregnancy, but I was having trouble bringing the baby down with my pushing. I used alternative positions in my first delivery with my legs up to my chest. My husband assisted by holding my head and holding my legs up, and I was able to bring the baby down well enough for the mid-forceps to be applied. In the second delivery, however, it seemed all my pushing was for naught. Nothing was happening in the nontraditional positions. We were about to give up when the doctor said, "Let me try something." He put me in the old-fashioned position with the stirrups. He must have had a significant intuition because the baby came flying out almost sooner than they could scrub. I delivered a 7-pound, 5-ounce girl, Madeline, with no episiotomy or forceps.

THE POSTPARTUM PERIOD

The most significant thing for me in the postpartum period was to be close to my baby immediately. I am sure that is true of all women, but I believe I felt a particular need because I had not felt most of the labor. I also had great doubts that I would be a good mother, which I am sure most women have, too. But I was still trying to overcome apprehensions about parenting with a disability. So I was very lucky they brought my babies to me right away, and I breastfed in the delivery room, which was very important for my bonding. I needed some help supporting the baby while I breastfed.

It took some time for me to feel I could be a good mother. For the first few days, I was even afraid to change Sammy's diaper. I can't explain it. I just felt terribly inadequate. I was lucky my husband took over until I felt up to it.

The hyperreflexive sweating was much more profound with my second pregnancy. These sweats, to me, are the most uncomfortable part of being spinal cord injured. This combined with the fullness of my breasts from nursing and the letdown reflex made me more uncomfortable and agitated than I care to remember. I was committed to nursing because I wanted to give my baby the immunological advantage. Retrospectively, I think I hung on too long. Sometimes I was shaking so much from the sweats I almost dropped her. Sometimes my sweat would be dripping on her as she fed. I believe it affected my early bonding because it is difficult to feel closeness when you are feeling so uncomfortable yourself. So I stopped breastfeeding her after 8 weeks. It was a great relief, and I felt much closer to her.

After my first pregnancy, I developed carpal tunnel syndrome, which required surgery on both wrists. I had them both done at once because one surgical procedure is as debilitating to a person who pushes a wheelchair as two. You cannot push a chair with one hand, so I wanted to get it over with. But I was extremely dependent during the recuperation and had to hire a personal assistant for the first time, in addition to child care assistance.

But there was a silver lining. This forced me into renting a motorized wheelchair, which I never would have otherwise done. I then discovered the great freedom a power chair gave me as a parent. Even before the baby was able to sit up on his own, I could hold him with one arm and drive all over the place. In the manual chair, with both hands occupied, I was very limited in what I could do with the babies in my lap until they developed their own balance. So there were a lot of new and frustrating limitations during this interim period. Having a power chair opened up a lot of freedom and richness for me and my babies that I would not have thought possible. I highly recommend it.

The key to my overcoming the insecurity as to whether I would be a good parent was once again sharing experiences with other women with disabilities. I was really pleased when I learned of an organization, Through the Looking Glass, which was starting to research the relationships formed between parents with disabilities and their children. I sent away for some of their materials and it was so validating to read about others who were experiencing what I was with my own children. For example, I lifted Sammy in and out of his crib by his clothing when he was little, and he would tuck his body into a little ball, which I always thought was really adorable. It may not have been the best way to lift, but I had no choice. An article I read described this very set of circumstances and said the child would adapt to being lifted this way by tuck-balling itself like a kitten. It was so reassuring to know that this was a normal way for a child to adjust to a parent with a disability.

In summary, women with disabilities going through pregnancy and delivery are much like anyone else. They have questions, they are going through physical changes, and they are struggling with emotional issues. I found that the most effective aspect in this regard was effective peer support. Having other people with disabilities to serve as role models, to provide emotional support, and to share practical tips on adjusting to pregnancy and parenting was indispensable. Medical professionals need to know how to find such people and be able to refer their patients accordingly.

Other counselors, such as genetic counselors, should be available and must have the proper sensitivity and awareness so pregnant women with disabilities will be able to make the right choices. It took a lot of different kinds of counseling for me to be able to work through a lot of my fears.

Physicians, when faced with a situation with which they have never dealt, need to acknowledge their own limits. They need to be willing to help gather information and share it with their patients. There is a great need for training materials that familiarize medical staff with all the aspects of dealing with disabled women. There should be material like this geared toward disabled women, too. It would make the transition to parenthood much easier.

Technology applications need to be thoroughly considered. In my case, it was a power wheelchair. For others, it may be some sort of device. There should be a comprehensive exploration as to how technology can make pregnancy and parenting easier.

Physical access is as important as ever. This applies not just to the physician's office, but to the person's home and the community in general. Optimal community access is obviously an important factor in developing strong, healthy relationships between parents with disabilities and their children, and in teaching their children how to relate with the other children of the world. This will be successfully accomplished to the extent that parents with disabilities and their children are able to participate in the kinds of activities that everyone else does.

Finally, there's dialogue. We need to bring together to thoroughly discuss this subject people from all walks of life, particularly the medical and research communities and the disabled community. I am always amazed at how much we can learn from one another, and I firmly believe that the 43 million disabled Americans are a vast untapped resource in terms of making physicians better at what they do. The more we can get together and talk about this, the better it will be for everyone.

~~~~~~

Sing a Song in Silence

Irving Kenneth Zola

*Y*our head is turned to one side and the flickering candle lights up your greying hair. You smile as I begin to caress you and let your hand rest on my shoulder. You look so peaceful.

Peaceful . . . I used to cringe when anyone described a relationship in those terms. And yet that's what I feel with you . . . peaceful, safe, comfortable. Can I really be in a relationship without turmoil . . . without longing . . . without pain? A part of me gets scared when I let this in, makes me feel it shouldn't be so easy.

You move your head without opening your eyes and I remember when we first met. It was an outdoor concert and I claimed that next to your Amigo was the only place I could park my wheelchair . . . and still hear. It was a lie. From the outset, we were very straightforward, careful to define the boundaries and problems . . . all before we ever touched. Both of us said we had a lifestyle that we wanted to continue. Both of us said we were too old to make long-term plans. Both of us said we didn't know what the word "love" meant.

But it's been a long time and here we are . . . still together. No commitments . . . and still we manage to see each other weekly.

We've talked about moving closer together but not together. You complained that it was too far to park and walk—sometimes you said waddle—from your car to my apartment. I matched you complaint for complaint. With my 60-plus years, bumping over even a 1-inch curb wasn't as easy as it once was.

And so we negotiate. No promises and yet when one of us is hurting, the other seems to know and is there.

When we first got together I used all the curbs and thresholds I had to bump over as an excuse for tiredness and a need to stay over. You countered that it was all downhill to my house.

You're beginning to make sounds like a purring kitten. I smile happily and want to say something. You told me once about another man who always spoke during lovemaking. I rarely do. I'm afraid I'll say the wrong thing. Besides tonight you told me we'd have to be extra quiet so we would not wake up your grandson.

I once tried to compose a poem for you but that didn't work. Another time I wrote you a letter but I tore it up. I did once sing you all the lyrics to "My Funny Valentine." You smiled and claimed I was trying to prove that I didn't have Alzheimer's.

I fear that after all our hesitations, all our fumblings, if I use the word love . . . I'll be reneging. If I use it then you'll think I'm just trying to overwhelm you . . . to extract forever-like promises.

When we first became lovers you said older women get very dry and like to go slower. I told you that older men aren't in such a hurry any more.

You reach down and touch my head. With both your hands you push me in deeper.

Why aren't there any words that do as well? Is "love" just something to fill the space when we can't think of anything else to say? But "care" and "appreciate" just seem so bland. Yet part of me wants to be bland . . . to be distant . . . to be independent.

I didn't even tell you about my birthday—or invite you to share it with me. I wasn't afraid you'd refuse, but just that you'd think I was asking more of you than you wanted to give. I did the same thing when I went in for those tests last year. Scared as I was, I didn't tell you or my children. I went alone.

A woman who knows me quite well once said that I need not put everything into words. Maybe I don't.

Your breathing is coming faster. Your lips part as if you're about to sigh. Feel me now. Feel my hands. Let my lips, my fingers, my tongue say what I won't let my words repeat.

Your hips rise off the bed and I hold onto your buttocks as if they were an anchor. And as I suck into you deeply, I fairly shout, "I love you . . . I love you," but only your vagina hears.

8

A Guide to Pregnancy, Labor, and Delivery for Women with Disabilities

Judith G. Rogers

The following is adapted from *Mother-To-Be: A Guide to Pregnancy and Birth for Women with Disabilities,* by Judith G. Rogers and Molleen Matsumura (1991), and discusses a few of the problems that affect the majority of pregnant women with disabilities.

Thirty-six women with a variety of disabilities were interviewed. (For anonymity, the women were given names in which the first letter corresponded with the disability. For example, Clara has cerebral palsy.)

The interviews conducted suggested that often it is the severity of disability, rather than the type, that helps to predict how difficult a pregnancy will be. For example, a woman who is quadriplegic because of cerebral palsy may have more in common with a woman who is quadriplegic because of spinal cord injury than with a woman with milder cerebral palsy. An interesting fact about the interaction of disability and pregnancy is that it may cause an exacerbation or a remission.

EMOTIONAL CONCERNS

Women with disabilities face both the same and additional emotional issues as women without disabilities. Women with disabilities

From Matsumura, M., & Rogers, J.G. (1991). *Mother-to-be: A guide to pregnancy and birth for women with disabilities.* New York: Demos Publications; reprinted and adapted with permission.

are in an unusual situation: Unlike most women, who experience social and emotional pressure to have children, *women without disabilities are under pressure not to have children.* The forces of social disapproval and, often, their own fears work against their having children. Even when abortions were illegal, they were relatively easily obtained by women with physical disabilities. Yet women with disabilities feel the same desire for raising children as other women. We support their right to choose motherhood.

Many women with disabilities still encounter negative attitudes toward their pregnancies. For women with disabilities, making the decision whether to have a baby involves answering three basic questions: 1) How will the pregnancy affect their disability? 2) How will their disability affect the course of pregnancy and the health and development of the baby? 3) How might the disability influence the tasks of child-rearing?

Some pregnancy problems are specific to, or made worse by, disabilities. For example, a women as she ages may be concerned not only about declining fertility, but also about declining physical abilities. Even for women whose disability is not progressive, concerns about aging are strengthened by the knowledge that disability adds to the usual stresses of aging.

As with all women, pregnancy in women with disabilities caused a gamut of emotions. Some were surprised and all were relieved that they could get pregnant. All were happy that their bodies worked the way they were supposed to. This is how all women feel, but it is intensified among those with disabilities. One interviewee said it was the first time her body worked the way it should.

For many women, how they felt about their pregnancy was affected by their family's response. Some parents were afraid of the physical effects pregnancy might have on their daughter. Sasha said she didn't enjoy her pregnancy as she should have because of her family's worry.

In the second trimester, the public becomes involved because the pregnancy shows. It tells all. Some enjoyed the stares because it shot down misconceptions about women with disabilities. One woman said how well she handled the stress depended on her mood. Frustrated by repeated comments of how brave she was, she retorted, "It wasn't any worse for me than for other women. In fact, my pregnancy was better than those of some of my able-bodied friends."

As with all couples, the primary relationship is affected by pregnancy. Sometimes, the pregnancy requires extra help from the spouses. But this, too, is intensified for the disabled woman. For one couple interviewed, the husband felt so overloaded that he left the marriage when his child was 18 months old. Therefore, it may be crucial to arrange for needed help.

Body image and sexuality are also affected by pregnancy. Some women enjoy how their body looks for the first time. Others feel they look more awkward. The first trimester brings relief that fertility/birth control are no longer issues. Some women lose interest in sexual relations because they feel sick, while others are afraid of harming the baby. During the second trimester, some women who experience pregnancy complications need to avoid sex because it can provoke labor. In the third trimester, many find sex uncomfortable and cumbersome.

INTERACTIONS OF DISABILITIES AND PREGNANCY

In interviews conducted between 4 weeks and 20 years after giving birth, all of the women said they had returned to much the same level of disability as had existed before pregnancy. No one felt that her disability had been permanently worsened or improved. (A few women, in informal conversations a few years after their interviews, wondered whether there had, in fact, been lasting effects. However, it was also possible that aging, or continuing disability processes, were responsible for the new problems these women were experiencing.)

Specific problems sometimes associated with disability, such as kidney dysfunction, can affect pregnancy and should be evaluated before conception. Also, some disability symptoms may be worsened by pregnancy. For example, a woman with respiratory problems may have more difficulty breathing during late pregnancy, when pressure from the uterus causes many women to become short of breath.

PREGNANCY DISCOMFORTS
COMMON TO WOMEN WITH DISABILITIES

Common discomforts of pregnancy that are uniquely affected by disability are listed below.

Urinary Discomforts

Urinary discomforts affect disabled pregnant women in several different ways.

1. As with pregnant women in general, women with disabilities experience increased frequency of urinary discomforts. However,

those with MS, for example, may have increased frequency due to pregnancy and to an exacerbation of their MS.

2. A few women without disabilities experience stress incontinence. This too is experienced by women with physical disabilities. It seems more prevalent with women who were already predisposed, for example, because of structural disabilities.

3. Because women with spinal cord injuries are already prone to bladder infections, a severe infection can cause pre-term labor.

As adaptations, some women have used disposable diapers and some have gone without underwear. Catheterization may become difficult. Occasionally, catheters may become obstructed with calcium crystals. One woman who had previously catheterized herself had difficulty doing so because of the pregnancy. In addition, she was constantly dripping. Because of these problems she went against her doctor's advice and used a Foley's catheter (a permanent catheter). Because her bladder lost its elasticity, she found it impossible to discontinue its use.

Mobility Difficulties

Mobility difficulties affected the majority of the pregnant women with disabilities, usually as early as the second trimester. Mobility also affects different activities of daily living. Some of the women interviewed found it difficult to rise from a chair or a toilet—many found if they used a raised toilet seat or an extra cushion, it became easier. Some also found it a "big hassle" to sit up from lying down. Some used an overhead trapeze to help. It is easier to move to a sitting position from lying on your side or when using a support or pillows or backrest.

Getting in and out of the bathtub was one of the most difficult maneuvers. It would be better to use a shower, but, if not available, use a chair or stool in the tub. Some women would get on their hands and knees and use a chair in the tub or a grasp bar to pull up. One woman avoided a bath because it was uncomfortable to transfer in and out and took sponge baths instead.

Transferring in and out of a car is difficult. One woman couldn't fit behind the steering wheel. Others found different ways to transfer to the car. One woman used a pillow, because it was easy to slide on and off.

Many interviewees mentioned their fears about falling during pregnancy. Ordinarily, they might worry because their disabilities made falling likely, or because falls could lessen their mobility. However, ever since Scarlett O'Hara's tumble down the stairs in

"Gone With the Wind," the idea that falls inevitably cause miscarriages has been a common misconception about pregnancy in 20th-
century America. This fear may become intensified in women with
disabilities.

Mobility problems bring up psychological problems, because
having a disability usually has a negative connotation. Some women
waited longer than they should have to start using a wheelchair and
thereby compromised their comfort and safety. These very women
switched to a wheelchair earlier than in their subsequent pregnancies. It is hard to break down the childhood message: "It is important to walk—walking is normal."

Fortunately, having time to adjust makes changes more palat-
able for women who are having a problem. One interviewee said, "If
I had to go immediately from not being pregnant to 8 months pregnant, it would have been impossible, but I managed because it was
gradual."

There are a few women whose mobility improved because of
pregnancy. A few women with rheumatoid arthritis found themselves free of joint pain. One said it had been an ordeal to walk from
one room to another, and it became enjoyable to walk.

Respiratory Discomforts

Respiratory discomforts also improved in some cases. One woman
said the baby acted like a corset: "The pressure made it easier for me
to breathe and cough." However, for some, the pressure of the uterus
on the diaphragm created difficulty, in some to the point of pain.
One who found it more difficult to talk took a breath more often to
compensate. One wheelchair user found breathing painful because
constant sitting caused her baby to ride higher. She relieved the pain
by changing position, by lying down. A recliner chair could also help
this problem.

Eating more often and eating smaller amounts seems to help,
because it avoids adding the extra pressure of a full stomach to the
pressure of the uterus. Another hint is to breathe in through the
nose and out through the mouth. It is important to find out how
much breathing may be compromised, because a lowered oxygen
level may endanger both the mother and fetus. A respiratory therapist may also have other helpful techniques for breathing.

Skin Condition

Skin condition has always been a worry for those with spinal dysfunction, leading to special concern for exacerbation during pregnancy. Although our sample was small, the majority of women expe-

rienced their best skin condition ever. One woman with spina bifida who had a constant problem throughout her life with a pressure sore on her foot was delighted that it cleared up for the first (and only) time while she was pregnant.

SPECIAL NEED FOR TEAMWORK

Because few obstetricians have extensive experience with disabilities, it is crucial for the obstetrician to confer with the patient's disability specialist. One interviewee who had arthritis felt that her OB had little knowledge of her disability. Once he began collaborating with her rheumatologist, he was able to order appropriate tests and adjust medications accordingly. Having previously felt uncomfortable, she then felt confident about the care she received. Sometimes medications used to treat pregnancy complications can exacerbate disability symptoms. For example, the drugs used for preeclampsia or pre-term labor may cause muscle weakness in women with myasthenia gravis or increase the risk of infections in women with lupus. It is not only important for the primary OB to talk to the disability specialist but also to partners and physicians who share care, as information may not be readily accessible on the patient's chart. It is also important that a doctor's personal attitudes not interfere with good medical practice. One woman with spina bifida had a supportive doctor, but the doctor's partner was appalled about her being a parent and coerced her into a tubal ligation at the time of delivery.

OFFICE PROCEDURES

Good communication is important with medical office staff as well. This is particularly true because what are simple office procedures for a regular patient may not be so for a pregnant woman with a disability. One common diagnostic measurement that can stump any good staff is how to weigh a woman who uses a wheelchair. Most obstetric scales are not suited for this situation. Some women who were interviewed weighed themselves elsewhere, on a freight scale, a laundry scale, a nursing home scale, and a vet scale. The common alternative of an attendant or husband weighing her- or himself and then weighing both together may not work. One woman who tried this method was afraid to gain weight, because she was afraid of injuring her husband. A diagnostic test that may be difficult to conduct is urinalysis because of inaccessible bathrooms, difficult transfer onto the toilet, or difficulty in self-catheterization. A common solution has been to bring a sample from home. Several problems can occur in connection with the pelvic exam. First is difficulty with transfer onto the examining table. If the woman doesn't have an attendant present, it is important that the patient inform the staff about her preferred transfer technique. One physician ended up buying a hydraulic examining table. Second, there is a risk with being alone in the room before or after the exam. Should problems arise, she may have no way of getting help. Even if all is well, she may be stranded on the table unable to dress or leave. It is also important to make sure adaptive equipment is easily available. There also may be a problem in conducting the pelvic exam or in interpreting it. Sometimes the fundus appears higher than should correlate with the length of the pregnancy. This happened to one interviewee who had lordosis, which affected the angle of the uterus and caused miscalculation of the due date. Finding a comfortable position for the exam may be hard, because some women have difficulty assuming the usual position. A few prefer to be on their side. Some women may need to have their feet held. Others find it more comfortable with their knees supported by the stirrups. There may be some difficulty doing an exam for a woman with a catheter. The catheter does not need to be removed, but the tubing should not be bent. A good hint is to put the leg bag on the table to help assure good drainage. Women with spinal cord injuries need to be protected from hyperreflexia. Blood pressure increase is common and, without timely intervention, carries the potential for a stroke. A simple preventive measure is to have the bladder and bowel empty. Thus it may be important to schedule the exam the day after her weekly or biweekly bowel program. An internal exam may also promote hyperreflexia, and some physicians have found that applying anesthetic gel to the vagina and speculum is helpful. Sometimes a pelvic exam may also set off muscle spasms in a limb. It is helpful to hold and brace the limb until the spasms subside. Good communication is helpful between patient and staff for a positive experience.

LABOR

It is not surprising that women wonder, "How will I know I'm really in labor?" Some women with disabilities may experience atypical symptoms, and many women who have disabilities that involve the loss of sensation may not have the experience they expected. The sensory nerves to the uterus are between T10 and T12, so women who have injuries below T12 will feel labor and those with injuries higher than T10 may still feel labor. Samantha was sure she would feel labor contractions despite her disability, an injury to T10–T12. She had been experiencing Braxton-Hicks contractions, and her midwife told her that her cervix was slightly dilated. However, she never felt early labor. It began in her sleep, and she suddenly woke up in the transitional phase. (Some women without disabilities have had similar experiences.) Other women were surprised when they *did* feel labor contractions.

Women with spinal dysfunction may experience labor differently from other women. Women who have some internal sensations, such as bladder fullness, noticing fetal movements, or Braxton-Hicks contractions, may feel something during labor, but *what* they will feel cannot be predicted. Stephanie, who "didn't expect to feel it that well" and thought, "The sensation would be sufficiently dull to take the edge off," was surprised when, "It hurt more than I expected." Sharon described a feeling of "pressure." Sheila said that when her second child was born, she felt "an uncomfortable tightening" and was able to time her contractions, although she did not feel contractions with her first child. For some with diminished sensation, the woman herself or a friend can rest a hand on the lower abdomen and wait to feel the first tightening or hardening of the uterus.

Women with spinal dysfunction may need to be alert for other signs or symptoms of labor. Sheila remembers that the night before she knew that labor had started, she felt an urge to urinate every 20–30 minutes, but never did pass much urine. However, her amniotic membrane ruptured in the morning, and she then realized she was in labor. Looking back, she realized that her urge to urinate must have been a response to labor contractions. Sheila remembers that just before her water broke, she looked down and noticed that "my stomach had an odd, lopsided shape." Sharon, too, commented, "I saw my stomach stick out, then fall." Because some women never do feel labor, we suggest that women with spinal dysfunction make a habit of looking or feeling for contractions a few times a day during the weeks preceding their due date.

For some women, hyperreflexia may be triggered by contraction pressure within the uterus. One interviewee had a severe headache at the beginning of labor, which dissipated when her water broke. During her second labor, she had a small leak, and the only symptom of her hyperreflexia was a slight headache that never escalated.

Generally, if labor doesn't progress, induction or augmentation will be used. However, labor must not be induced or augmented in women with spinal cord injuries at or above T6. The longer and stronger contractions of induced labor seem to increase the risk of hyperreflexia.

While the inconvenience of an IV may be minor for able-bodied women, it is more of a problem for women with disabilities. Clara, who is hemiplegic, commented, "I'm really glad I didn't need an IV when I was in labor. Whenever I have surgery, they have to put the IV in my unaffected arm, because it's too hard to get a good vein on the other side. Then it's really hard for me to change position." An IV during labor may also disrupt the sense of equilibrium. One woman said, "It was difficult to move because I felt off balance." In addition, a woman with a disability may need extra care during transfers to protect the IV line.

Transition is a difficult time for many women because contractions are spaced so closely together. When Samantha talked about this phase of her labor, she explained, "The contractions were right on top of each other—unlike my other labors, where I seemed to have some space between contractions. It was *very* intense." Samantha's remark is especially significant because this labor, her third, occurred after her spinal cord injury.

Finding a good position during labor can be challenging for patients with disabilities. Sitting, reclining, and side-lying are especially useful for some. Sharon, with a spinal cord injury, can usually turn onto her side by herself, but she felt she needed to be careful because of the epidural catheter in her back, so she needed help turning onto her side. Another woman needed help because the IV in her arm made it difficult to change position. For some women, an ordinary hospital bed was helpful; Stacy grasped the hand rails to help herself turn. Using the controls of the bed, a woman can get into a comfortable seated position, or move to a reclining position as a first step toward a side-lying position. When Faith had her third child, she was in labor sitting in her wheelchair. She explained, "My husband was sick and he couldn't help me transfer, so it was easier to just stay in my chair till I went to the delivery room. When they needed to do an exam, I just went over to a bed and somebody propped my legs up on the side of the bed."

Range of motion exercises throughout the labor may reduce clonus or muscle spasms, which commonly occur during transition. Besides massaging the cramped muscle, the coach can try holding and bracing the leg. Bracing is especially useful for very severe cramps and spasms that some women with disabilities experience. Christina had severe leg spasms during transition, and her three coaches took turns holding her legs. One coach would hold each leg while the third coach rested. Clara's worst spasms, which occurred during delivery, were so strong that her second coach could not hold her leg, but her husband managed to by bracing Clara's foot against his chest and using both hands to turn it outward, away from the spasm.

Faith found an original way to relieve muscle spasms. During labor, she spent part of her time kneeling against a bean bag chair. She said, "Leaning against the bean bag was very comfortable. Then I started having spasms—my legs jumped with every contraction. We spread a sleeping bag on the floor and I got on all fours on the sleeping bag. The pressure on my knees stopped the spasms." Faith's method might not work for all women, but it is worth trying if other methods of relieving spasms do not work.

Some practitioners consider the urge to push as the hallmark of transition, but this can be misleading. This urge, or sometimes a feeling of rectal fullness, seems to be caused by the fetal head pressing against the rectal nerve. Only half of the interviewees with spinal cord injuries experienced an urge to push. Jennifer remembers asking a nurse who had just checked on her, "When should I call you?" and the nurse replied, "When you feel like pushing." Stacy, despite her spinal cord injury, reported, "My need to push was too strong to control."

DELIVERY

One special concern of women with disabilities at this stage is the transfer from a labor room to a delivery room. It can be helpful to have labor and delivery in the same room. Otherwise, it is a good idea for the woman's attendant to show the hospital staff how she normally transfers. Sheila had an unusual reaction to the pressure of the fetal head—her legs became numb. She said, "Usually I can do a standing pivot transfer, but I couldn't do it then. My legs went numb and they were limp as spaghetti."

For many women with disabilities, side-lying or partially reclining positions work well for delivery. Some women may also need help in holding up their legs. Christina, with cerebral palsy, used a delivery table, but could not use the stirrups because she could not bend her knees. Instead, two nurses helped, each one holding one leg out to the side. Sharon used the stirrups part of the time and had her legs held by a nurse part of the time. Others found the delivery table and stirrups helpful and even comfortable. Celeste chose a side-lying position because she had difficulty spreading her legs. While lying on her side, a nurse held up her top leg and the delivery went well. Samantha, who gave birth at home, sat more comfortably with her husband behind her and leaning on him for support. She held her thighs and someone else supported her lower legs.

Women with spinal cord injuries may not feel the urge to push due to fetal position, regional anesthesia to prevent hyperreflexia, or the disability itself. Sharon, who had felt no urge to push, bore down three or four times as instructed, and delivery was then completed with forceps. Sheila, who couldn't push, was "able to feel the baby slip down."

Because the flaccid abdominal muscles of the woman with a spinal cord injury cannot help voluntary pushing, the author suspects that the strength of the stomach muscles is less important to the delivery than the strength of uterine contractions. Some women in the general population have difficulty giving birth, which is clearly related to weak, tired, or uncoordinated uterine contractions. What is most important is that women with spinal cord injuries are often able to give birth vaginally, often without assistance, because of the strength of the uterus.

CESAREAN SECTION

Because the need for c-sections often can't be predicted, good communication before the need arises is essential. C-sections pose special complications for women with disabilities. Given prior limitations, surgery may significantly affect mobility in the ability to transfer, change position, or walk. Some women found their balance was impaired and required a period of time to return. A woman with Friedreich ataxia said, "It took 3 to 4 months to bounce back after the birth of my first baby by c-section." Although her disability is progressive, Faith was able "to bounce back in 3 or 4 weeks" after the vaginal birth of her second child. Decreased mobility can, in turn, lead to emboli when women cannot exercise and to respiratory infections in women with breathing difficulties. Surgical recovery may contribute to flare-ups of lupus or MS because of the extra stress on the body.

In case a c-section is necessary, a cesarean preparation course will improve readiness for the procedure. Given the disability, consultation may be advisable for the patient, anesthesiologist, and disability specialist. Faith had general anesthesia because the anesthesiologist was uncomfortable about the interaction of a regional anesthesia (spinal) and her disability, Friedreich ataxia. Faith felt more devastated by the cesarean because she was unconscious. As with other women with disabilities, general anesthesia could have been avoided if her anesthesiologist had been more knowledgeable.

Recovery is another important step. Women who have had a regional anesthesia are usually observed for the return of sensation and motion. However, for women who have spinal cord injuries, sensation and motion cannot be used to verify recovery from anesthesia. Instead, muscle tone and reflexes below the level of the injury should be evaluated and compared with the pre-surgical state. Sometimes a woman is aware of certain special needs because of her disability. For example, one interviewee is unable to lie flat on her back. She needed to make arrangements to recover in a different position, either on her side or with a pillow for support.

Transfers may require special care. Several interviewees were jolted when transferred, which pulled on their incision. There are several procedures to ease transfers. Pain medication should be given $1/2$ hour before transfer. The woman with a disability needs to talk to the nursing staff prior to surgery to inform them of the best way to handle the transfers.

Catheterization was uncomfortable for most women. Some felt it caused stress incontinence because the catheter stayed in longer than usual or longer than absolutely necessary.

POSTPARTUM RECOVERY

Postpartum nurses also need information about the woman's disability. For example, many people with spinal cord injuries are taught a "clean" method of self-catheterization for home use that is less rigorous than the standard sterile hospital technique. Because hospitals require the latter to prevent nosocomial infections (infections acquired in the hospital), misunderstandings can be avoided by explaining to the patient the temporary need for a different technique. A nurse from the local rehabilitation unit may be able to provide helpful pointers.

CHILDCARE ISSUES

Because women with disabilities may have a special fear about the health of their babies, it is important for them to see their newborns as soon as possible for reassurance that all is well.

Holding the baby is difficult for some women. Even if they are not tired or shaking, they may feel insecurely balanced on the narrow delivery table, or fearful of dropping the baby because of poor hand control. A little help from the father or nursing staff can ensure that the first moments after birth are joyous ones.

Breastfeeding has some special considerations for disabled women. Are medications problematic for the baby? Which is physically easier—preparing bottles or proper positioning of the baby for breastfeeding? Will total breastfeeding be tiring and lead to an exacerbation of disability symptoms?

Despite the fears of many, mothers with disabilities and their babies generally adapt well to each other's needs and limitations. For example, all five of Portia's children learned to crawl to her wheelchair and cling to her arm so she could lift them into her lap. Their skill was strikingly illustrated when she babysat for a neighbor's child who could not follow suit.

CONCLUSION

Some of the women interviewed did not experience any more difficulty in pregnancy, labor, and delivery than the average woman. Regardless of whether the women found their pregnancies more difficult than average, none of the interviewees said that they regretted their decision.

~·

Tell Me...Tell Me

Irving Kenneth Zola

Now I was the one who was nervous. Here we were alone in her room thousands of miles from my home.

"Well, my personal care attendant is gone, so it will all be up to you," she said sort of puckishly, "Don't look so worried! I'll tell you what to do."

This was a real turnabout. It was usually me who reassured my partner. Me who, after putting aside my cane, and removing all the clothes that masked my brace, my corset, my scars, my thinness, my body. Me who'd say, "Well, now you see 'the real me'." How often I'd said that, I thought to myself. Saying it in a way that hid my basic fear—that this real me might not be so nice to look at . . . might not be up to "the task" before me.

She must have seen something on my face, for she continued to reassure me, "Don't be afraid." And as she turned her wheelchair toward me she smiled at me that smile that first hooked me a few hours before. "Well," she continued, "first we have to empty my bag." And with that brief introduction we approached the bathroom.

Anger quickly replaced fear as I realized she could get her wheelchair into the doorway but not through it.

"Okay, take one of those cans," she said pointing to an empty Sprite, "and empty my bag into it."

Though I'd done that many times before it wasn't so easy this time. I quite simply couldn't reach her leg from a sitting position on the toilet and she couldn't raise her foot toward me. So down to the floor I lowered myself and sat at her feet. Rolling up her trouser leg I fumbled awkwardly with the clip sealing the tube. I looked up at her and she laughed, "It won't break and neither will I."

I got it open and her urine poured into the can. Suddenly I felt a quiver in my stomach. The smell was more overpowering than I'd expected. But I was too embarrassed to say anything. Emptying the contents into the toilet I turned to her again as she backed out. "What should I do with the can?" I asked.

"Wash it out," she answered as if it were a silly question. "We try to recycle everything around here."

Proud of our first accomplishment we headed back into the room. "Now comes the fun part . . . getting me into the bed." For a few minutes we looked for the essential piece of equipment—the transfer board. I laughed silently to myself. I seemed to always be misplacing my cane—that constant reminder of my own physical dependency. Maybe for her it was the transfer board.

When we found it leaning against the radiator I reached down to pick it up and almost toppled over from its weight. Hell of a way to start, I thought to myself. If I can't lift this how am I going to deal with her. More carefully this time, I reached down and swung it on the bed.

She parallel parked her wheelchair next to the bed, grinned, and pointed to the side arm. I'd been this route before, so I leaned over and dismantled it. Then with her patient instructions I began to shift her. The board had to be placed with the wider part on the bed and the narrower section slipped under her. This would eventually allow me to slip her across. But I could do little without losing my own balance. So I lay down on the mattress and shoved the transfer board under her. Then first one foot and then the other I lifted toward me till she was at about a 45° angle in her wheelchair. I was huffing but she sat in a sort of bemused silence. Then came the scary part. Planting myself as firmly as I could behind her, I leaned forward, slipped my arms under hers and around her chest and then with one heave hefted her onto the bed. She landed safely with her head on the pillow and I joined her wearily for a moment's rest. For this I should have gone into training, I smiled silently. And again, she must have understood something as she opened her eyes even wider to look at me. What beautiful eyes she has, I thought, a brightness heightened by her very dark eyebrows.

"You're blushing again," she said.

"How can you tell that it's not from exhaustion?" I countered.

"By your eyes . . . because they're twinkling."

I leaned over and kissed her again. But more mutual appreciation would have to wait; there was still work to be done.

The immediate task was to plug her wheelchair into the portable recharger. This would have been an easy task for anyone except the technical incompetent that I am.

"Be careful," she said. "If you attach the wrong cables you might shock yourself."

I laughed. A shock from this battery would be small compared to what I've already been going through.

But even this attaching was not so easy. I couldn't read the instructions clearly, so down to the floor I sank once more.

After several tentative explorations, I could see the gauge registering a positive charge. I let out a little cheer.

She turned her head toward me and looked down as I lay stretched out momentarily on the floor, "Now the real fun part," she teased, "You have to undress me."

"Ah, but for this," I said in my most rakish tones, "we'll have to get closer together." My graceful quip was, however, not matched by any graceful motion. For I had to crawl on the floor until I could find a chair onto which I could hold and push myself to a standing position.

As I finally climbed onto the bed, I said, "Is this trip really necessary?" I didn't know what I intended by that remark but we both laughed. And as we did and came closer, we kissed, first gently and then with increasing force until we said almost simultaneously, "We'd better get undressed."

"Where should I start?" I asked.

"Wherever you like," she said in what seemed like a coquettish tone.

I thought it would be best to do the toughest first, so I began with her shoes and socks. These were easy enough but not so her slacks. Since she could not raise herself, I alternated between pulling, tugging, and occasionally lifting. Slowly over her hips, I was able to slip her slacks down from her waist. By now I was sweating as much from anxiety as exertion. I was concerned I'd be too rough and maybe hurt her but most of all I was afraid that I might inadvertently pull out her catheter. At least in this anxiety I was not alone. But with her encouragement we again persevered. Slacks, underpants, corset all came off in not so rapid succession.

At this point a different kind of awkwardness struck me. There was something about my being fully clothed and her not that bothered me. I was her lover not her personal care attendant. And so I asked if she minded if I took off my clothes before continuing.

I explained in a half-truth that it would make it easier for me to get around now "without all my equipment." "Fine with me," she answered and again we touched, kissed, and lay for a moment in each other's arms.

Pushing myself to a sitting position I removed my own shirt, trousers, shoes, brace, corset, bandages, and undershorts until I was

comfortably nude. The comfort lasted but a moment. Now I was embarrassed. I realized that she was in a position to look upon my not-so-
beautiful body. My usual defensive sarcasm about "the real me" began
somewhere back in my brain but this time it never reached my lips.
"Now what?" was the best I could come up with.

"Now my top . . . and quickly. I'm roasting in all these clothes."

I didn't know if she was serious or just kidding but quickness was
not in the cards. With little room at the head of the bed, I simply could
not pull them off as I had the rest of her clothes.

"Can you sit up?" I asked.

"Not without help."

"What about once you're up?"

"Not then either . . . not unless I lean on you."

This time I felt ingenious. I locked my legs around the corner of
the bed and then grabbing both her arms I yanked her to a sitting
position. She made it but I didn't. And I found her sort of on top of me,
such a tangle of bodies we could only laugh. Finally I managed to push
her and myself upright. I placed her arms around my neck. And then,
after the usual tangles of hair, earrings, and protestations that I was
trying to smother her, I managed to pull both her sweater and blouse
over her head. By now I was no longer being neat, and with an apology
threw her garments toward the nearest chair. Naturally I missed . . .
but neither of us seemed to care. The bra was the final piece to go and
with the last unhooking we both plopped once more to the mattress.

For a moment we just lay there but as I reached across to touch
her, she pulled her head back mockingly, "We're not through yet."

"You must be kidding!" I said, hoping that my tone was not as
harsh as it sounded.

"I still need my booties and my night bag."

"What are they for?" I asked out of genuine curiosity.

"Well my booties—those big rubber things on the table—keep
my heels from rubbing and getting irritated, and the night bag . . .
well that's so we won't have to worry about my urinating during the
night."

The booties I easily affixed, the night bag was another matter.
Again it was more my awkwardness than the complexity of the task.
First, I removed the day bag, now emptied, but still strapped around
her leg and replaced it with the bigger night one. Careful not to
dislodge the catheter, I had to find a place lower than the bed to attach
it so gravity would do the rest. Finally the formal work was done. The
words of my own thoughts bothered me for I realized that there was
part of me that feared what "work" might still be ahead.

She was not the first woman with a disability I'd ever slept with but she was, as she had said earlier, "more physically dependent than I look." And she was. As I prepared to settle down beside her, I recalled watching her earlier in the evening over dinner. Except for the fact that she needed her steak cut and her cigarette lit, I wasn't particularly conscious of any dependence. In fact quite the contrary, for I'd been attracted in the first place to her liveliness, her movements, her way of tilting her head and raising her eyebrows. But now it was different. This long process of undressing reinforced her physical dependency.

But before I lay down again, she interrupted my associations, "You'll have to move me. I don't feel centered." And as I reached over to move her legs, I let myself fully absorb her nakedness. Lying there she seemed somehow bigger. Maybe it was the lack of muscle tone if that's the word—but her body seemed somehow flattened out. Her thighs and legs and her breasts, the latter no longer firmly held by her bra, flopped to her side. I felt guilty a moment for even letting myself feel anything. I was as anxious as hell but with no wish to flee. I'm sure my face told it all. For with her eyes she reached out to me and with her words gently reassured me once again, "Don't be afraid."

And so as I lay beside her we began our loving. I was awkward at first, I didn't know what to do with my hands. And so I asked. In a way it was no different than with any other woman. In recent years, I often find myself asking where and how they like to be touched. To my questions she replied, "my neck . . . my face . . . especially my ears . . ." And as I drew close she swung her arms around my neck and clasped me in a surprisingly strong grip.

"Tighter, tighter, hold me tighter," she laughed again, "I'm not fragile . . . I won't break." And so I did. And as we moved I found myself naturally touching other parts of her body. When I realized this I pulled back quickly, "I don't know what you can feel."

"Nothing really in the rest of my body."

"What about your breasts?" I asked rather uncomfortably.

"Not much . . . though I can feel your hands there when you press."

And so I did. And all went well until she told me to bite and squeeze harder, then my arm began to shake. Feeling the quiver she again reassured me. So slowly and haltingly where she led, I followed.

I don't know how long we continued kissing and fondling, but as I lay buried in her neck, I felt the heels of her hands digging into my back and her voice whispering, "Tell me . . . tell me."

Suddenly I got scared again. Tell her what. Do I have to say that I love her? Oh my God! And I pretended for a moment not to hear.

"Tell me . . . tell me," she said again as she pulled me tighter. With a deep breath, I meekly answered, "Tell you what?"

"Tell me what you're doing," she said softly, "so I can visualize it." With her reply I breathed a sigh of relief. And a narrative voyage over her body began; I kissed, fondled, caressed every part I could reach. Once I looked up and I saw her with her head relaxed, eyes closed, smiling.

It was only when we stopped that I realized I was unerect. In a way my penis was echoing my own thoughts. I had no need to thrust, to fuck, to quite simply go where I couldn't be felt.

She again intercepted my own thoughts—"Move up, please put my hands on you," and as I did I felt a rush through my body. She drew me toward her again until her lips were on my chest and gently she began to suckle me as I had her a few minutes before. And so the hours passed, ears, mouths, eyes, tongues inside one another.

And every once in awhile she would quiver in a way which seemed orgasmic. As I thrust my tongue as deep as I could in her ear, her head would begin to shake, her neck would stretch out, and then her whole upper body would release with a sigh.

Finally, at some time well past 1 we looked exhaustedly at one another. "Time for sleep," she yawned, "But there is one more task— an easy one. I'm cold and dry so I need some hot water."

"Hot water!" I said rather incredulously.

"Yep, I drink it straight. It's my one vice."

And as she sipped the drink through a long straw I closed my eyes and curled myself around the pillow. My drifting off was quickly stopped as she asked rather archly, "You mean you're going to wrap yourself around that rather than me?"

I was about to explain that I rarely slept curled around anyone and certainly not vice versa but I thought better of it, saying only, "Well I might not be able to last this way all night."

"Neither might I," she countered, "my arm might also get tired."

We pretended to look at each other angrily but it didn't work. So we came closer again, hugged, and curled up as closely as we could, with my head cradled in her arm and my leg draped across her.

And much to my surprise I fell quickly asleep—unafraid, un-smothered, and more importantly, rested, cared for, and loved.

9

The Adoption Option

Colleen Starkloff

Our experience with domestic adoption, although expensive and psychologically exhausting, did result in our finally being able to have our three wonderful children. Through it all I could not help but believe that it has got to be easier to be pregnant!

As I speak with friends who have disabilities and who want to adopt children, I know that they will need time, money, and lots of energy, in addition to emotional drive, in order to surmount the numerous barriers to domestic adoption that they will face. I would like to address those barriers, because unless they are reduced, the future will remain bleak for prospective adoptive parents.

The first problem is a source of children. The number of American women wanting to adopt is growing, attributable in large part to the fact that more women in America today are having their careers first and then starting their families and are experiencing problems with fertility. Therefore, the competition is fierce from nondisabled people wanting to adopt, and people with disabilities and their non-disabled spouses are not considered as first choices by social workers. This discrimination is doubled when a couple, both of whom have disabilities, wishes to adopt. Triple the discrimination if a single person with a disability wants to adopt. Suffice it to say that the more severe the disability of one or both partners, the greater the discrimination they face when trying to adopt.

Other factors also influence the low number of children available. Abortion is an obvious factor. Lack of support of adoption as an acceptable solution to an unwanted pregnancy on the part of families and society in general leads many young girls and women to choose abortion or to keep their babies.

Policies about not placing biracial children in white homes keeps many of these children in foster care instead of getting them into homes where they will be loved and accepted.

Laws protecting parents' rights to their children often pose a serious interference when agencies try to free foster children for adoption. For example, in the state of Missouri, a child who is in foster care cannot become free for adoption on the basis of neglect by the parent, unless the parent has neglected the child for 6 months. Neglect in foster care means no contact with the child by the natural parent during that time. However, one single phone call or postcard from the parent to the foster home constitutes interest in the child on the part of the parent, and, therefore, a new neglect period of 6 months must begin. Also, at least one natural parent must show up in court to sign a termination of parental rights document in order to free a child for adoption. Then the other parent is "advertised" for a period of time before he or she can be considered to have abandoned the child and his or her parental rights terminated by the court. What happens too often is that the birth mother will not show up for her court date and no one seems to know where she is. It can take weeks or months for the adoption agency to get another court date, and the baby or child lingers in foster care.

Other barriers needing resolution include the high cost of adoption. Ten thousand dollars and more is not an unusual cost for an adoption of a domestic child. There are tax credits for adopting a "special needs child" or a child with some disability but no tax exemptions for adoption of a child with no disability.

Insurance will not cover the medical costs related to adoption. For example, we have family coverage and maternity benefits are included. None of the medical costs for prenatal care or delivery for our second and third children were covered by our insurance because I was not pregnant.

Attitude on the part of adoption agency social workers is another problem. The assumptions that physical limitations equate with inability to parent are simply not true, but just telling some agency social workers that is often not enough. However, there are many parents with disabilities who have raised or are raising their children successfully who are most willing to share their tricks of the trade. It is a matter of collecting and sharing this information through a common medium.

Obviously, not every social worker needs an attitude adjustment when it comes to placing children with a parent or parents with disabilities. There are some who can sing great praises about the social workers who helped them. Unfortunately, such social workers are a rare breed.

Another problem that seems to go unmentioned too often is the lack of persistent follow-up counseling for birth mothers. Giving up a baby is a very difficult decision to come to for many, and to live with for most, without competent psychological support. Many young women and girls give up their babies for lots of reasons: lack of family support, lack of money, no husband, the pregnancy interrupts the pursuit of a career, they don't want children, they are on drugs, they want the children to have opportunities they cannot give them—it runs the gamut. But sometimes after they have given the baby up, it hits them. Without strong counseling support, the impact of their decision can cause irreparable psychological damage. I speak on their behalf because if three of these women had not given their babies up for adoption, I would not be a mother today. I am grateful to all three of them and to all of the women who give up their babies. I have recently become aware of how few of them take the psychological support that is offered them by their agency and of the serious repercussions some of them experience. Some OBs may find the opportunity to recommend adoption to someone with an unwanted pregnancy. I hope that they will also insist on follow-up counseling to make sure that the decision really rests well with the birth mother, and she can go on with her life without the guilt, shame, and longing that often present themselves.

I recognize that the problems I have mentioned are the same for nondisabled couples who wish to adopt children. But the existence of these problems only magnifies the problems that people with disabilities face when we try to adopt children. We are usually the last option chosen by an agency for placement of a child. We need to work to solve the general problems of adoption in order to increase our chances of success.

Some of the solutions I would like to propose are as follows:

1. Development of videotapes that can be used to teach social work, rehabilitation, and medical students about the parenting abilities of people with disabilities. (These could also be helpful to people with disabilities who want tips on parenting techniques.)
2. Changes in foster care laws that would free children for adoption more quickly
3. Tax deductions for costs directly related to the adoption of children
4. Insurance coverage for medical costs related to adoption

10

The Adoptive Process
Challenges and Opportunities for People with Disabilities

Glen W. White and Nancy L. White

People with physical disabilities frequently face barriers when trying to have their own children. This may be due to a number of factors. For example, some disabilities may affect the ability to procreate. The male is usually the one affected by a secondary condition of infertility due to a primary disabling condition such as spinal cord injury or diabetes. Male sexual dysfunction problems may include impotence and inability to produce viable semen for insemination.

Another possible barrier to biologic families is the potential for a parent with an inherited disability to pass on disability-related genetic traits of the condition to his or her progeny (e.g., Huntington's disease or cystic fibrosis).

A number of options exist to accommodate a person with a disability who desires a family. Such options might range from finding a partner who already has children to determining if one's semen can be recovered and used for artificial insemination. This chapter focuses on another alternative: adoption.

For people with disabilities who wish to increase their family size through this option, the adoption process can pose a formidable challenge. Prospective adoptive parents are placed through a series of interviews, parental competency tests, and in many cases, fingerprint and background checks. This chapter briefly explores the adoption process for people with disabilities and addresses why individuals with disabilities may choose to adopt and the typical channels used for adoption. The various types of child placements available and how to find the right adoption agency are also examined.

THE ADOPTION PROCESS

Orientation Meeting

Most adoption agencies have regularly scheduled adoption orientations that specify agency eligibility criteria and relevant information on adoption policies, process, and cost. Often these meetings are designed to assist clients in determining whether adoption is a possible option for them.

Home Study

As the name suggests, the home study is an evaluation of the appropriateness of the prospective adoptive parents' home for placement of an adoptive child. During this process, an assigned caseworker from the adoption agency becomes familiar with the prospective parents, their home environment, and extended family-life relationships. As part of the home study, numerous papers documenting each applicant's major life events such as birth and marriage certificates, divorce records, medical statements from personal physicians, notarized copies of financial statements, and verification of employment may be requested for the caseworker's files.

The home study often requires personal interviews with prospective adoptive parents. During these interviews, the caseworker discusses with potential adoptive parents their reasons for adoption and also evaluates the applicants' needs and strengths and extended family feelings about an adoptive placement. For individuals with a disability who plan to adopt, the issue of disability will most likely come up during the interview. The caseworker may query an applicant with a disability on how he or she perceives that the disability will affect his or her parenting, or how it will affect the adoptive child as he or she grows and develops. The issue of financial support is also addressed. All potential adoptive parents disabled or not, are asked about the available resources that they have to raise a child who may be placed in their home.

Later in the adoptive process, demographic and biologic histories are obtained from the applicants. Evaluations are then conducted to determine the applicants' capacity to parent and how supportive the home and extended family environment is for raising children.

Once the caseworker has given her or his approval, the assignment of a child is made to the adoptive parents, if one is available for placement. The parents may then receive a picture of the child and, if available, a brief medical and social history. Some time after this process, the child is placed in the adoptive parents' home.

The finalization of adoption is made through a court hearing, and a petition to adopt is tendered to a municipal judge. This often takes place in a closed courtroom or the judge's personal chambers. If all investigations and legal documents are in order, the judge orders a decree of adoption. After such a decree, the state issues a new birth certificate for the adopted child, stating his or her new name and the names of the adoptive parents.

INTERNATIONAL ADOPTION

With an international adoption, applicants must not only meet their local adoption agency requirements, but they may also be required to meet the requirements of the adoption agency in the country from which they are adopting. Adoption of children from other nations is an option frequently chosen due to the relative availability of these children compared to children in the U.S. However, many countries are tightening their restrictions for adoption or are making adoption prohibitively expensive.

REASONS FOR ADOPTION

Although there are no data to support this assertion, there is a high probability that would-be parents are not spending years on waiting lists to receive an adoptive child just to claim another tax deduction, or for the opportunity to change dozens of dirty diapers, or to be the recipient of a hearty sneeze when their child is eating oatmeal.

Like their counterparts without disabilities, many would-be parents with disabilities may want to adopt a child to bring a sense of fulfillment to their lives. This fulfillment may be manifested in various forms, such as in the opportunity to instill the parental values into a young child's life that allow growth and development, or in extending the family name, or perhaps because of loneliness and a desire for a reciprocal relationship where one can love and be loved.

In the general population, prospective parents most frequently choose the adoption option because they are unable for various reasons to procreate (Chase, 1990; Mazor & Simons, 1984). Similarly, prospective parents with disabilities may be unable to produce biologic children due to secondary conditions that result from their disability. However, there are new techniques developed that reduce impotence (Donatucci & Lue, chap. 26, this volume) and facilitate ejaculation of semen from men with spinal cord injuries (Halstead & Seager, chap. 27, this volume). Zasler (1991) suggests that such techniques may well increase the chances for men with spinal cord injuries to have biologic children.

In some family units, one parent may have a disabling condition that could potentially be passed on to a biologic child. In such cases, the family is often advised to obtain genetic counseling concerning family planning. Genetic counseling and test results may suggest that having a child biologically would put the birth child at-risk for inheriting the parent's disabling condition. For example, Usher's syndrome is a genetically inherited disability characterized by severe hearing loss and gradual tunneling and later loss of vision. When one or both potential parents have been diagnosed with Usher's syndrome and decide to have children, the offspring are at a high risk for developing this condition. Parents with genetically related disabling conditions may choose adoption in order to increase their family size.

TYPES OF ADOPTION

There are several approaches that can be taken in adopting children. The following approaches describe those most frequently selected by families seeking adoption.

Public Agencies

This approach is usually through a city, county, or state division of social services. Adoptive services through public agencies may be less costly than services from private agencies, but the waiting list for children can be very long.

Private Agencies

Private agencies usually have more restrictions about where they will place adoptive children. For example, some religious agencies will only place children in homes of the same denomination. Other private agencies have developed specialized services such as international adoptive placement services. Compared to public agencies, private agencies are usually faster in child placements, but clients can expect to pay hefty agency fees. Some private agencies offer a sliding fee scale based on income level to help provide child placement for families.

Independent

The independent approach usually involves working through physicians or lawyers to secure a child. Due to the potential for illegal activity, such as "black market" babies, more states are passing legislation to ban independent adoption arrangements. There is an increasing trend for childless couples to nationally advertise (e.g., *USA Today*) their desire to adopt a child in exchange for paying for all of the biologic mother's medical expenses related to childbirth.

Interstate Compact on Placement of Children

Some states have an interstate compact that allows parents from one state to adopt a child from another state. Under present adoption laws, no child can be sent across state lines without approval from the interstate compact office of each appropriate state.

Adoptive Arrangements

When arranging for child placements, there is an increasing trend to discuss whether the adoption will be on an open basis, where biologic and adoptive parents are known to each other, or on a closed basis, where the arrangements are made anonymously. Each of these arrangements is discussed below.

Open In this arrangement, the adoptive and birth parents meet and share information (e.g., medical histories, religious affiliations) openly. Under some arrangements, the birth mother (and father) can decide with whom the child will be placed. This may cause placement problems for individuals with disabilities who are seeking to adopt, if the birth parent prejudges or does not understand the capabilities of people with disabilities.

Unidentified (Closed) The adoptive arrangement in this case is confidential. It frequently involves the exchange of necessary information such as birth parents' medical histories. The purpose is to protect anonymity for both the birth and adoptive parents. Some states are now allowing the adoption files to be opened if petitioned to do so by the adoptive child. However, the birth parents are often contacted first to give their consent to reveal their identities to the adoptive child.

Desperately Seeking the Right Adoption Agency

When considering selection of an adoption agency, it must be recognized that not all adoption agencies offer equivalent services, nor are they right for each parent's needs or situation. Individuals with disabilities should carefully consider this point.

Each adoption agency has specific criteria for the home situations in which it will place children. Such criteria often include age, marital status, fertility status, religion, and ethnic orientation.

Individuals with disabilities who are interested in becoming adoptive parents should investigate each agency's criteria in view of their own situation. Other issues should also be addressed when selecting and working with an adoptive agency. First, albeit simplistic, is the agency site accessible? Part of the adoption process may mean coming to the agency for several interviews and information sessions, so it is necessary that the agency be accessible. The Americans with Disabilities Act (ADA) requires public and private service agencies to provide accessible public accommodations.

Another issue of great importance is the adoptive agency's attitudes toward potential adoptive parents with disabilities. People with disabilities applying at adoptive agencies should be alert for any patronizing behavior. One way to determine whether adoption agencies are sensitive and willing to work with people with disabilities is to ask if they have had any adoption applications from other individuals with disabilities and how many placements were made. If placements were made to adoptive parents with disabilities, a request may be made to obtain permission to meet with the adoptive families.

The person with a disability should also consider other questions when selecting an adoption agency. Is the agency empathetic toward special needs populations? Does the caseworker understand or value the consumer empowerment philosophy vital to independent living? Does the adoptive agency take the role of expert, who always knows best, in every situation, including working with clients who have disabilities? Again, the Americans with Disabilities Act (ADA) is an excellent tool to assist clients with disabilities to negotiate with adoptive agencies should they feel discriminated against during the adoptive process.

Finally, when examining the services an adoption agency offers before and during the adoptive process, the type of post-placement services that the agency offers should not be overlooked. Such post-adoptive services can be a valuable tool in assisting both parents and adoptive children. These services might include post-adoption peer support groups or problem-solving groups to assist parents in obtaining support, information, or resources needed to make their family function more effectively. Some adoption agencies offer post-adoptive cultural activities for children placed from other countries. For example, Children's Home Society of Minnesota has placed many children from Korea into homes throughout Minnesota and the U.S. Each year the society sponsors a summer camp for children who were adopted from Korea and their siblings. The camp's purpose is to give a sense of cultural heritage for Korean children who are adopted.

Choosing the Adoptive Child

The availability of Caucasian American infants has severely diminished in recent years due to factors including teen-age mothers opting to keep their babies, increased birth control, and legalized abortion. The waiting period for these infants is several years. Some agencies have such long waiting lists for Caucasian infants that they no longer accept applications.

Infants and toddlers from other countries, including Korea, Colombia, India, and the Philippines may be more readily available to individuals seeking adoption. Additionally, healthy African-American or African-American/white infants in the U.S. are more available than their Caucasian counterparts, with an estimated waiting period of 6 months–1 year. Most agencies attempt to place children with families of similar race or ethnicity. This is also the trend of recent federal laws. For example, the Indian Child Welfare Act of 1978 requires that native American families are located for native American children before non-native American families can be considered for adoptive placement.

Another classification of child that might be considered for adoption is the special needs or hard-to-place child. These children include those who: 1) need to be placed in an adoptive home with one or more of their siblings; 2) are older children, usually pre-adolescent; 3) are of minority or mixed race; and 4) have existing disabilities or medical conditions that may or may not be correctable. Such conditions include heart defects, cerebral palsy, seizure disorders, missing limbs, cleft palate and/or lip, burns, severe malnutrition, visual and/or hearing impairments, emotional disorders, and mental retardation or developmental disabilities.

CONCLUSION

The adoption process offers one possible strategy for people with physical disabilities to increase their family size. To newcomers, the adoption process appears to be an easy and straightforward procedure. Those who have participated in the adoption process, however, can describe a range of scenarios ranging from frustration, heartbreak, and disappointment to the more pleasurable and successful outcomes of having infants or children placed in their homes.

Persons with disabilities who wish to adopt must not only endure all of the red tape and bureaucratic procedures that their non-disabled counterparts undergo, but they must also develop a plan to address potential barriers they are likely to encounter. Frequently, the most significant barrier is the financial cost of the adoption process. According to the U.S. Census (1985) figures, approximately 50% of all adults with disabilities had annual incomes, from all sources, of $4,000 or less. Due to their limited incomes, many people with disabilities could not think of participating in the adoption process. Perhaps, adoption costs could be partially underwritten by private foundations or church groups to assist potential adoptive parents with disabilities who have low incomes.

Attitudinal barriers present another formidable challenge that prospective parents with disabilities must overcome. As individuals with disabilities face hostile and prejudiced attitudes about their disabilities and their potential for parenthood, they must educate the agency about their disability and distinguish the fact that the severity of a person's disability has little to do with his or her parenting skills. This education should be augmented with personal and systems advocacy of the civil rights mandated to people with disabilities under the Americans with Disabilities Act. Applicants with disabilities who apply for adoption should be vigilant that they receive treatment and consideration of adoptive services equal to what other nondisabled applicants receive.

As these two formidable challenges suggest, the road to adoption is not an easy one. However, those who select adoption as their strategy to have infants or children, and are tenacious in following the process to completion, will have a reasonable chance of success.

AUTHORS' NOTE

The authors have personally found the adoption option challenging and rewarding and have had the privilege of raising two wonderful children from Korea. In addition, they have had the opportunity to assist several other friends, with and without disabilities, in adopting children from other countries.

REFERENCES

Americans with Disabilities Act of 1990 (ADA), PL 101–336. (July 26, 1990). Title 42, U.S.C. 12101 et seq: *U.S. Statutes at Large, 104,* 327–378.
Brindley, G.S. (1986). Sexual and reproductive problems of paraplegic men. *Oxford Reviews of Reproductive Biology, 8,* 214–222.

Chase, M.E. (1990). *Waiting for baby: One couple's journey through infertility to adoption.* New York: McGraw-Hill.

Griffith, E.R., Tomko, M.A., & Timms, R.J. (1973). Sexual function in spinal cord injured patients: A review. *Archives of Physical Medicine and Rehabilitation, 54,* 543–649.

Mazor, M.D., & Simons, H.F. (Eds.). (1984). *Infertility: Medical, emotional, and social considerations.* New York: Human Sciences Press.

United States Census Bureau. (1985). *U.S. census of population 1980: Selected characteristics of persons with a work disability by state: 1980* (PC 80-S1-20 Supplemental report). Washington, DC: Government Printing Office.

Zasler, N.D. (1991). Sexuality in neurologic disability: An overview. *Sexuality and Disability, 9,* 11–27.

A Father's Gift

Irving Kenneth Zola

*W*e sat beside one another as we had many times before, looking absently at "The Show of Shows" on TV, a father and a son without much to say. I was 18 and he was 48, but the gap was more than years. I was the new college boy and he was the high school dropout. I was the family success and he the failure. So many times I'd heard him described that way—so often that I'd begun long ago to distance myself from him. Not that I didn't love him. I did. It's just that . . . well, we had nothing in common anymore.

"You look worried," he said, interrupting my thoughts.

"Hmm," I answered noncommittally.

"Is it the operation?"

"Well," I hesitated. Did I really want to discuss this with him?

"I know we don't talk much nowadays," he continued.

"Oh Dad!" I snapped back.

"No, no," he went on, "I know it's true. And besides I know it's not easy for you to talk about."

He was right. It wasn't easy to talk about. It was only 2 years since I'd had polio. Barely a year since I'd been walking again. And now the doctors had scheduled an operation.

They said it would help stabilize my leg. But all I could think of was that I'd be in a cast for 6 months—immobile, dependent, and unmanly once more.

"Is there anything I can do?" he asked.

"No, I don't think so," I answered quickly.

"Well . . ." he began, "It looks like you'll be pretty confined for several months."

"Yes, I guess I will," I nodded.

"You're 18, right?"

"Yes," I answered, wondering what he was getting at.

"It's a long time since I was that . . . but not that long."

"So!" I said unsympathetically.

"I know this isn't easy but I was wondering if you'd ever been with a woman."

"Dad!" I blushed.

"I'm just asking."

"Well . . . sure . . . sort of."

"Look, I know I don't have an education like you but I do know that being with a woman can't have been that easy for you."

He knows a lot, I thought to myself. Of the things I didn't feel good about, sex was at the top of the list. I had just begun to date again and it was damn awkward, not just the crutches and the limping but the real fear. For months with polio I'd been impotent. And now, though I did get sexually aroused, I still wondered about myself.

"You don't have to tell me the details. That's not important. Or even if you have screwed someone . . . but sex is more than making it in the back seat of a car."

I smiled at the apt summing up of my experience.

"What I thought was . . . that maybe if you wanted, I could arrange something for you."

"You could?" I answered both in excitement and disbelief.

"Yes, I can," he laughed. "After all, I might not be much but I've been around."

I grimaced at the self-deprecation but added, "Ah, yes . . . I would."

"Then it's a deal," and he got up from the couch and came across the room to hug me. And as we held each other, I tried hard to hold back my own tears.

He said nothing and sniffled himself as he turned to go.

"Ah, don't worry . . . I'll . . . uh . . . arrange it and ah . . . she understands . . . and she'll be gentle."

And he did and she was.

11

Mothers with Disabilities

Anne Finger

Because I am a writer of fiction and creative nonfiction, I am going to begin this chapter by relating several stories. At first, the relationship between these stories and the topic at hand may seem tangential, and my way of going about arriving at truths about disabled mothering quirky, but I trust that by the end of this chapter, the insights that arrive from this method will make sense.

The first story: I took part in organizing a literary reading given by the English Department at Wayne State University, where I teach. The next day, I had to return the key to the auditorium where the reading had been held to the Communication Department. Getting off the elevator in my wheelchair, I asked someone standing in the hallway where the Communication Department was. "I'll take you there," she volunteered.

"You don't need to do that. Just tell me where it is."

But she insisted, and led me down the hallway, to an office. "Here you are," she said, and smiled at me.

"I'm from the English Department," I said to the woman behind the desk. "I'm returning the auditorium key that we used for the reading last night."

"Let me check you off the list," the woman behind the desk said.

That seemed a bit odd: Surely there aren't that many people who borrow keys? And no, my name wasn't on the list. After much confusion, it turned out that I wasn't in the Communication Department after all; the helpful soul in the corridor had seen my wheelchair and taken me, not to the Communication Department, but the Communication Disorders Clinic. (An interesting irony here: lack of communication, the question of whose communication was disordered.) And when I said to the woman behind the desk, "I'm from the English Department. I'm returning the auditorium key we used for the reading last night," she simply had not heard me. I was in a wheelchair, therefore I must be a patient. My words were not heard. I was going to say that my body spoke more loudly than my voice, but after all, it wasn't my body speaking; rather, it was her assumption about what my body said.

I am in a shop near campus. I ask the price of a scarf. "Sixteen dollars—with your student discount," the woman behind the counter says. I'm almost 40 years old. I wear make-up. I dress like a professor, but still, people hold the door for me, and say, "Good luck on your exams!"

I go into a campus building that is "wheelchair accessible." There are ramps leading up to doors with electric eyes that open them automatically; there are bathrooms with pictographs on them: "male," "wheelchair" on one; "female," "wheelchair" on the other. (Do not fail to notice the gendering of language here: male, female, disabled; masculine, feminine, neuter.) The lecture hall is well designed: seats with writing paddles for left-handers, space at the back (of course, at the back) for wheelchair users to sit. Only the lecture platform isn't accessible.

I heard about an orthopedically disabled woman who swam daily at a public pool throughout her pregnancy. Because she didn't like "pregnant" bathing suits, she wore a bikini, her belly roundly, proudly displayed. After she gave birth, she walked into the pool with her new baby. A lifeguard who had seen her nearly every day throughout her pregnancy asked, "Whose baby is that?" "Mine." "You were pregnant?" What cannot be imagined cannot be seen.

I taught an introductory fiction class in which we read Johanna Russ's short story, "Autobiography of My Mother," a piece in which Russ imagines her mother in a variety of "unmotherly" situations: she imagines meeting her mother when she is 35 and her mother is 2. She joins her mother in a Chinese restaurant when her mother is 19 and she is not born yet; skating together, both 11, braids flying; the two of them going out together, waiting under street lights, pretending to be prostitutes. As a way of responding to the story, I asked my students to imagine their mothers as nonmothers, to write about the women their mothers would have become if they had not given birth to children, to imagine the lives of their mothers apart from them. It was a task they seemingly found impossible: They wrote about the things their mothers said to them, the things their mothers cooked for them, the way they nagged them. To imagine the woman apart from the mother seemed an impossible assignment.

In the women's studies discussion group at school, the question is asked of us, 30 professional women sitting around a table, "Do we feel that we have to pretend to be men in our academic lives?" An answer pops into my mind: "No, I'm too busy pretending to be a woman."

What can we learn from these stories? What do we hear in the voice that says, "Where's the Communication Department, please?" and is not heard? The architect who cannot imagine that we would ever ascend to the stage, the passersby who look at me and read: student.

Silence? No, I speak. Deafness? I reject it, not just on the grounds of it being a politically incorrect metaphor, but more because it lets those who do not hear me off the hook: After all, they have the ability to hear. No, it is something else: They do not hear because they cannot imagine the range of things I could say, am saying. They cannot imagine that a woman in a wheelchair could be on the fourth floor of Manoogian for any other reason than to go to the Communication Disorders Clinic: They cannot imagine me outside of the role of patient/victim/object of pity.

And then there are those mothers of my students, those mothers who can bake chocolate chip cookies and have jobs that they sandwich between childcare and taking kids to ballet classes and the dentist, mothers who nag them to do their homework and pick up their coats, but who cannot be imagined as childless, living in one-bedroom apartments with five cats or alone with their husbands in quiet houses, or at 19, turning down the proposal from your father, going to live in New York or on an island in the Aegean.

And what of me, sitting in that sterile conference room, wearing a dress that I bought from a catalog, a catalog that has never shown a woman who looks like me in its pages, feeling that I have to pretend to be a woman?

There is an absence here that doubles and triples: The woman with disabilities who cannot be imagined apart from her disability, the mother who cannot be imagined apart from her motherhood, the woman who experiences her femaleness as a guise.

Hanna and Rogovsky (1986) asked college students without disabilities to draw associations with the phrase "disabled woman." The students virtually never thought of a mother, although this was a common association for the word "woman" alone. While men with disabilities were assumed to have become disabled through involvements in accidents and war, women's disability, in these students' associations, was attributable to disease. Women with disabilities were assumed to be passive, dependent, despairing, "almost lifeless."

In fact, some of the students in this study handed their papers back in blank. They could not associate anything with the phrase "disabled woman."

We should not be surprised that a silence that exists in our personal lives exists also in the academic literature: A literature search for "disability and parenting" brings forth a few references on the computer screen. But when you read the articles, they invariably focus on the effects on a child of having a disabled parent—never on the effects on a disabled person of being a parent (Attard, 1988; Pomerantz, Pomerantz & Colca, 1990; Thurman, 1985).

Never mind that the word parent is rarely, if ever, broken down into its constituent parts: mother and father. Consider even the simplest meanings of those words: the meanings that come first in the dictionary and first in our minds. "To father" is to impregnate a woman, pass along one's genes, a discrete act, a biological fact. "To mother," on the other hand, is to nurture, to rear, to engage in an ongoing process. "Parenting" assumes that two people share the work and joy of childrearing. Even when a particular couple works out equitable child care arrangements, vastly different role expectations, economic power, and socialization between women and men remain. This can be even more exacerbated by the presence of disability in one or both partners (Asch & Fine, 1988).

Yet the few references we find about disability and parenting resolutely ignore the intersections of gender and disability. Gilhool and Gran (1985), in their discussion of custody issues for parents with disabilities, note cases in which mothers with disabilities lost custody to nondisabled fathers or other relatives, and one case in which a father with a disability was awarded custody rather than his nondisabled ex-wife, without ever considering the part that gender—especially women's lower wages and perceptions of the mothering role versus the fathering role—may have played in these cases.

Those questions that I want answered: What was her experience of pregnancy? How did she get the medical care she needed—and not get medical care she didn't need? Why did she decide to have a child? What sort of physical adaptations did she make in the home environment? How did having a child affect her psychologically? Those questions are not even asked.

I was asked to address strategies for change in this chapter, and I began to make a list of things that would make life better for disabled mothers: adequate income, support services, education of medical personnel about our bodies and our lives. I found myself imagining instead what life could be like for mothers with disabilities, not in a perfect world, but in a better one. For it seems that our task must be partly one of imagination. Imagination is not a substitute for political action, but without a vision of what we are moving toward, we cannot hope to formulate strategies for change. Let us imagine then, the life of a disabled woman not in a utopia, but in a better world.

Imagine a mother with rheumatoid arthritis. She wakes up in the morning with aching joints. But no one has ever dichotomized her body into "good" and "bad"—no smiling physical therapist has ever said to her, "Now can you raise your bad leg for me, dear?"; no doctor has ever mused out loud, "Now your right arm. . . that's your good arm, isn't it?" She has not been taught to despise what is weaker, apart from the norm. She feels pain. Make no mistake about it: her joints ache. But let us imagine that in this better world, there is something to do with pain besides get rid of it: Pain can be experienced, known.

Let us imagine that reproductive freedom is a reality for this woman. She received sex education that acknowledged her existence as a disabled woman, acknowledged the existence of sexual pleasure. When she was living as a heterosexual, she had access to safe and effective birth control, funded abortion. Now, she lives as a lesbian in a world that welcomes her presence, acknowledges that there are many different kinds of families, many ways to be a parent.

Her child is crying. She goes to him. His crib doesn't require four strong limbs to lower the side: She picks up her son.

She opens the morning paper: A blind woman appears in a soft drink advertisement, her head thrown back, in one of *those* poses: you don't need to be Sigmund Freud to see the sexual associations. She takes her daughter to a daycare center where the children learn sign as a second language. Because her energy levels are low, and the amount of time she must spend dealing with her personal needs relatively high, she works 6 hours a day. But income support systems no longer require you to fit into one of two categories: either disabled, unable to work, and eligible for medical and income benefits; or else disabled but able to squeeze yourself into job standards designed for the nondisabled. She makes a living wage, gets the medical benefits she needs, without having to pay for them with exhaustion, physical pain, without having to give up her life beyond work.

While we imagine this future for mothers with disabilities, let us not forget that for the vast majority of mothers with disabilities, life is very, very far from this vision. Women with a broad range of disabilities have found themselves faced with threats to custody rights. It is not uncommon for children to be taken from parents with disabilities, who often can cope, or certainly could cope, were adequate support services provided. And the foster care to which these children are sent is far more expensive than support services to the family would be. For women with disabilities as a whole, the overwhelming reality of poverty, discrimination, and social disapproval mean that the very act of entering into motherhood, while it is a badge of normalcy for women without disabilities becomes a mark of deviance for women with disabilities.

REFERENCES

Asch, A., & Fine, M. (1988). *Women with disabilities: Essays in psychology, culture, and politics.* Philadelphia: Temple University Press.

Attard, M.T. (1988). Point of view: Mentally handicapped parents: Some issues to consider in relation to pregnancy. *British Journal of Mental Subnormality, 34*(1)(66), 3–9.

Gilhool, T.K., & Gran, J.A. (1985). Legal rights of disabled parents. In S.K. Thurman (Ed.), *Children of handicapped parents: Research and clinical perspectives* (pp.11–34). Orlando: Academic Press.

Hanna, W.J., & Rogovsky, B. (1986). *Women and disability: Stigma and "the third factor."* Unpublished paper, College of Human Ecology, University of Maryland, College Park.

Pomerantz, P., Pomerantz, D.J., & Colca, L.A. (1990). A case study: Service delivery and parents with disabilities. *Child Welfare, 69*(1), 65–73.

Thurman, S.K. (Ed.). (1985). *Children of handicapped parents: Research and clinical perspectives.* Orlando: Academic Press.

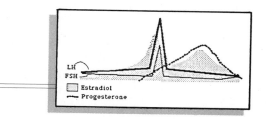

III

CLINICAL ISSUES

12

Reproductive Disabilities
An Overview of Congenital Factors

Joe Leigh Simpson

Reproductive disabilities may be either congenital or acquired. Most clinical progress toward diagnosing and treating these reproductive disabilities has been made from investigating congenital disabilities, but the same principles apply to acquired reproductive disabilities. The purpose of this overview is to review the spectrum of reproductive disabilities and the principles underlying their management.

CLASSIFICATION

For heuristic purposes, reproductive disabilities may be classified as those in which only a single organ system is involved (gonadal, genital, or ductal) and those in which multiple organ systems are involved (Table 1). Discussion of disorders in which multiple organ systems are involved—male pseudohermaphroditism, true hermaphroditism, and some cases of female pseudohermaphroditism— are beyond the scope of this chapter. Instead, discussion is confined to single organ system abnormalities. Elsewhere, the author has reviewed all of these disorders in detail (Simpson, 1976, 1992; Simpson & Golbus 1992; Simpson & Rebar, 1990), where extensive references are provided.

OVARIAN FAILURE DUE TO OVARIAN ABNORMALITIES: CLINICAL FEATURES

Gonadal disabilities in females can result either from primary abnormalities of the ovaries per se or from secondary abnormalities of

Table 1. Classification of reproductive disabilities

I. Involvement of single organ system
  Gonadal (ovary or testis)
    Primary failure due to gonadal failure
    Secondary failure due to gonadotropin deficiency
  Genital (isolated hypospadias in males, female pseudohermaphroditism due to adrenal hyperplasia in females)
  Ductal
II. Involvement of multiple organ systems
  Female pseudohermaphroditism (some forms)
    Genital ambiguity such that female sex-of-rearing is in doubt in 46,XX individuals
  Male pseudohermaphroditism
    Genital ambiguity such that male sex-of-rearing in doubt in 46,XX individuals
  True hermaphroditism
    Presence of testicular and ovarian tissue in a single individual (i.e., histologic definition irrespective of chromosomal complement)

the hypothalamic-pituitary system that lead to deficiency of the appropriate trophic signals necessary for ovulation.

Clinical Features of Primary Ovarian Failure

In ovarian dysgenesis, the gonads traditionally are said to exist in the form of streak gonads usually 2–3 cm long and about 0.5 cm wide. The streaks are devoid of germ cells, accounting for the common term *gonadal dysgenesis.* These streaks are located in the position ordinarily occupied by the ovary. A streak gonad is characterized histologically by interlacing waves of dense fibrous stroma, devoid of oocytes but otherwise indistinguishable from normal ovarian stroma. Individuals with gonadal dysgenesis show a spectrum of karyotypes: 45,X; 46,XX; 46,XY; various mosaics; and X or Y structural aberrations.

The absence of oocytes in monosomy X is the result of increased oocyte atresia, not failure of germ cell formation. Indeed, 45,X embryos and 45,X neonates have germ cells. Inasmuch as germ cells are present in 45,X embryos, it is not too surprising that occasional (3%–5%) 45,X individuals menstruate spontaneously. Indeed, several fertile 45,X individuals have been reported.

In individuals with gonadal dysgenesis, secondary sexual development usually does not occur. Pubic and axillary hair fail to develop in normal quantity. Although well differentiated, the external genitalia, the vagina, and the mullerian derivatives (uterus and cer-

vix) remain small. As is true for virtually all individuals with gonadal dysgenesis, estrogen and androgen levels are decreased; FSH and LH are increased.

In 45,X individuals, gonadal dysgenesis is accompanied by somatic anomalies of Turner syndrome: epicanthal folds, high arched palate, low nuchal hair line, webbed neck, shield-like chest, coarctation of the aorta, ventricular septal defect, renal anomalies, pigmented nevi, lymphadenoma, hypoplastic nails, and cubitus valgus. Inverted nipples and double eyelashes (distichiasis) may be present as well. No feature is pathognomic, but, in aggregate, these anomalies form a spectrum of anomalies more likely to exist in 45,X individuals than in normal 46,XX individuals.

The external genitalia and streak gonads in 46,XX individuals are indistinguishable from those in gonadal dysgenesis secondary to a sex chromosomal abnormality. Likewise, the endocrine profiles do not differ. However, individuals with XX gonadal dysgenesis are normal in stature. Most cases are the result of a mutant autosomal recessive gene, but phenocopies for XX gonadal dysgenesis also are recognized.

Gonadal dysgenesis can also occur in 46,XY individuals. In XY gonadal dysgenesis, affected individuals are phenotypic females who show sexual infantilism and bilateral streak gonads. The gonads may undergo neoplastic transformation (20%–30% prevalence). At least one form of XY gonadal dysgenesis results from a mutant X-linked recessive gene. Rarely, sporadic cases may result from deletion of TDF on the Y short arm.

OVARIAN FAILURE DUE TO OVARIAN ABNORMALITIES: TREATMENT

Treatment of women with ovarian failure has long been possible through hormonal replacement therapy. Discussed in detail in standard texts of obstetrics and gynecology, synthetic estrogens can be provided readily to women deficient in endogenous production. This should be initiated at the time of expected puberty or whenever gonadal failure becomes evident. With proper replacement therapy, women with ovarian failure look and feel like other women. They enjoy normal sexual relationships and normal libido.

The difficulty arises with respect to the inability of these women to have their own children. Fortunately, this is now possible through donor in vitro fertilization or donor oocyte transfer (gamete intrafallopian tube transfer). The basic principle is that a fertile donor must contribute oocytes. This became possible when excess

46,XX oocytes became available through in vitro fertilization procedure. Prior to widely available cryopreservation, it was not considered good practice to freeze embryos. Given these circumstances, it was reasonable to offer otherwise superfluous embryos to infertile women with an intact uterus (e.g., ovarian failure). Initial successes were very encouraging, in fact, even better than for infertile couples who present for in vitro fertilization (Sauer, Paulson, & Lobo, 1990). This presumably reflects not only the younger age of ovarian failure recipients but also their relative lack of pelvic pathology. (Disorders such as fallopian tube blockage often necessitate in vitro fertilization in the donor.) At any rate, successful pregnancy can be achieved through donor embryos. Hormonal maintenance must be provided exogenously during the time in which the corpus luteum is expected to function, but after about 10 weeks of gestation, no exogenous support is necessary.

Alternatives to donor embryo programs have been developed recently. Donors may contribute oocytes (Sauer, Paulson, & Lobo, 1992). Donor oocytes may also be placed along with the sperm of the recipient's husband in the recipient's fallopian tubes (donor GIFT, or gamete intrafallopian tube). Donor oocyte use is the converse of artificial insemination by male donors, a long accepted clinical practice.

OVARIAN FAILURE SECONDARY TO GONADOTROPIN DEFICIENCY: CLINICAL FEATURES AND TREATMENT

Deficiency of gonadotropin (FSH and LH) without deficiencies of other pituitary trophic hormones and without associated somatic anomalies is a rare cause of hypogonadism. Affected females show primary amenorrhea and lack secondary sexual development. Affected males are poorly virilized and infertile. Ovaries show numerous primordial follicles but no oocytes. If no somatic anomalies are present, the autosomal recessive trait isolated gonadotropin deficiency is, by definition, considered to be present. If somatic anomalies exist (especially hyposomia), other conditions would exist. Usually the diagnosis will be Kallmann syndrome.

Treatment for women with hypogonadotropic hypogonadism is generally successful. Exogenous estrogen and progestins are necessary to produce secondary sexual development. Thereafter, clomiphene citrate can theoretically induce ovulation in women with hypothalamic disorders. However, women who have pituitary disorders traditionally have required exogenous gonadotropins (hMG followed by hCG), for these act directly upon the ovary. More recently, evidence that the etiology of hypogonadotrophic hypogonadism often involves deficient production or secretion of pulsatile GnRH has led to recommendations for treatment with pulsatile GnRH (Layman, 1991) subcutaneously or intravenously administered until a preovulatory follicle is observed on ultrasound, after which hCG is given to induce ovulation. Irrespective, ovulation can usually be successfully induced (80%–90%) and, following fertilization, pregnancy maintained.

FEMALE GENITAL ABNORMALITIES

In female pseudohermaphroditism, genital differentiation is not that expected for 46,XX individuals; however, ovaries are present and fertility possible. Individuals generally present with genital abnormalities at birth.

General Considerations in Adrenal Hyperplasia

The most common causes of genital abnormalities are the syndromes of adrenal hyperplasia. These result from deficiencies of the various enzymes required for steroid biosynthesis (Figure 1). Deficiencies of 21-hydroxylase, 11β-hydroxylase, and 3β-ol-dehydrogenase produce female pseudohermaphroditism. In all, the common pathogenesis involves decreased production of adrenal cortisol. Cortisol regulates secretion of ACTH through a negative feedback inhibition mechanism. If cortisol production is decreased, ACTH secretion is not inhibited. Elevated ACTH leads to increased quantities of steroid precursors, from which androgens can be synthesized. Be-

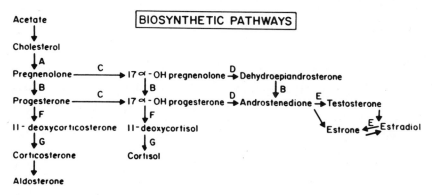

Figure 1. Summary of important adrenal and gonadal biosynthetic pathways. Letters designate enzymes required for the appropriate conversions: A, 20ð-hydroxylase, 22ð-hydroxylase, and 20,22-desmolase; B,3β-ol-dehydrogenase; C, 17ð-hydroxylase; D, 17,20-desmolase; E, 17-ketosteroid reductase; F, 21-hydroxylase; and G,11β-hydroxylase. (From Simpson, J.L. [1976]. *Disorders of sexual differentiation: Etiology and clinical delineation* [p. 158]. New York: Academic Press; reprinted by permission.)

cause the fetal adrenal begins to function during the third month of embryogenesis, excessive production of adrenal androgens will virilize external genitalia. Mullerian and gonadal development remain unaffected because neither is androgen dependent.

Females deficient for 21- or 11β-hydroxylase show clitoral hypertrophy, labioscrotal fusion, and displacement of the urethral orifice to a location more nearly approximating that of a normal male. Extent of virilization may vary among individuals with the same type of enzyme deficiency. Wolffian derivatives (vasa deferentia, seminal vesicles, epididymides) are rarely present, probably because fetal adrenal function begins too late in embryogenesis to stabilize the wolffian ducts. Mullerian derivatives develop normally, as expected in the absence of the nonandrogenic hormone AMH (antimullerian hormone). Ovaries likewise develop normally. Areolar hyperpigmentation may occur, presumably because ACTH has melanocyte stimulating properties. In fact, hyperpigmentation suggests the diagnosis of 21- or 11β-hydroxylase deficiencies in males, whose genitalia are normal at birth. If not ascertained at birth, males usually pass undetected until approximately 2 years of age, when pubic hair develops and increased statural growth is observed.

Treatment

Treating women with isolated genital abnormalities is quite simple in principle. The uterus is normal; thus, pregnancy and childbearing can be normal. Any clitoral reduction necessary for cosmetic purposes can be accomplished with no loss of sexual function, given properly designed operations. Thus, sexual relations and libido should be normal.

In treating adrenal hyperplasia, attention must be given in the neonatal period to administration of cortisol, correction of hyperkalemia, and restoration of fluid–electrolyte balance. Salt-retaining hormones (e.g., fluorinated hydrocortisone) may be necessary. With control of excess androgen precursors, ovulation and pregnancy should occur normally. As discussed elsewhere (Speiser, Laforgia, & Kato, et al., 1990), our group and others have made the diagnosis of 21-hydroxylase deficiency in utero and successfully administered dexamethasone to the pregnant woman to prevent genital virilization in the genetically abnormal fetus.

FEMALE DUCTAL ABNORMALITIES: CLINICAL FEATURES AND TREATMENT

Anomalies of the distal female reproductive tract represent a heterogeneous group of malformations resulting from abnormal development of the mullerian ducts. Many less severe anomalies do not adversely affect reproduction, whereas others may increase fetal wastage. Fertility itself seems unaffected in patients with uterine malformations. The development of secondary sexual characteristics is virtually always normal, and ovulation generally occurs normally.

Imperforate Hymen

Although an imperforate hymen does not involve the genital ducts, it must often be considered in the differential diagnosis of anomalies of the mullerian system. Ordinarily, the central portion of the hymen is patent (perforate), thereby allowing outflow of mucus and blood. If the hymen is imperforate, mucus and blood accumulate in the vagina or uterus (hydrocolpos or hydrometrocolpos). An imperforate hymen may be suspected because a bulging membrane, often bluish, may be visible at the introitus. However, the diagnosis may not seem so simple on physical examination. Ultrasound may be helpful in verifying the presence of a uterus. Surgical correction is rather simple.

Transverse Vaginal Septum

Transverse vaginal septa may occur at several locations and may be complete or incomplete. This condition probably results from failure of the urogenital sinus derivatives and mullerian duct derivatives to fuse or to canalize. The septa are usually about 1 cm thick and located near the junction of the upper third and lower two thirds of the vagina; however, they may be present in the middle or lower third of the vagina. If no perforation exists, mucus and menstrual fluid lack egress; thus, hydrocolpos or hydrometrocolpos may develop. Other pelvic organs are usually normal.

Resection of the septa with mucosal reanastomosis generally obviates future problems with conception. If either a transverse vaginal septum or an imperforate hymen is undiagnosed following onset of menstruation, endometriosis may arise secondarily and interfere with subsequent fertility.

Mullerian Aplasia

Aplasia of the mullerian ducts leads to absence of the uterine corpus, uterine cervix, and upper portion of the vagina. A short vagina (1–2 cm) probably is derived exclusively from invagination of the urogenital sinus. Despite primary amenorrhea, secondary sexual development is normal. The differential diagnosis includes imperforate hymen, transverse vaginal septum, vaginal atresia, and the syndromes of androgen insensitivity.

Renal anomalies are associated with mullerian aplasia more frequently than expected by chance. The most frequent renal anomalies are pelvic kidney, renal ectopia, and unilateral renal aplasia. Vertebral anomalies are also relatively common. Thus, assessment of the renal system by ultrasound or excretory urography are obligatory, as is assessment for vertebral anomalies.

Incomplete Mullerian Fusion

During embryogenesis, the mullerian ducts are paired structures. Subsequently, fusion and canalization produce the upper vagina, uterus, cervix, and fallopian tubes. Uterine anomalies may occur if the sequence of events that normally converts the bilateral mullerian ductal system into a single female reproductive tract is arrested (Figure 2).

If the two mullerian ducts fuse incompletely, a bicornuate uterus may result. Hysterosalpingography, laparoscopy, or hysteroscopy may be required to differentiate a bicornuate from a septate uterus. The ability of women with a bicornuate uterus to conceive is believed to be equal to that of the general population. However, incidence of spontaneous abortion is increased. Women with bicor-

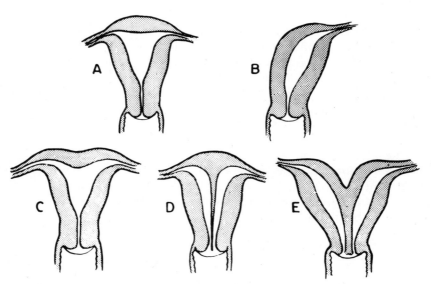

Figure 2. Diagrammatic representation of some Mullerian fusion anomalies: A = normal uterus, fallopian tubes, and cervix; B = uterus unicornis (absence of one uterine horn); C = uterus acuratus (broadening and medial depression of a portion of the uterine septum); D = uterus septus (persistence of a complete uterine septum); and E = uterus bircornis unicollis (two hemiuteri, each leading to the same cervix). (From Simpson, J.L. [1976]. *Disorders of sexual differentiation: Etiology and clinical delineation* [p. 352]. New York: Academic Press; reprinted by permission.)

nuate uteri also show an increased likelihood of premature labor and an abnormal fetal position during labor (fetal lie). However, women with bicornuate uteri may be permitted to conceive without surgery because term pregnancies often result; however such women should be counseled regarding the risk of pregnancy loss and the desirability of surgical correction should pregnancy losses occur.

Complete lack of fusion of the mullerian ducts results in uterus didelphys. In the 75% of cases in which there are separate uteri and two cervical ostia, there also exists a longitudinal vaginal septum. Pregnancies in these women also may end in spontaneous abortion. The frequencies of premature labor and abnormal fetal positions (fetal lie) are increased.

In the septate uterus, the uterine cavity is divided either partially or completely by a longitudinal septum. Fetal wastage is high, although, again, fertility per se is not affected. Women with septate uteri also manifest increased frequency of postpartum hemorrhage and intrauterine adhesion formation, perhaps because the placenta attaches to a relatively avascular septum and leads to placenta accreta. Excision of uterine septa is indicated in women with histories of repeated pregnancy loss.

Incomplete mullerian fusion also may be one component of several genetically determined malformation syndromes. One especially important condition with respect to disabilities is the hand-foot-uterus syndrome, an autosomal dominant disorder in which affected females not only have a bicornuate uterus, but also certain malformations of the hands and feet.

Conclusions Concerning Treatment

Likelihood of successful childbearing in women with isolated uterine anomalies naturally reflects the specific condition. In women who lack a uterus, childbearing is obviously not possible although sexual development and sexual relationships may be completely normal. The ovaries of these women are normal, leading to the possibility of such women: 1) undergoing oocyte aspirations to be followed by, 2) fertilization in vitro with the sperm of their husband, and finally 3) transfer of the embryo to a recipient uterus. This would seem to be a highly justified form of surrogacy. According to media reports, this has been accomplished in at least one case. The mother of the patient with mullerian aplasia was said to be the recipient. However, surrogacy is, of course, exceptional.

More conventionally achieved outcomes are possible for most of the other uterine anomalies discussed above. We noted that in transverse vaginal septum, simple division of the septum can result in a normal vaginal canal, permitting fertilization, pregnancy, and delivery. In mullerian defect fusion, childbearing may or may not be compromised. If it is, surgery can often reunify uteri, although there may persist a tendency to premature labor and early pregnancy loss. Still, in all these ductal abnormalities, external genitalia and gonads are normal. Thus, sexual relationships and libido are normal.

TESTICULAR FAILURE DUE TO TESTICULAR ABNORMALITIES: CLINICAL FEATURES AND TREATMENT

Testicular failure in males is analogous to that in females both in etiology and in treatment. Failure may occur as result of: 1) abnormalities of the gonads per se, usually as a result of 47,XXY Klinefelter syndrome or germ cell aplasia; or 2) abnormalities of the hypothalamus or pituitary that lead secondarily to testicular dysfunction.

Clinical Features

Klinefelter syndrome   Males with at least one Y chromosome and at least two X chromosomes have Klinefelter syndrome. Most cases are 47,XXY, but the phenotype may also be associated with 46,XY/47,XXY, and 49,XXXXY complements. The most characteristic features are seminiferous tubule dysgenesis and androgen deficiency. Somatic anomalies sometimes coexist. The presence of a chromosomal abnormality and elevated gonadotropins readily differentiates Klinefelter syndrome from hypogonadotropic hypogonadism (see below).

Germinal Cell Aplasia   In this condition, seminiferous tubules lack spermatogonia, and the testes are slightly smaller than average. However, Leydig cell function is normal; thus, secondary sexual development is normal. In germinal cell aplasia, FSH is elevated, but LH is normal. Tubular hyalinization and sclerosis usually do not occur. Occasionally, a few spermatozoa are present, but affected individuals usually are sterile. Despite infertility, androgen therapy is unnecessary because secondary sexual development is normal.

Anorchia   Males (46,XY) with bilateral anorchia have unambiguous male external genitalia, normal wolffian derivatives, no mullerian derivatives, and no detectable testes. Unilateral anorchia is usually asymptomatic and not extraordinarily rare, but bilateral anorchia is very uncommon. Despite the absence of bilateral testes, the phallus is well differentiated. Pathogenesis presumably involves atrophy of the fetal testes after 12–16 weeks gestation, by which time genital virilization has occurred. Vasa deferentia terminate blindly, often in association with the spermatic vessels. The diagnosis should be applied only if testicular tissue is not detected in the scrotum, the inguinal canal, or the entire path along which the testes descend during embryogenesis.

Treatment

Treatment of males with Klinefelter syndrome or bilateral anorchia requires hormone replacement therapy. This can be done quite easily, allowing normal male development, sexual relationships, and libido. Hormonal replacement therapy is generally not necessary in males with germ cell aplasia. With respect to childbearing, sterility is typical. Artificial insemination is the only obvious option, although one exceptional possibility arises in monozygotic twins. A testis could be transplanted from the unaffected monozygotic twin to his twin affected with bilateral anorchia.

TESTICULAR FAILURE DUE TO HYPOGONADOTROPHIC HYPOGONADISM

The most common form of hypogonadotropic hypogonadism in males is Kallmann syndrome, defined above. Isolated hypogonadotropic hypogondism also occurs in both males and females. A third condition—isolated LH deficiency—has only been reported in males.

Isolated LH Deficiency

Males with normal or nearly normal spermatogenesis who fail to undergo normal sexual development are said to be "fertile eunuchs." LH secretion is deficient. Affected individuals have high-pitched voices, poor muscle development, and scanty beard growth. Their testes have normal numbers of germ cells, but practically no Leydig cells. Sperm counts are usually normal. In isolated LH deficiency, testosterone therapy is usually necessary for virilization and normal sexual relations. Administration of hCG and testosterone has occasionally resulted in fertility, although artificial insemination remains the more conventional option.

Treatment

Treating hypogonadotropic hypogonadism in males has not proved as satisfactory as in females. However, the principles are similar. Hormonal replacement therapy (testosterone) may be necessary. If necessary, virilization can be achieved readily, assuring normal libido and sexual relations. In the past either clomiphene citrate or, more often, FSH plus hCG, have been administered to induce spermatogenesis. GnRH therapy is also successful (Whitcomb & Crawley, 1990) and can also be used to induce puberty (virilization). If spermatogenesis is not induced, artificial insemination is available.

ABNORMALITIES OF MALE GENITAL DEVELOPMENT: CLINICAL FEATURES

Genital abnormalities in males can involve either isolated hypospadias or microphallus, or genital abnormalities associated with complex conditions (multiple organ system abnormality, such as male pseudohermaphroditism). Hypospadias only are discussed below.

Hypospadias

In hypospadias, the external urinary meatus terminates on the ventral aspect of the penis, proximal to its usual site at the tip of the glans penis. Hypospadias can be classified according to the site of the urethral meatus: glans penis, penile shaft, penoscrotal junction, or perineum. Testicular hypoplasia frequently coexists in severe hypospadias (penoscrotal or perineal).

Microphallus

A phallus less than 2 cm long at birth (microphallus) is heterogeneous in etiology, but fetal testosterone deficiency appears to be the most common cause. In the human male fetus, placental hCG stimulates testosterone synthesis during the critical period of male differentiation (8–12 weeks gestation). Only later does fetal pituitary LH modulate testosterone synthesis and continued phallic growth. Microphallus can also occur in individuals with congenital hypopituitarism and isolated growth hormone deficiency, as well as those with isolated gonadotropin deficiency alone. Thus, growth hormone appears to be important in phallic development. Testicular failure beginning after genital differentiation can also result in microphallus at birth.

ABNORMALITIES OF MALE GENITAL DEVELOPMENT: TREATMENT

Genital reconstruction for simple hypospadias is possible, but not always as easy as genital surgery in the female. In fact, in severe hypospadias, a decision must sometimes be made whether rearing as a male is appropriate. If not, raising individuals with hypospadias as females may lead to more satisfactory outcomes.

Although problems in sperm deposition can interfere with fertility in perineal hypospadias, this is rarely a problem for glanular or coronal hypospadias. As noted, more severe forms of hypospadias (e.g., perineal) tend to be associated with an increased frequency of testicular failure. In such cases, hormonal replacement therapy and artificial insemination may be necessary.

Microphallus usually responds to testosterone, once propriety of treatment is determined.

MALE DUCTAL ABNORMALITIES: CLINICAL FEATURES AND TREATMENT

Ductal abnormalities in males are less common than those in females. The principal conditions include absence of the vas deferens and fusion defects involving the epididymis and vas deferens.

Wolffian Aplasia

Absence of wolffian derivatives (wolffian aplasia) may or may not be associated with absence of the upper urinary tract. Complete agenesis of both the wolffian duct derivatives implies resorption of wolffian elements after the wolffian duct has reached the cloaca. Even if absence of wolffian derivatives is accompanied by upper urinary tract anomalies, the gonads only are rarely involved. More frequently, the upper urinary tract is normal in individuals who lack an epididymis, vas deferens, and seminal vesicle, or who lack only the ductus epididymis and proximal portion of the vas deferens. If the defect is bilateral, the patient is infertile; if the defect is unilateral, the patient usually is asymptomatic. Absence of the vas deferens is associated with cystic fibrosis (Anguiano, Amos, Oates, et al., 1991). It is possible that mutations at this locus are even the usual cause, even in asymptomatic individuals.

Failure of Fusion of Epididymis and Testis

This defect involves failure of fusion of the testicular rete cords and the mesonephric tubules that form the ductuli efferentia. Spermatozoa cannot exit from the testis, and if this condition is bilateral, infertility results. One or both testes may fail to descend.

Treatment

Surgical treatment of male ductal abnormalities is still quite new. Some surgical corrections have been attempted, but successes are limited and even controversial. Sperm have also been aspirated prior to the obstruction, capacitated in vitro and then used for insemination in vitro or in vivo. Again, success is arguable, but reported.

REFERENCES

Anguiano, A., Amos, J., Oates, R., et al. (1991). Cystic fibrosis (CF) gene mutations in males with congenital bilateral absence of the vas deferens (CBAVD). *American Journal of Human Genetics, 49*(4), 22.

Layman, L.C. (1991). Idiopathic hypogonadotropic hypogonadism: Diagnosis, pathogenesis, genetics and treatment. *Adolescent & Pediatric Gynecologist, 4,* 111.

Sauer, M.V., Paulson, R.J., & Lobo, R.A. (1990). A preliminary report on oocyte donation extending reproductive potential to women over 40. *New England Journal of Medicine, 323,* 1157.

Sauer, M.V., Paulson, R.V., & Lobo, R.A. (1992). Reversing the natural decline in human fertility: An extended trial of oocyte donation to women of advanced age. *Journal of the American Medical Association, 268,* 1275.

Simpson, J.L. (1976). *Disorders of sexual differentiation: Etiology and clinical delineation.* New York: Academic Press.

Simpson, J.L. (1992). Genetics of sexual differentiation. In J. Rock, & S.E. Carpenter (Eds.), *Pediatric and adolescent gynecology.* New York: Raven Press.

Simpson, J.L., & Golbus, M.S. (1992). *Genetics in obstetrics and gynecology* (2nd ed.). Philadelphia: W.B. Saunders.

Simpson, J.L., & Rebar, R.W. (1990). Normal and abnormal sexual differentiation and development. In K.L. Becker (Ed.), *Principles and practice of endocrinology and metabolism* (pp. 710–739). Philadelphia: J.B. Lippincott.

Speiser, P.W., LaForgia, N., Kato, K., et al. (1990). First trimester prenatal treatment and molecular genetic diagnosis of congenital adrenal hyperplasia (21-hydroxylase deficiency). *Journal of Clinical Endocrinology and Metabolism, 70,* 838.

Whitcomb, R.W., & Crawley, W.F., Jr. (1990). Clinical review 4: Diagnosis and treatment of isolated gonadotropin-releasing hormone deficiency in men. *Journal of Clinical Endocrinology Metabolism 70,* 3.

13

Spousal Relationships and Disability

Nancy M. Crewe

Disability invariably affects intimate relationships, often in complex ways. Some of the effects may be positive, such as a drawing together of family members, perceived personal growth, and changes in values that serve to emphasize the importance of interpersonal relationships. However, the negative effects may include stress, which can lead to health problems in the spouse (Kester, Rothblum, Lobato, & Milhouse, 1988), financial upheaval, loss of valued activities, and assumption of unwanted tasks and responsibilities.

Reactions to disability are complex because the people and situations that produce them are complex. Even the title of this chapter, "Spousal Relationships and Disability," may engender quite different expectations in the mind of each reader. It may raise the image of a young homemaker with multiple sclerosis and her spouse of 7 years, or a 35-year-old single man with spinal cord injury, who is considering the possibility of marriage for the first time. Disability also could affect the relationship of a young couple who give birth to a child with severe cerebral palsy. A lesbian couple in which one person has experienced traumatic brain injury in an automobile accident could provide another example of a relationship affected by disability. The relationship of an elderly couple might be profoundly affected by Alzheimer's disease. The topic of spousal relationships and disability could encompass the impact on a middle-age couple of dependent and chronically ill parents.

Considering the diversity of circumstances, no simple generalizations can be made, but this chapter attempts to: 1) summarize some of the variables that moderate the impact of disability on spousal relationships, 2) review research on marital relationships and disability, and 3) offer recommendations for rehabilitation services.

RELEVANT VARIABLES

Several dimensions, inherent in the examples provided above, affect any conclusions to be drawn about the impact of disability on marriage. They include the following:

1. Role of the person with the disability—Is the individual a spouse or another family member? When a spouse has a disability, both gender and the role that person plays within the family may be important in determining the effect of the disability on the marriage. Alternatively, a child with a disability may engender different effects than an aging parent or other relative.
2. Characteristics of the relationship—Such factors as the duration of the relationship and the stage of life of the partners are significant moderators. A correlated factor is the age of the spouses—are they young, middle-age, or elderly? Another factor that must be considered is the sequence of marriage and disability. Did the disability come into an existing marriage, or did the marriage occur among persons with disabilities?
3. Characteristics of the disability—Is the disability stable or progressive? Does it involve cognitive dysfunction or physical disability alone?
4. Characteristics of environmental support—Who beside the spouse is involved in helping with the extra work created by the disability? Is respite care available? Are financial resources adequate?

THE EFFECT OF DISABILITY ON MARRIAGE AND DIVORCE

The literature contains conflicting reports about the correlation between disability and rates of marriage and divorce. Perhaps the most reliable data are available on individuals with spinal cord injury, because of the existence of a national database. DeVivo and Fine (1985) reported on the marital status of 276 individuals who sustained spinal cord injury between 1973–1980 and compared their rates of marriage and divorce with the general U.S. population. The researchers found that their sample experienced substantially fewer marriages and significantly more divorces than would be expected according to the base rates for age. The lower incidence of marriage is likely to be seen among many groups with early onset disabilities, and a substantial proportion of these individuals remain single throughout their lives. The reasons are speculative, but they may well include reduced social opportunities, financial disadvantage, attitudinal barriers, and physical restrictions. In DeVivo and Fine's sample, no demographic variables were reliably related to marrying, but several significant correlates of divorce were identified. The authors reported that women, younger individuals, people who had been previously divorced, and African-Americans had a higher likelihood of being divorced after spinal cord injury.

Comprehensive data on other disability groups are hard to find. Tew, Laurence, Payne, and Rawnsley (1977) reported on marital stability of families in Britain following birth of a child with spina bifida. They found the divorce rate for families with a surviving child was nine times higher than the general rate for the local population over a comparable time period. They also indicated that the divorce rate in families where the child with spina bifida died was three times higher than the general base rate. Most vulnerable were marriages where the child was conceived before wedlock; in 50% of those cases the spouses divorced. Among families with a surviving child, divorce was initiated by the fathers. All such fathers in their sample remarried, but only one of the mothers did so. The mothers in this study all had custody of the children.

Our own research (Crewe, Athelstan, & Krumberger, 1979; Crewe & Krause, 1988) also suggests that married women who become disabled are particularly vulnerable to divorce. This longitudinal study of persons with spinal cord injury began in the early 1970s and has continued for almost 2 decades. More than 80% of persons with spinal cord injury are male, so the number of women in our study was relatively small. However, it was striking that among our initial subjects, six out of the seven women who had been married at the time of spinal cord injury were divorced within the first few years afterward.

THE MINNESOTA STUDY OF
MARRIAGE AND SPINAL CORD INJURY

Because the longitudinal study, referred to as the Minnesota Spinal Cord Injury Study, includes marriage as a primary topic of interest, it is discussed here in some detail. In 1973, a study was undertaken of 256 individuals who had services from the University of Minnesota or from an affiliated clinic at the Sister Kenny Institute. Subjects provided information about themselves using the Life Satisfaction Questionnaire (LSQ), an instrument that was developed for the original study in 1974 that has been expanded and used in the subsequent follow-up studies. The LSQ and the methodology of the Minnesota Study are described in some detail in an earlier publication (Crewe & Krause, 1990). Briefly, the LSQ includes information related to date and type of spinal cord injury, need for assistance with activities of daily living, dating and social activities, marital and family status, work activities, educational level and school involvement, sitting tolerance and need for medical services, rating scales of satisfaction with various aspects of life, and a 10-point rating scale of the individual's present personal adjustment to spinal cord injury and that projected in the future. During the 1985 follow-up study, a series of items were added that rate the importance of various problems in the subjects lives. In addition, the LSQ has provided continuity in the three longitudinal studies that have been conducted to date; the first study (1974) included face-to-face in-depth interviews with a subsample of 100 individuals and their spouses or significant others.

The 1985 follow-up study included as many of the 256 subjects in the 1973 sample (sample one) as could be located (179 were known to be alive). In addition, a new sample (sample two, $N = 266$) of persons with more recent injuries was added to the pool. The response rate was extremely high (56% of sample one and 78% of sample two).

In 1989, the two samples were again followed, and responses were received from 135 (88%) of sample one and 151 (78%) of sample two. Response percentages were calculated after deducting subjects who were deceased or who could not be located.

Data were analyzed to answer a number of marriage-related questions including the following:

1. Are there measurable differences between married and single subjects on measures of demographic characteristics, life satisfaction, social and work activities, and reported problems?
2. Are there significant differences that can be observed in the marriages that survived the spinal cord injury and in those that took place after the injury?
3. Among persons who are single at the time of a spinal cord injury, is it possible to predict who will later marry and who will remain single?

To answer the first question, data from the combined 1989 follow-up study (Crewe & Krause, 1992) were analyzed. Age and marital status were significantly related, with single subjects being younger, both at the time of injury and at the time of follow-up (mean age at follow-up was 37.6 years for single subjects, 45.1 years for married subjects, and 44.7 for separated, widowed, or divorced individuals. A higher proportion of individuals with quadriplegia were single (48.7%) compared with individuals with paraplegia (32.7%). An identical proportion of men and women in the sample were single (42.6%). Thirty-four percent of women were married compared with 46.3% of the men, with the difference reflecting more women who were separated, widowed, or divorced. Because of the small numbers of women in the sample, however, that difference was not statistically significant.

Married subjects were more likely to be employed (51.1%) than single persons (37.0%). The many Life Satisfaction Questionnaire ratings and problem ratings were factor analyzed to reduce the number of variables in the analysis, thereby reducing the chance of spurious significant results. The life satisfaction ratings were reduced to two factors. The first, involving social life, functional adjustment, and control over one's life and recreational opportunities, is one that could be expected to vary with marital status, but no significant relationship was found. Married people did score higher on the second factor, however, reflecting greater satisfaction with employment and finances.

The problem ratings produced three factors. Married people rated the first factor, which included loneliness, depression, and boredom, as less troublesome than did the single or separated/widowed/divorced group. The second problem factor, which included items related to personal dependence and family conflicts, was rated as more serious for those in the separated/widowed/divorced group than for either the single or married subjects. No significant difference was found on the third factor, which included health problems and pain.

These findings indicate that some differences can be documented between groups based on marital status and that those differences generally favor people who are married. In many areas of behavior and life satisfaction, however, no consistent differences could be identified between single and married people. Earlier observations from the interviews and the first LSQ survey (Crewe et al., 1979) suggested that some significant distinctions related to marital status may have been masked by the fact that the married group included both individuals who had been married at the time of their injuries and those who were married at a later time. Criteria for inclusion in the study required that all subjects be at least 2 years post-injury, so the marriages that had ended soon after injury were not represented in the sample. As a result, the surviving marriages demonstrated strength and commitment, but they also included noticeable areas of loss and regret. Spouses in pre-injury marriages were much more likely to be providing personal care than spouses in post-injury marriages even when the level of injury was constant. Individuals in pre-injury marriages also appeared to be much less likely to be working compared with those in post-injury marriages.

Additional data related to this issue were collected in the 1985 follow-up study, which included 33 married individuals from sample one and 89 married individuals from sample two. These 122 individuals were classified into either pre-injury ($N = 46$) or post-injury ($N = 76$) marriage groups. Seventy-eight percent of the pre-injury group were male compared with 87% of the post-injury group (no significant difference). The injury level of the two groups was also similar with 59% of those in the pre-injury group having cervical injuries, compared with 56% in the post-injury group. However, significant differences were evident in age, with those in the pre-injury marriage group older, both at the time of onset (39 years compared with 20 years for the post-injury marriage group) and at the time of follow-up (53 years compared with 38 years). Those in the post-injury marriage group had a longer duration of spinal cord injury (18 years compared with 13 years in the pre-injury group). As a result, all analyses involving continuous variables utilized analysis of covariance, with age at these two time points as covariates.

Significant differences were found between the groups on many emotional and behavioral measures. Individuals in post-injury marriages were more active socially, had higher educational attainment (14.4 years versus 12.6 years), and were far more likely to be working; 79% of those under 65 in the post-injury marriage group were employed, compared with 30% of comparable subjects in the pre-injury marriage group.

Many significant differences were also identified among the life satisfaction variables. Again, after controlling for the effects of age, individuals in post-injury marriages were significantly more satisfied with their living arrangements and sex lives ($p < 0.001$), with their social lives and general health ($p < 0.01$), and with their emotional adjustment and sense of control of their lives ($p < 0.05$). It was interesting that, despite the wide discrepancy in employment rates between the two groups, they did not differ in terms of satisfaction with employment or financial means or in terms of their family relationships, recreational opportunities, or general life opportunities.

Ratings of personal adjustment and life satisfaction tended to be high across both groups. On a 10-point scale with 10 representing the best possible adjustment to spinal cord injury, ratings were significantly higher for younger people, but no statistically significant difference could be attributed to the timing of marriage. Similarly, age was more frequently related to the rated severity of problems. Among a list of 13 problem areas, only loneliness was significantly less troublesome for individuals in post-injury marriages than for those married before injury, whereas four problem areas were significantly related to age (pain, lack of transportation, dependency, and inadequate community accessibility).

What could account for the differences that were identified between the marriages that survived spinal cord injury and those that took place sometime after the individual experienced the disability? Perhaps the differences begin with the tendency of the rehabilitation system to identify the individual with a spinal cord injury as the patient and to see the spouse as his or her caregiver and part of the support system. The spouse may provide needed care early after the spinal cord injury and may find it difficult to break these patterns as the individual becomes more independent. Furthermore, the government systems that provide financial support for personal care assistance may not pay spouses to provide help, so the spouse may be caught in the stressful situation of attempting to provide personal assistance as well as maintain the household and an outside job. A conflict also may exist between providing intimate physical care and maintaining a sexual and romantic relationship important to the health of a marriage. It is easy to see that these stressors could have a negative impact, particularly on pre-injury marriages.

Further evidence for the importance of a balanced relationship comes from Urey and Henggeler (1987), who compared the interaction and communication patterns of 44 couples. One half of the couples in the sample were in distressed marriages and one half were in nondistressed marriages. One half of the couples in each group had a partner with a spinal cord injury. The researchers found that similar processes were operating in the functioning of the couples with and without spinal cord injury. Marital happiness was related to satisfaction with the *exchange* of instrumental affective positive behaviors and with more positive marital communication patterns.

Another special issue for individuals in pre-injury marriages is that of loss and change. The onset of disability results in functional limitations that may lead to omission of activities or changes in the way that they are carried out. Married couples in which one spouse has a severe physical disability must find ways to cope with functional limitations, but loss of valued activities may be more painful than doing without activities that were never shared.

As noted in the third research question raised by the Minnesota Study, the possibility that individuals who attract a spouse following injury may be an unusual and highly selected subsample of the population with spinal cord injuries must be taken into account. Accordingly, data gathered in 1974 were used to compare individuals who were single in 1974 and who were married by the 1985 follow-up study with those who were single in 1974 and who were not married by 1985 (Crewe & Krause, 1992). One variable, work status, stood out as a potent predictor. Among the people who were single and working in 1974, almost half had married by 1985, whereas fewer than 20% of those who were not working had married by 1985. Looking at the same data from another perspective, of the 31 people who went from single to married status between 1974 and 1985, 80% had been employed in 1974.

Among the other distinctions that more frequently charac-terized the group that married were the following: they went out more often socially, they rated their overall adjustment as higher, and they scored higher on a cluster of life satisfaction items involv-ing social life, sex life, and general health. It is apparent, then, that individuals who marry after spinal cord injury do have some person-al advantages that set them apart from their fellows with spinal cord injuries who remain single. These studies also suggest that the expe-rience of marriage serves to enhance life satisfaction and produc-tivity.

MARRIAGES INVOLVING COGNITIVE DISABILITIES

The impact of cognitive and personality changes on spousal rela-tionships is almost certainly more troublesome than physical dis-ability alone. Rosenbaum and Najenson (1976) reported on the life patterns and emotions of Israeli wives whose husbands had sus-tained either brain injury or spinal cord injury. The wives whose husbands had sustained traumatic brain injury (TBI) reported drastic and upsetting changes, especially in relationships with their hus-bands, in-laws, and friends. The wives reported personal symptoms closely related to depression. They described their husbands as more childlike, self-oriented, and dependent than did the wives of hus-bands with spinal cord injury. Wives of husbands with head injury reported a substantial increase in contact with their in-laws, but they did not feel close or supported. The husband's parents appeared to be overly protective in response to their son's injury, whereas the husband's dependency was extremely distressing to the wives. The couple saw fewer friends and became progressively more isolated. Both the husbands with head injury and the husbands with spinal cord injury played a reduced role in raising the children. There was a drastic decrease in sexual activity for both groups, although the authors speculate that different factors were responsible in the two groups. The wives of the men with TBI reported disliking contact with their husbands, whereas the wives of men with spinal cord injury reported more impairments in physical functioning as the reasons for change.

Mauss-Clum and Ryan (1981) also studied marriages that involved men with traumatic brain injury. They reported that almost one half of the wives identified with the statement, "I'm married, but I really don't have a husband." Referring to the same disability, Zeigler (1987) stated that the healthy spouse not only mourned specific losses the partner has experienced but also her own specific loss of a partner. Many feel trapped by guilt, expectations, and reality. She said that the mourning process may lead to either divorce or remaining and assuming the role of a caregiver. Lezak (1978) followed up a sample of individuals with head injury and also noted substantial changes in marital relationships. She indicated that accepting the fact that the previous relationship is permanently changed may be emotionally freeing to the spouse.

RECOMMENDATIONS FOR REHABILITATION SERVICES

In families where a spouse makes a good, albeit incomplete, recovery, professionals and others may be tempted to reassure the spouse there is much to be grateful for. They may point out that many are worse off and that they may even grow from the experience. Yet, coming from any outsider, these reassurances are too simple.

Featherstone (1981) is a professional educator who gave birth to a child with a severe disability. In describing her family's experience, she outlined the ways in which professionals can be of maximum service to husbands and wives touched by disability. The first resource she emphasized was information, offered directly and with a minimum of jargon. Many people who have lived through the onset of severe disability have horror stories to tell about misguided predictions (e.g., "Your son will always be a vegetable") or the avoidance of painful truth. Second, Featherstone listed respect. She points out that self-confidence can be badly shaken during such a crisis and that the difference in power between families and professionals can seem overwhelming. This is one of the reasons that many persons with disabilities prefer to seek information from peers. The consumer movement in health care and rehabilitation has significantly heightened the awareness of the need to treat patients and families with openness and respect, and we must be continually sensitive to the difference in perspective between insider and outsider. Another way in which professionals can offer respect is to help spouses avoid slipping into the stereotyped roles of caregiver and recipient of care. In all intimate relationships, problems may result if one person is asked over time to give much more than he or she receives. Relationships are balancing acts. Featherstone uses the analogy of a seesaw. The reciprocal shifting needs and contributions of the partners keep the relationship in motion. If the balance is lost, the relationship becomes frozen, with one partner perpetually up in the air and the other stuck on the ground. Rehabilitation should help individuals with a disability to recognize, believe, and live out the fact that they have as much to contribute to their marriages as their partners.

The third contribution that professionals can make to families affected by disability is services, according to Featherstone. These families are thrown into a confusing and tangled system of services, and they need help to find out what is available and how to obtain it. She states that studies have often shown that people fail to utilize services available to them until they are at the point of physical and emotional exhaustion. If we can coordinate services so that they are available more readily, so much the better. Cleveland (1976) studied families that included an adolescent with spinal cord injury and found that family satisfaction with available help depended greatly on whether someone was available to coordinate the many services needed from diverse sources.

The fourth professional contribution noted by Featherstone was emotional support. She pointed out that with a trusted professional, she could surrender a little bit of the responsibility that she felt for being in charge of the care of her child and allow herself to be cared for.

In conclusion, disability *does* affect intimate relationships. It would be futile and fatuous to deny the disappointments and frustrations that disability causes. At the same time, disability is woven into the fabric of a relationship as surely as any other crucial characteristics of the partners. If the relationship is good, the disability is a part of that goodness. Without it, the individuals would be different and so would the relationship; that is why the disability may be accepted by partners and even embraced.

REFERENCES

Cleveland, M. (1976). *Family adaptation to the permanent disablement of a son or daughter.* Unpublished doctoral dissertation. University of Minnesota, Minneapolis.

Crewe, N.M., Athelstan, G.T., & Krumberger, J. (1979). Spinal cord injury: A comparison of preinjury and postinjury marriages. *Archives of Physical Medicine and Rehabilitation, 60,* 252–256.

Crewe, N.M., & Krause, J.S. (1988). Marital relationships and spinal cord injury. *Archives of Physical Medicine and Rehabilitation, 69,* 435–438.

Crewe, N.M., & Krause, J.S. (1990). An eleven-year follow-up of adjustment to spinal cord injury. *Rehabilitation Psychology, 35,* 205–210.

Crewe, N.M., & Krause, J.S. (1992). Marital status and adjustment to spinal cord injury. *Journal of the American Paraplegia Society, 15,* 14–18.

DeVivo, M.J., & Fine, P.R. (1985). Spinal cord injury: Its short-term impact on marital status. *Archives of Physical Medicine and Rehabilitation, 66,* 501–504.

Featherstone, H. (1981). *A difference in the family.* New York: Penguin Books.

Kester, B.L., Rothblum, E.D., Lobato, D., & Milhouse, R. (1988). Spouse adjustment to spinal cord injury: Long-term medical and psychosocial factors. *Rehabilitation Counseling Bulletin, 32,* 4–21.

Lezak, M. (1978). Living with the characterologically altered brain injured patient. *Journal of Clinical Psychiatry, 39,* 592–598.

Mauss-Clum, N., & Ryan, M. (1981). Brain injury and the family. *Journal of Neurosurgical Nursing, 4,* 165–169.

Rosenbaum, J., & Najenson, T. (1976). Changes in life patterns and symptoms of low mood as reported by wives of severely brain-injured soldiers. *Journal of Consulting and Clinical Psychology, 44,* 881–888.

Tew, B.J., Laurence, K.M., Payne, H., & Rawnsley, K. (1977). Marital stability following the birth of a child with spina bifida. *British Journal of Psychiatry, 131,* 79–82.

Urey, J.R., & Henggeler, S.W. (1987). Marital adjustment following spinal cord injury. *Archives of Physical Medicine and Rehabilitation, 68,* 69–74.

Zeigler, E.A. (1987). Spouses of persons who are brain injured: Overlooked victims. *Journal of Rehabilitation, 53,* 50–53.

14

Genetic Counseling and Evaluation of Recurrence for People with Physical Disabilities

Samuel A. Rhine

Any couple in which one partner has a physical disability might have concerns during pregnancy because many physical disabilities have a genetic etiology. For the same reason, parents and siblings of a person with a physical disability might have questions and concerns about the genetics of their children. Likewise, the children of an individual with a physical disability might have concerns about the genetics of their offspring. This chapter looks at the "What are the chances it could happen again?" concerns for the person with a physical disability and for his or her parents, siblings, and children.

5% + X

Approximately 5% of all babies born in the U.S. have some type of disability (Jones, 1988). The number of 5% is defined by any child who has: 1) a mental disability, 2) a physical disability, or 3) a requirement of corrective surgery. Using these three criteria includes about 1 in every 20 babies, or 5%. This translates to mean any couple who conceives has about a 5% chance of their baby having a disability.

153

In certain couples, for all sorts of different reasons, this 5% chance is increased. For instance, a couple with a child with Down syndrome who conceives again usually have an additional 1% chance, since the recurrence for most cases of Down syndrome is about 1 in 100 (Jones, 1988). This means that for the second pregnancy, they have 5% + 1% or a 6% chance. Another couple, with a child with spina bifida, may have up to a 5% + 7% or 12% chance, since the recurrence risk for spina bifida runs from 4%–6% (Buyse, 1990; Jones, 1988). If both parents carry the gene for cystic fibrosis, which is caused by an autosomal recessive gene, the occurrence or recurrence chances are 1 in 4, or 5% + 25%. If one parent has Huntington's disease, which is caused by an autosomal dominant gene and is passed to 50% of the children, it is 5% + 50%. If a woman is pregnant and drinking 4–6 drinks per day, there is about a 30%–50% chance for fetal alcohol syndrome, or 5% + 30% to 5% + 50% (Jones, 1988). Some rarer genetic conditions can be 5% + 75% or even 5% + 100%.

Our main focus of attention in this chapter is to identify the various factors (x values) that affect the reproductive decision-making of the individual with a physical disability. The x value is the occurrence risk for a couple with no previous disabilities in their family, or the recurrence risk for a couple with a child with a disabling condition. Determining the x value is the special job of those with expertise in genetics, and genetic counseling is probably a procreative concern of the person with a physical disability.

GENETIC AND ACQUIRED

How does a genetic counselor "solve for x" for a particular couple seeking information before having a child? The key to determining the x value for any couple is to understand the cause of the concern. The causes of physical disabilities fall in two broad categories: genetic and acquired.

Genetic issues involve genes and chromosomes and are often inherited, or familial. Familial means the situation "runs through the family" and can be observed in multiple generations. However, not all genetic traits are familial. For instance, Down syndrome is usually not inherited but usually appears only one time in the family history. It is genetic because it involves genetic material, the chromosomes, but it has the potential to be inherited only when a chromosome translocation is involved, which occurs in about 2.5% of all cases of Down syndrome (Jones, 1988). Genetic issues can almost always be traced to the fertilized egg at conception. A problem may exist in the sperm cell from the father or in the ovum from the mother. Sometimes the particular combination of a particular ovum and sperm cause a problem. Genetic problems within the egg at conception are termed intrinsic and fall into three categories: cytogenetic (chromosomal), monogenic (single gene inheritance), and multifactorial (embryologic developmental errors). An extensive family history, along with a detailed physical exam, often help to confirm the diagnosis of a genetic condition.

"Acquired" is a very general term used in medicine to designate a condition that is caused by something in the environment. Acquired means that the disability is acquired during the course of the pregnancy if it is congenital, or acquired sometime during the lifetime of an individual if it is not congenital. Acquired disabilities are due to the effect of an environmental factor outside the fertilized egg, and, therefore, they are extrinsic. During pregnancy, acquired problems might involve DATA (drugs, alcohol, or tobacco abuse), PPC (poor prenatal care), STDs (sexually transmitted diseases) and other infections, TAP (teenage parents), and L&D (difficulties in labor and delivery). In addition, socioeconomic status is often a major contributing factor, because it often involves many of the above areas of concern. Some acquired factors cause severe disabilities that are recognized at delivery, such as fetal alcohol syndrome. Other acquired factors lead to a greater chance of a low birth weight (LBW) baby. Low birth weight means that the baby's birth weight is below 2,500 grams (5½ pounds) (Rubenstein & Federman, 1992). LBW is the primary cause of infant mortality (death within the first year of life) and the primary cause of infant morbidity (medical problems) in the U.S. (Rubenstein & Federman, 1992). LBW is also a leading cause of neurodevelopmental problems in newborns, often resulting in cerebral palsy and/or seizures.

After birth, acquired disabilities include those caused by infections (polio), accidents (spinal cord injury), stroke (brain injury), or late onset diseases such as amyotrophic lateral sclerosis (ALS), Alzheimer's disease (AD), or multiple sclerosis (MS).

As a general rule, the x value for a genetic disability is a greater concern than for an acquired disability. Because there is an inherited connection to many genetic disabilities, the x value can range from 1%–100%. With an acquired disability, the x value is usually negligible, if the particular environmental factor can be eliminated or avoided in subsequent pregnancies or throughout the lifetime of the individual.

There are also many cases when the cause of a particular physical disability is never found. We do not know if it is genetic or acquired. In those cases, the x value is a guess and ranges from 2% to 25%.

An example of a genetic disability versus an acquired disability can be illustrated by Jodie and David, two enthusiastic young people each born with the inability to hear. Jodie's deafness is genetic in origin and is caused by an autosomal recessive gene aberration. David's deafness was acquired when his mother contracted Rubella during pregnancy. This is an example of one case genetic, one case acquired, both manifesting in a very similar way. For Jodie's parents, the chances of genetic deafness would be 5% + 25% for any subsequent pregnancies; for David's parents, the chances of acquired deafness for any subsequent pregnancies were essentially 5% + 0%. Since David's mother has now had Rubella, she has immunity to the infection and therefore would not likely contract it again. Jodie has recently finished her Ph.D. from Gallaudet University, and David has a degree from Purdue University.

GENETIC DISABILITIES

Cytogenetics is the study of chromosomes and represents the first category of genetic concerns. Most chromosome problems are so severe that the pregnancy results in miscarriage. Fetuses with chromosome problems that go to term and are delivered are likely to have multiple congenital anomalies, including mental retardation (Jones, 1988). These individuals rarely reproduce, and, therefore, individuals with chromosome aberrations are not addressed in this chapter.

Monogenic traits, which are caused by a single pair of genes, represent the second category of genetic concerns. Next, the three main modes of inheritance and their x values are outlined. The first mode of inheritance is autosomal recessive (AR), where both parents are unaffected but both are carriers for a single dose of the abnormal gene. The affected child, either male or female, receives a double dose of the abnormal gene, which occurs 25% of the time, hence the chance for occurrence of AR is 5% + 25%.

The second mode of inheritance is autosomal dominant (AD), where one parent has the condition or disease, and it is passed to half of the children, male or female, hence 5% + 50%. Sometimes an autosomal dominant gene will show up in one person in a family as a new mutation, never seen in the family before. It will then be passed from that person to half of his or her children.

The third mode of inheritance is X-linked recessive. The abnormal gene is carried by the mother who is unaffected, but the inheritance works in such a way that the abnormal trait is passed to half of her male children. Therefore, the inheritance is 5% + 50% if the baby is a boy, 5% + 0% if the baby is a girl. Half of the girls will be carriers like their mother and have a 50% chance of passing the abnormal gene to their sons in the next generation.

It can be complicated to determine which mode of inheritance is responsible for a particular trait in a particular family. In the catalog of single-gene diseases, McKusick (1990) lists a total of 4,937 separate human medical conditions caused by single genes. Sometimes, reaching the correct diagnosis and, therefore, the correct x value can be very difficult. Below are some examples of physical disabilities that illustrate the difficulty in diagnosis and the importance of seeking proper genetic counseling expertise.

Friedreich ataxia (FA) is a relatively rare, hereditary spinocerebellar degenerative condition usually resulting in moderate to severe physical disability. It is usually inherited as an autosomal recessive trait. However, there is a form of FA that presents with congenital glaucoma, which is a recessive trait, and another form of FA that presents with optic atrophy and sensorineural deafness, which is an autosomal dominant condition (McKusick, 1990).

Multiple sclerosis (MS) is usually recognized as an autoimmune disease in which an individual's immune system destroys the myelin sheath around the nerve fibers. Autoimmune diseases are thought to occur when an environmental factor, such as a virus, acts upon a predisposing inherited dominant gene and initiates the disease process. MS is strongly connected to an inherited predisposing dominant gene of the immune system, HLA-Dw2 (McKusick, 1990). However, McKusick (1990) also lists a condition very similar to MS, disseminated sclerosis, as a dominant trait and a MS-like condition known as Pelizaeus-Merzbacher disease as a dominant trait. Rheumatoid arthritis is another autoimmune disorder closely associated with the predisposing dominant gene HLA-Dw4 or HLA-Cw3. Myasthenia gravis is listed among the autoimmune diseases, but McKusick (1990) has four other listings, one dominant and three recessive which are not autoimmune conditions. There are 10 different types of muscular atrophy, both dominant and recessive. The muscular dystrophy (MD) category has 23 types, which include dominant, recessive, and X-linked recessive. The most common forms of MD, the pseudohypertrophic progressive forms, known as the Duchenne and Becker types, represent two different forms of the same X-linked recessive gene so that they are usually evidenced in males.

Amyotrophic lateral sclerosis (Lou Gehrig's disease) is inherited in about 10% of cases. The inherited form is caused by a dominant gene on chromosome 21. The other 90% of the cases are acquired. Likewise, Alzheimer's disease is familial in about one third of affected individuals and acquired in the other two thirds. (McKusick, 1990).

Some human genetic traits are determined by genes that do not reside on the 46 chromosomes found in the nucleus of the cell. They are on a chromosome, chromosome M, which is a circle of DNA found in the energy-producing mitochondria in the cell cytoplasm. Since mitochondria are inherited from the mother via the egg, and none are received from the father via the sperm, these traits exhibit matrilineal inheritance. This second category of genetic traits are passed from the mother to all of her children but never from the father. Certain ophthalmologic and neuromuscular diseases are known to be caused by genes on the mitochondrial chromosome, some of which might lead to a physical disability. These include Leber's hereditary optic atrophy, myoclonic epilepsy, ragged red muscle, and Kearns-Sayre syndrome (Wallace, 1992). These gene defects cause a loss in mitochondrial energy production, which can ultimately lead to cell death and loss of neural or muscular function.

The third category of genetic traits is termed multifactorial. As the name implies, many factors are involved, both genetic and environmental. The genetic component is termed polygenic and is thought to involve many genes working in concert, instead of a single pair of dominant or recessive genes.

Many of the multifactorial traits are evidenced as structural errors in the newborn, which result from some early malformation of the embryo. These include congenital heart defects, neural tube defects (NTDs), cleft lip and/or palate, congenital hip dislocation (CHD), pyloric stenosis, and hypospadias, among others.

Of greatest concern in this chapter are neural tube defects, in particular, spina bifida. NTDs result from embryologic problems in the closure of the spinal tube of the developing fetus during the 4th week of pregnancy. Parents of a child with a NTD or an individual with a NTD have a significant x value to consider as part of their family planning. McKusick (1990) lists three types of NTDs that are connected with single genes, so a detailed genetic counseling evaluation is recommended for the family with a previous NTD. In addition, NTDs can also be acquired, resulting from maternal hyperthermia, vitamin deficiencies (especially folic acid), the use of seizure control medications, or cocaine abuse.

Another factor that can complicate genetic counseling and determination of the x value is assortative mating. When each partner has a disability, then two separate causes of two separate conditions must be taken into consideration in determining x. Questions as to whether both disabilities are genetic, or both are acquired, or one is genetic and the other acquired, or one cause is known and the other is not, make these situations difficult for the genetic counselor and the individuals planning a family.

ACQUIRED DISABILITIES

Acquired physical disabilities are, by definition, not genetic and not inherited, so the x value is very close to zero *if* that particular environmental factor can be avoided during future pregnancies. It is also important to keep in mind that acquired problems can happen to any couple during any pregnancy.

The problems of drugs, alcohol, and tobacco abuse during pregnancy are a very special concern. Alcohol consumption during pregnancy is now recognized as the leading cause of mental retardation in the U.S. (Streissguth et al., 1991). The emotional and psychological stress for an individual who is dealing with both a physical handicap and pregnancy might predispose some to alcohol use during the pregnancy (Rubenstein & Federman, 1992). These are individuals who may need to develop support teams to help with those and other pressures during the pregnancy.

Smoking during pregnancy may cause fetal injury, premature birth, and low birth weight. Cocaine, marijuana, and other drugs are known to be associated with numerous problems in newborns (Chasnoff, 1991). Another major acquired concern is known as the "I'll quit when I get pregnant" syndrome. It involves individuals who are 8, 10, or more weeks pregnant before they realize it. Since they were not expecting to be pregnant, and did not realize they were pregnant, they have continued drinking during those early critical weeks of pregnancy when the fetus was forming. Sometimes the unborn baby is destined to have mental retardation before the mother has realized she is pregnant!

Some prescription medications are dangerous during pregnancy. Of particular concern are medications for seizure control, since seizures sometimes accompany physical disabilities. The list of seizure control medications that can affect the unborn baby include: phenytoin, (hydantoin effects), trimethadione, valporic acid, carbamazepine, and phenobarbital (Jones, 1988). Any woman who is taking one of these medications needs to be evaluated by her obstetrician, her neurologist, and, ideally, a genetic counselor before pregnancy. Sometimes the medication can be changed or the amount modified to minimize the risk to the fetus.

Other medications of concern are the anticoagulant warfarin and the acne medication retinoic acid. Ideally, no medications would be taken during pregnancy. If a woman must take medication, its safety should be evaluated by her doctor before pregnancy.

Acquired problems may also occur during labor and delivery (Verduyn, chap. 21, this volume). The patient with physical disabilities should be consulting closely with her obstetrician before and during the pregnancy to ensure adequate preparation for potential problems.

GENETIC COUNSELING

It is the intention that this short and somewhat superficial overview of the numerous causes of physical disabilities gives the reader an idea of the complexity of deciphering information about genetic and acquired disabilities. Any individual with a physical disability with a known genetic cause or unknown cause should certainly consult with a professional genetic counselor to confirm the diagnostic information and to evaluate the x value. In addition, the genetic counselor is able to provide information about the numerous prenatal tests that are available. Over 450 different medical conditions can now be diagnosed before birth (Weaver, 1989). In some cases, prenatal therapy is available so that an affected fetus can be treated before birth. It is even possible to remove the fetus from the uterus in order to perform prenatal surgery to correct some malformations (Longaker et al., 1991).

It is too much to expect that a medical practitioner with no specialty in genetics can provide comprehensive information that parents need to make their reproductive decisions. No one would expect an orthopedist or a neurologist to also be a specialist in genetics. An individual with a physical disability who is planning a pregnancy should therefore consider consulting a professional genetic counselor or counseling team.

REFERENCES

Buyse, M.L. (Ed.). (1990). *Birth defects encyclopedia.* Cambridge, MA: Blackwell Scientific Publications.
Chasnoff, I.J. (Ed.). (1991). *Clinics in perinatology* (Vol. 18, No. 18). Philadelphia: W.B. Saunders.
Jones, K.L. (1988). *Smith's recognizable patterns of human malformation* (4th ed.). Philadelphia: W.B. Saunders.

Longaker, M.T., Golbus, M.S., Filly, R.A., Rosen, M.A., Chang, S.W., & Harrison, M.R. (1991). Maternal outcome after open fetal surgery. *Journal of the American Medical Association, 265,* 737–741.

McKusick, V.A. (Ed.). (1990). *Mendelian inheritance in man* (9th ed.). Baltimore: Johns Hopkins University Press.

Rubenstein, C., & Federman, D.D. (Eds.). (1992). *Medicine.* New York: Scientific American.

Streissguth, A.P., Aase, J.M., Clarren, S.K., Randels, S.P., LaDue, R.A., & Smith, D.F. (1991). Fetal alcohol syndrome in adolescents and adults. *Journal of the American Medical Association, 265,* 1961–1967.

Wallace, D.C. (1992). Mitochondrial genetics: A paradigm for aging and degenerative disease. *Science, 256,* 628–632.

Weaver, D.D. (1989). *Catalog of prenatally diagnosed conditions.* Baltimore: Johns Hopkins University Press.

15

Parenting by Fathers with Physical Disabilities

Frances Marks Buck

Since the inception of rehabilitation, approximately in the 1940s, knowledge and practice regarding psychological, social, and sexual aspects of physical disability often have been guided initially by theory, clinical observation, and even mere speculation. Burgeoning psychosocial research since the 1970s has shown that clinical "wisdom" at best leaves much to be desired, and at worst reflects negative stereotypes of professionals that may unduly affect rehabilitation interventions (Trieschmann, 1988). Theories of adjustment, presumed emotional reactions to disability, marital satisfaction and stability, and sexuality are but a few examples where research later failed to confirm professional beliefs about the nature and extent of psychosocial sequelae to disability (Trieschmann, 1988).

Currently, armchair psychology, with its negative bias in the absence of empirical data, is nowhere more evident than in the area of parental disability. Most professional publications posit that physical disability has a deleterious impact on the parental role and children's well-being. Yet, the few studies conducted to date do not support professionals' dire assumptions that a father's role is impaired by physical disability.

HISTORICAL OVERVIEW

A comprehensive review of the research literature on parental disability in 1979 concluded that, "Like the non-disabled person, the individual with a physical disability goes to school, works, plays, travels, serves in the community, loves, makes love, and marries. Yet, one significant aspect of living is missing—parenthood" (Buck, 1980, p. 1). In contrast to empirical research, articles of opinion regarding disability in a parent were numerous. With few exceptions (Buck, 1980; Burnett, 1973; Nordqvist, 1970), the prevailing opinion at that time was that physical disability disrupts the parental role and poses a severe threat to normal child development and adjustment. Personality, adjustment, sex-role development, body image, physical health patterns, athletic ability, interpersonal relationships, and parent–child relations all were speculated to be adversely affected by parental disability (Anthony, 1970; Bene, 1977; Bray, 1970; Bruhn, 1977; Christopherson, 1968; DiCaprio, 1971; Gibson & Ludwig, 1968; Heslinga, Schellen, & Verkuyl, 1974; Hilbourne, 1973; Kossoris, 1970; Olsen, 1970; Romano, 1976; Thomason & Clifford, 1972). Two literature reviews summarize in detail these theoretical and speculative effects of disability on the parental role and children's adjustment as well as research available in 1980 (Buck, 1980; Buck & Hohmann, 1983).

Over a decade later, little has changed. Except for research published by Buck (1980) and Buck and Hohmann (1981, 1982, 1984) on relationships between spinal cord injury in fathers and children's personality, behavior, and attitudes, no empirical studies have been done. New publications continue to be characterized by clinical lore, anecdotal reports, theoretically driven descriptions, and counseling strategies for parents with disabilities. And, most articles continue an apparent bias, in the absence of data, that parental disability engenders problems for families (Bishop & Epstein, 1980; Glass, 1985; Hanna & Edwards, 1988; Kennedy & Bush, 1979; Kopala & Egenes, 1984; Power, 1980; Power & Dell Orto, 1980; Romano, 1984; Strasberg, 1991).

Although no new research has appeared, some changes have emerged, many of which are positive. Until the 1980s, disability routinely was viewed to negatively affect the parental role. While many publications continue this view, a few have urged professionals against presuming without data that paternal disability has deleterious effects on parenting (Buck & Hohmann, 1983; Greer, 1985). As Buck and Hohmann (1983) wrote, we "need to discourage reliance on opinions and biased research that reflect all of the prejudice and negative stereotypes of the disabled as found in the general population" (p. 233). Greer (1985) points to the tendency to attribute problems in children to any characteristic of a parent that is unique and states, "One must question whether one factor, in this case a physical disability, is the overwhelming influence some would have us believe, when we consider the almost infinite number of factors affecting an individual" (p. 135).

In addition to questioning whether having a disability necessarily prevents adequate parenting, authors have emphasized the critical need for empirical studies. Gaps in empirically based knowledge, important questions for future research, and methodological strategies to examine disability in parents have been identified more clearly (Buck, 1980; Buck & Hohmann, 1983; Coates, Vietze, & Gray, 1985; Thurman, Whaley, & Weinraub, 1985). Underscored in these demands for research is the necessity for evaluating and minimizing the investigators' own biases about parental disability, ensuring that appropriate comparison groups are utilized, and recognizing that many factors affect children's development and welfare beyond the salience of a father's disability (Buck, 1980; Buck & Hohmann, 1983; Coates et al., 1985; Greer, 1985; Thurman et al., 1985).

A third change during the 1980s was a movement toward increased protection of the legal rights of parents with disabilities regarding adoption and custody issues (Gilhool & Gran, 1985). Perhaps most outstanding in its reversal of past legal trends with respect to parental disability was a landmark decision by the Supreme Court of California in 1979. A decision by the lower court granting custody to a nondisabled mother because of the father's spinal cord injury was overturned. On the basis of testimony given at the time, including Buck and Hohmann's research, Justice Mosk wrote (Buck & Hohmann, 1983, p. 236):

> We are called upon to resolve an apparent conflict between two public policies: the requirement that a custody award serve the best interests of the child and the moral and legal obligation of society to respect the civil rights of its physically handicapped members, including their right not to be deprived of their children because of their disability. Of the present day capabilities of the physically handicapped, these policies can both be accommodated. The trial court herein failed to make such an appraisal, and instead premised its ruling on outdated stereotypes of both the parental role and the ability of the handicapped to fill that role. Such stereotypes have no place in our law.

Other legislative and judicial decisions have emerged that protect the rights of parents with disabilities to have and rear children (Gilhool & Gran, 1985), and barriers to adoption have lessened. The Americans with Disabilities Act of 1990 safeguards further the parental rights of persons with disabilities.

In summary, little data-based information on disability in fathers and its implications is available, and most professionals rely on clinical judgments and isolated case descriptions from which to draw conclusions about the impact of paternal disability on children. Previous reviews of research, theoretical views, and implications for research and clinical practice regarding parental disability remain pertinent today (Buck, 1980; Buck & Hohmann, 1983; Thurman, 1985). Because of this author's view that reliance on opinion or theory in the absence of data is professionally unacceptable and potentially harmful to those with disabilities, this chapter focuses on information gleaned from research that meets basic requirements of research design.

DISABILITY IN THE FATHER

Relationships between disability in fathers and children's adjustment have been examined systematically in only three studies (Arnaud, 1959; Buck, 1980; Olgas, 1974). All three used a comparison group of children whose fathers were not disabled, but in only two were objective measures employed (Buck, 1980; Olgas, 1974). Several variables theorized by rehabilitation professionals to moderate the influence of parental disability on children also have been examined. Severity of the father's disability (Buck & Hohmann, 1982), employment status of the father with a disability (Buck & Hohmann, 1984), financial resources of the father (Buck & Hohmann, 1984), and the father's parenting style (Buck, 1980) have been addressed. Buck (1980) also studied adjustment of children reared by fathers with disabilities as a function of children's gender.

Discussion of paternal disability and children's adjustment is organized according to the issues that have been researched empirically: 1) type of disability, 2) gender of the children, 3) severity of the father's disability, 4) employment status of fathers with disabilities, 5) financial resources of the fathers, and 6) parenting styles of fathers with disabilities.

Type of Disability in the Father

Only multiple sclerosis (Arnaud, 1959; Olgas, 1974) and spinal cord injury in fathers have been investigated (Buck, 1980; Buck & Hohmann, 1981). One study showed problems in children as a function of paternal disability (Arnaud, 1959).

Studies of parenting by fathers with multiple sclerosis (MS) yielded conflicting results (Arnaud, 1959; Olgas, 1974). Arnaud (1959) compared 7- to 16-year-old children of fathers with and without MS on measures from the Rorschach, a subjective test of psychological adjustment. He predicted and found that children of fathers with MS showed higher levels of body concern, dysphoria, hostility, constraint in interpersonal relations, dependency longings, and false maturity. Contrary to prediction, higher levels of anxiety in the children whose fathers had MS were not shown. However, the reliability, validity, and generalizability of these findings are quite compromised by several methodological pitfalls. Objective measures were not used, and the comparability of groups was not ensured. The potential effects of experimenter bias in Rorschach administration, scoring, and interpretation were not addressed.

In a better designed study, Olgas (1974) examined body image using both objective (Body-Cathexis scale, semantic differential) and subjective (Draw-A-Person) measures. Sixty-two children of 33 fathers with MS were compared to 60 children of 35 fathers without MS. The children were 7–11 years old. Olgas predicted on the basis of identification theory that children of fathers with MS would show more body image distortion than children of fathers without MS. Results showed that children of fathers with MS had body images as positive as the comparison children on the individual measures and on a combined score of the three measures.

Similarly, spinal cord injury (SCI) in fathers is not associated with problems in the long-term adjustment patterns of children (Buck, 1980; Buck & Hohmann, 1981). In a national sample, adult children, reared from age 2 or younger by fathers with SCI, were compared with adult children raised by fathers without SCI. Subjects were matched on sex and father's age, education, geographic area of residence, and disposable family income. Seven objective tests assessed the major areas of psychosocial adjustment, personality, sex-role identity, body image, values, interpersonal relationships, physical health patterns, athletic pursuits, recreational activities, and parent–child relations, which had been speculated in the literature to be affected by parental disability. Six measures were standardized tests, and one was a newly developed self-report questionnaire. Three control procedures assessed the accuracy of self-reports. Mean scores on the Minnesota Multiphasic Personality Inventory (MMPI) Lie scale (Dahlstrom, Welsch, & Dahlstrom, 1972) and Bem Social Desirability scale (Bem, 1974) indicated that subjects were not distorting their self-reports in a socially desirable direction, nor did the two groups differ significantly. Ratings by friends or relatives who knew subjects well were compared to self-ratings to assess both social desirability and self-deception. Self-reports were comparable to friends' ratings of subjects.

Overall, no evidence was found that SCI in fathers affected parent–child relations or normal development of children (Buck, 1980; Buck & Hohmann, 1981). Adult children of fathers with SCI were as psychologically well-adjusted as children reared by fathers without SCI as indicated by MMPI and 16 Personality Factor Questionnaire (16PF) (Cattell, Eber, & Tatsuoka, 1970) scale scores. Only one significant difference emerged. Children of fathers with SCI were slightly more reserved in emotional expression than comparison children. On open-ended questions, these adult children attributed their well-being to learning values and coping styles from their fathers with SCI that enabled them to lead full and happy lives.

Contrary to what many rehabilitation professionals speculate, sex role orientation, body image, and values were not found to be adversely affected by "identification" with a father with a disability. No significant differences emerged on body image (Body-Cathexis scale, Secord & Jourard, 1953) or gender role identity (Bem Sex Role Inventory, Bem, 1974, 1977). Most children as adults showed appropriate sex typing or were androgynous, and they were satisfied with the appearance and functioning of their bodies. Children of fathers with SCI shared many similar terminal values (idealized end-states) and instrumental values (idealized modes of conduct) with comparison children (Rokeach Value Survey, Rokeach, 1973). Only six values were differentially ranked by the two groups. On terminal values, children reared by fathers with SCI valued more highly "a world at peace" and "national security," perhaps because many fathers in the study were spinal cord injured during World War II. Instrumental values of children of fathers with SCI were somewhat more conventional; they placed higher value on "clean," "obedient," and "responsible" than comparison children. "Logical" was more important to children reared by comparison fathers.

Three attitudinal differences also were found. Compared to children of fathers without SCI, children with fathers with SCI tended to "judge negatively people who complain about physical complaints" but were not likely to "feel sorry for people who are physically disabled." They also were less likely to "couch tragedy in a humorous way" than comparison children.

Children did not learn "sick role" behavior from fathers with SCI or become overly concerned with their physical health. Nine measures of somatic symptoms, frequency of medical care, and wellness behaviors failed to differentiate children of fathers with and without SCI. Contrary to what many authors had suggested, children's interest, participation, and choices of athletic/recreational activities were not disrupted by SCI in fathers. Indeed, these children reported greater participation in athletics than comparison children. Perhaps contributing to this finding was that, despite limitations in physical mobility, fathers with SCI participated as much as fathers without disabilities in recreational and sports activities with their children.

Children's friendships, dating patterns, and social comfort revealed no associations with SCI in fathers. Nor was evidence found that during childhood and adolescence children experience stigmatization from peers by virtue of the father's disability, as is so often cited in the literature.

Prevalent in the literature had been the concern that a father's ability to assume and to adequately perform the parental role is constrained markedly by physical disability. Buck's (1980) data did not support this notion. On three factors describing parental attitudes and behaviors (Attention, Loving-Rejecting, and Casual-Demanding), fathers with SCI did not differ from fathers without SCI. Fathers with SCI, and their wives, were perceived by children as warm, affectionate, helpful, and able to create an environment where children felt loved and respected. They were able to discipline effectively their children no differently than fathers without SCI. Much research in the general population has shown these factors to be related to many aspects of child adjustment. In this study, the demonstrated ability of fathers with SCI to parent effectively corresponds with the findings that their children were well-adjusted psychologically, socially, and physically.

Similarly, additional aspects of parent–child relations identified in the literature were not found to be deleteriously affected by paternal disability (Buck, 1980; Buck & Hohmann, 1981). Fathers with SCI did not relegate decision-making or child-rearing responsibilities to mothers, nor did they "lose control" of children. Children did not feel that fathers with SCI received more attention from mothers at their expense because the father had a disability. Nor were fathers with SCI more protective of children for fear of accidents. Some differences did emerge in discipline practices, but they were not negative in nature. Fathers with SCI used "withdrawal of privileges" as a means of discipline more often than fathers without SCI. They also expressed affection both physically and verbally more often than comparison fathers.

Several behaviors and attitudes expressed toward parents differentiated children of fathers with and without SCI. Children responded more quickly and willingly to both their mother's and father's requests when the father had SCI. Children reported helping fathers with SCI more than fathers without SCI, but they did not resent it. Of import was the finding that children held significantly more positive attitudes toward fathers with SCI than fathers without SCI, as measured by love, respect, and pride in the father. However, they did feel more protective of both their fathers and mothers when the father had SCI.

Thus, extant empirical data shows that men with SCI and MS can be effective fathers, and disability is not necessarily associated with adverse effects for children (Buck, 1980; Buck & Hohmann, 1981; Olgas, 1974). Only in the least methodologically sound study were ill-effects of parental disability found, as so often is theorized (Arnaud, 1959).

Gender of Children with Fathers with Disabilities

The differential influence of paternal disability on daughters versus sons has been addressed in two studies (Buck, 1980; Olgas, 1974). Olgas predicted but did not find differences in body image between 7- to 11-year-old sons and daughters of fathers with MS. She concluded that fathers with MS were able to foster positive self-concepts in both sons and daughters.

Similarly, Buck (1980) found that SCI fathers were as effective in fostering the development and adjustment of their sons as their daughters. Few differences emerged as a function of the child's gender on many measures of personality, behavior, and attitudes. Both sons and daughters of fathers with SCI scored within normal limits on MMPI and 16PF measures of personality and adjustment. Sex of child and SCI in fathers interacted on only three traits on the 16PF and none on the MMPI. Sons were more tough-minded, self-reliant, and realistic than were daughters of fathers with SCI (Factor I). Sons also scored as more conventional and practical in outlook than daughters of fathers with SCI (Factor M). In contrast, daughters of fathers without SCI were slightly more tough-minded as well as unconventional in outlook than were sons. Adult sons of fathers with SCI felt slightly less self-assured than daughters did, whereas the opposite pattern occurred in comparison children (Factor O). However, mean scores of the groups were in the normal range on these measures.

Physical health patterns were similar for sons and daughters of fathers with and without SCI with one exception. An interaction emerged on number of psychosomatic symptoms, but it was due to the deviant number of problems reported by comparison daughters. SCI in fathers did not affect participation in athletics of sons more than daughters.

Most aspects of friendship and dating patterns of children of fathers with and without SCI were similar regardless of gender. Only one significant finding emerged. Although seldom occurring and not necessarily negative, sons of fathers with SCI felt that dates tended to treat them differently after meeting their father more often than did daughters, while the reverse was reported by comparison children.

Regardless of their children's gender, fathers with SCI were similar in parenting styles, as defined by Loving versus Rejecting, Permissive versus Restrictive, and Attention factors on the Roe Parent–Child Relations Questionnaire (Roe & Siegelman, 1963). Some attitudinal differences among children were found as a function of gender. Daughters of fathers with SCI felt more self-conscious about their fathers in public than sons did, but comparison sons were more self-conscious than comparison daughters. Sons of fathers with SCI were more likely to blame fathers when upset by an event than daughters were. Daughters were more likely than sons to blame their fathers in a similar situation when the father did not have a disability.

Severity of Disability

It often has been presumed that the more incapacitating the father's disability, the more difficult it is to fulfill the parental role and the more disruptive the effects on children. To date, only preliminary data are available on this question (Buck & Hohmann, 1982), and conclusions are limited by the small sample size. Severity of disability was examined by comparing a matched sample of adult children raised by fathers with paraplegia and quadriplegia on objective measures of adjustment, personality, health status, interpersonal relationships, and parent–child relations. Overall, increasing severity of paternal disability was not associated with more problems in parenting ability or children's well-being. Only six significant findings emerged on more than 165 measures, and these seemed to be due more to specific physical limitations of quadriplegia than to psychological effects of paternal disability.

Psychological adjustment and personality styles of children were similar irrespective of severity of the father's disability. Children of fathers with quadriplegia and paraplegia were satisfied with their body appearance and functioning. Their sex-role orientations were appropriately sex-typed or androgynous. Although not significant, there was a trend for children of fathers with paraplegia to place higher value on "loving," whereas children of fathers with quadriplegia tended to view "independent" as more important to them. Athletic and recreational activities were comparable among children of fathers with quadriplegia and paraplegia.

Measures of children's physical health showed no relationship with severity of paternal disability. No differences were found in number of medical visits, frequency of physical symptoms, or how well they took care of themselves preventively.

No evidence was found to support the often speculated negative consequence to children of "being pitied, ridiculed, and ostracized by peers" because of a parent's disability, even when severe. Children of fathers with paraplegia and quadriplegia did not differ in their social relationships or in their comfort in social situations. The study found that, compared to children of fathers with paraplegia, those of fathers with quadriplegia felt their friends tended to respond differently, although not negatively, to them after meeting the father. Children of fathers with quadriplegia valued emotional sensitivity and persistence in accomplishing goals in their friends more highly than did children of fathers with paraplegia. It seems that children learned to value traits they observed in their fathers, since individuals with quadriplegia likely exert more effort to succeed on tasks, and there was a trend for them to be more loving than fathers with paraplegia.

Severity of disability affected some aspects of parenting behaviors. Fathers with quadriplegia were described as more permissive in child rearing practices than fathers with paraplegia, as measured by the Roe Parent–Child Relations Questionnaire (Roe & Siegelman, 1963). Although not significant, children tended to view fathers with quadriplegia as more loving than fathers with paraplegia. However, measures of parental discipline, decision-making, involvement in family activities, and attitudes showed few differences as a function of the severity of the father's disability. Not surprising, given neurologic limitations, was the finding that fathers with paraplegia used spanking to discipline children more often than did fathers with quadriplegia.

Employment of Fathers with Disabilities

A major role ascribed to fathers has been that of family provider and breadwinner. Given the high incidence of unemployment among individuals with disabilities, the presumed "role reversal" of being unemployed and at home often has been cited to explain the negative influence of paternal disability on children. In the only study testing this assumption, results did not confirm this presumption (Buck & Hohmann, 1984).

Adult children of unemployed fathers with SCI ($n = 22$) were compared to children whose fathers with SCI were employed full or part time during the children's formative years ($n = 23$). Although not significant, employed fathers, their wives, and children were on the average 2 years older than their cohorts. The 2-year age difference probably accounts for the finding that children of employed fathers had completed 2 more years of education, since 40% in each group were still students. Employed fathers also were more educated than unemployed fathers. Other than these demographic differences, only six significant findings emerged between children of employed and unemployed fathers with SCI.

Unemployment in fathers with SCI was not shown to have undesirable consequences for children, as speculated, because it "creates role ambiguity and role reversal" in the family structure. Children's scores on the MMPI and 16PF, Body-Cathexis scale, and sex-role inventory indicated satisfactory psychological adjustment, body image, and sex role typing. Two significant differences were found on the 16PF where children with employed fathers scored as brighter and as more self-controlled than children of unemployed fathers. However, these results could be due as much to the age and education advantage of the children with employed fathers as to the father's employment status per se. Value systems of the two groups of children were similar, with only one difference found among 36 values measured. Children placed higher value on "ambitious" when the father worked, perhaps due to modeling of employed fathers' behavior.

Neither physical health patterns nor recreational and athletic activity levels were related to employment of fathers with SCI. Employment of fathers also had little impact on children's interpersonal relationships, despite predictions in the literature that social stigmatization is worsened by fathers not fulfilling traditional male role functions. Only one difference emerged, in which children of employed SCI fathers valued emotional sensitivity in their close friends more than did children with unemployed fathers.

Of particular interest in this study was that data did not support theoretically driven hypotheses that unemployment and disability cause damage to the power structure of the family (Anthony, 1970). Both groups of fathers were active in child-rearing, as assessed by measures of discipline patterns, decision-making, and participation in social, educational, and recreational activities of the mothers and fathers. Only one statistically significant finding emerged across 50 measures of parent–child relations, and it is paradoxical and difficult to explain. Children perceived that fathers who were employed spent more time at home than unemployed fathers.

Financial Resources of Fathers with Disabilities

Another moderating variable thought to affect the parental role of fathers with disabilities is the lack of stable, adequate financial resources, due to low income and high costs of medical care, special transportation, accessible housing, and personal attendant care. However, results of the study by Buck and Hohmann (1984) were notable again for the absence of significant findings, although financial security had more impact than did severity of disability and employment status of fathers with disabilities.

The role of financial resources was tested by comparing children who were raised by service-connected fathers with SCI (high, stable income) with those reared by nonservice-connected fathers (low, less secure income). The annual income of service-connected fathers was nearly double that of nonservice connected fathers and was payable for life. The two groups differed on several demographic variables, a methodological limitation affecting the comparability of groups. Fewer children (8.3%) in financially secure families were married compared with those in low-income families (57.9%), although the latter group was about 1 year older. Fathers with SCI with higher incomes were better educated; 45.8% had college educations compared with only 5.3% of low-income fathers. Mothers in the high-income group also had more education. More service-connected fathers were employed. Although the financial upheaval of a new disability may pose stress on families, the long-term adjustment patterns of children were not adversely affected by marginal incomes of fathers with SCI. As adults, children with both high- and low-income fathers were well-adjusted and showed appropriate sex-role identities and body images. Some differences emerged among children as a function of the father's financial security, but scores were within the normal range of variation. With this caveat in mind, there appeared to be some advantages for children of higher family income in the areas of intellectual development, values, family recreation and social interests, and physical health patterns.

Children of high-income fathers with SCI were brighter intellectually and more worldly and sophisticated than children of low-income fathers, as measured on the 16PF. Children in financially secure families also placed more importance on the values "self-respect," "true friendship," and "intellectual" than children in low-income families. These findings may reflect greater exposure to educational, social, and cultural pursuits afforded by ample income and fostered by better educated parents. Indeed, it was found that both mothers and fathers in the financially secure group participated more in these kinds of activities with their children than low-income parents.

Although psychological well-being was not affected by financial security, two of nine measures of physical health patterns showed significant differences. Children of high-income fathers reported more somatic complaints than the low-income group. However, they also reported taking better care of their health through preventive measures, such as not smoking, maintaining physical fitness, eating a balanced diet, and being within normal weight limits.

Most indices of parenting by fathers with SCI were not related to financial status. Both high- and low-income fathers with SCI scored similarly on dimensions of parent behavior (Loving-Rejecting, Casual-Demanding, and Attention). Only four specific indices of parent behavior and children's attitudes toward parents were significantly associated with financial security. Contributing financially to the household was related to discipline roles assumed by fathers with SCI. Fathers with high incomes were more often the primary disciplinarians in the family (fathers = 54.2%, mothers = 25%, both = 20.8%), whereas mothers assumed this role more often in less financially secure families (fathers = 15.8%, mothers = 47.4%, both = 36.8%). However, this pattern did not emerge with respect to who made family decisions. It also was found that high-income fathers and mothers were more active with children in cultural and recreation activities than low-income parents. Interestingly, children felt more protective of their mothers, but not fathers, in low-income than in high-income families.

In sum, financial resources had more impact for the family than either employment or severity of disability in fathers. But, low income in the context of paternal disability did not pose problems per se, since psychosocial adjustment, physical health, interpersonal relations, and measures of parent–child relations were within normal limits. Rather, there appear to be some advantages that stem from having adequate and secure financial resources, which apply to the general population as well (Coates et al., 1985).

Parenting Styles of Fathers with Disabilities

Considerable research in the general population has pointed to two basic dimensions of parental behavior and attitudes that are related to many areas of children's adjustment. One critical determinant of development is the degree to which parents are loving or rejecting, with loving defined by behaviors that are accepting, approving, affectionate, helpful, understanding, child-centered, and warm. A second factor identifies restrictive versus permissive discipline style, in which a restrictive parent sets many rules and regulations, is strict in enforcing them, demands unquestioning respect, and uses power-assertive discipline. In the literature on paternal disability, scant attention has been paid to the mediating role of parenting

style. Rather, the presence of disability has commanded more attention than the father's behavior.

In light of this apparent neglect to consider parenting behavior
by the father, not just disability, Buck (1980) examined the importance of paternal behavior versus disability for children's adjustment. Using the Roe Parent–Child Relations Questionnaire (Roe &
Siegelman, 1963), matched groups of 45 fathers with SCI and 36
fathers without SCI were classified as Loving or Rejecting and Casual or Demanding. Children's personality and behavior were examined as a function of both paternal disability and paternal behavior.

Children's long-term adjustment was related more to the father's parenting behaviors than to whether he had a disability. Over
twice as many variables were associated with the parenting behaviors of fathers (34) as with his disability status (15). Consistent with
research on child development, children of loving fathers scored as
more well-adjusted than children of rejecting fathers. Fewer variables, as expected from prior studies, were related to casual versus
demanding behavior of fathers. Parenting style and disability status
of the father interacted on 10 measures of children's personality and
behavior. Areas of children's adjustment in which the father's disability status interacted with parenting behavior are the primary
focus of this review.

While Loving-Rejecting behavior of fathers in general showed
significant relationships with children's adjustment, as measured
on the MMPI (F, Hypochondriasis, Psychopathic Deviate Scales), no
interactions with paternal disability emerged. However, children of
loving and rejecting fathers differed on two 16PF personality traits,
depending on the father's disability status. Children whose fathers
with SCI were loving tended to be more sensitive, intuitive, and
tender-minded than those with rejecting fathers. In contrast, children with loving fathers scored as more tough-minded than those
with rejecting fathers when the father was without SCI. Children of
fathers with SCI scored as more worldly, shrewd, and socially astute
when the father was loving, whereas children of comparison fathers
were more naive and unpretentious when the father was loving. No
significant interactions emerged in sex roles, body image, physical
health patterns, recreation, social relationships, or parent–child
relations.

Casual versus demanding paternal behavior showed fewer relationships with children's adjustment than did Loving-Rejecting behavior. On the MMPI and 16PF, no main effects were found, and
only one interaction was significant. Children of fathers with SCI
who were permissive scored higher on the Hypochondriasis scale

than children of fathers with SCI who were restrictive, with the reverse pattern found in children of comparison fathers. A similar pattern also was found on a measure of frequency of psychosomatic symptoms experienced per month. Thus, it appears that children feel less free to acknowledge physical complaints when the father has a disability and is perceived to be restrictive than when he does not have a disability.

While children of fathers with SCI generally participated more in athletic activities than comparison children, no interactions with parental behavior were found. Choice of activities, however, was associated with parental behavior. Children of fathers both with and without SCI who were loving engaged in more non-dangerous activities than when the father was rejecting.

Interpersonal relationships revealed no differences as a function of SCI in the father, but five measures were related to Loving versus Rejecting and Casual versus Demanding behavior of fathers. Paternal disability and behavior interacted on one item. Children of both loving and rejecting fathers with SCI did not differ in the extent to which they valued similar morals and religious beliefs in their peers, but comparison children placed more importance on similar morals when the father was loving versus rejecting.

Contrary to the disability literature, but consistent with research in the general population, fathers' behavior has more impact than disability on relationships between parent and child. Eleven measures of parent–child relationships were associated with SCI in fathers, many of which were positive, as discussed earlier. In contrast, 23 were related to paternal behavior. A few areas showed interactions between SCI in fathers and parenting behavior.

Children of fathers without disabilities attributed more problems to their mother's influence when the father was rejecting than when he was loving. But, when the father had a SCI, children were no more likely to blame their mother when upset if the father was rejecting versus loving. Casual versus demanding paternal behavior interacted with disability status of the father in three areas of parent–child relationships. Mothers used spanking more often when the father with SCI was permissive than when he was restrictive. In contrast, mothers spanked less often when the comparison father was permissive than restrictive. One wonders if the mothers with husbands with SCI attribute the father's permissiveness more to his disability than to his preferred parenting style and thus felt they had to compensate. Without the salience of a disability, mothers were more comfortable being consistent with the father's approach. The finding that mothers with husbands with SCI in general used spanking more than comparison mothers supports this hypothesis. Second, while fathers with SCI expressed affection verbally more often than comparison fathers, an interaction also emerged. Fathers with SCI expressed affection verbally even more often when permissive in child-rearing style, compared to fathers without SCI who were more affectionate verbally when they were demanding. Third, children of permissive fathers with SCI reported feeling less self-conscious about their mothers in public than when the father was demanding. The reverse held true for children of fathers without SCI. Again, one wonders about the salience of disability in affecting children's attributions. In the general population, being restrictive is consistent with the traditional male role model and thus may not be perceived as "different." However, greater concern about the perceptions of others is felt when the father has both a disability and is viewed to be "demanding."

CONCLUSIONS AND IMPLICATIONS

Two main conclusions are apparent from this review. First, there is a dearth of empirically based information about disability in fathers. Much of what is known comes primarily from studies by Buck and Hohmann. While a beginning, this research has methodological limitations. All the sample fathers were veterans, most results were based on self-reports, and only long-term outcomes of children raised by fathers with SCI were examined. Second, what objective information does exist fails to support the beliefs and expectations often espoused by professionals that disability interferes with effective parenting by fathers. Studies using comparison groups and objective measures of children's adjustment fail to document deleterious effects on children as a result of being raised by a father with a disability (Buck, 1980; Buck & Hohmann, 1981; Olgas, 1974).

Implications for Research

Clearly, much research is needed to understand the process and outcome of parenthood among persons with disabilities. Areas for future research and suggested methodological strategies have been identified previously (Buck, 1980; Buck & Hohmann, 1983; Coates et al., 1985; Greer, 1985; Thurman et al., 1985). Those specific recommendations remain valid. The following discussion focuses on a general rationale for research.

Parenting by fathers with disabilities can best be understood within the general context of parent–child relations, rather than in isolation. Until the 1970s, little attention was paid to the father's role. He was the forgotten contributor, whose role primarily was breadwinner, recreation leader, and, occasionally, disciplinarian (Biller, 1971; Hamilton, 1977; Lamb, 1975). Accumulating research has documented the importance of the father in parenting. Competence, achievement motivation, self-esteem, success, internal locus of control, and creativity have been related to behavioral patterns of the father (Buck, 1980; Hamilton, 1977). Adjustment and behavior disorders are associated with absence of the father from the home and with inadequate parenting. It is imperative that investigations of the impact of disability on parenting and child development be considered in light of what is known generally about father–child relationships.

Many factors other than paternal disability per se affect children's adjustment and parenting ability by fathers. Future research would benefit from a less simplistic approach of examining one variable—paternal disability—and only circumscribed outcomes for children. A theoretical model is needed to provide a meaningful and coherent rationale that: 1) identifies the environmental, parental, and child variables affecting both the process and outcome of parenting by persons with disabilities; and 2) specifies important independent, dependent, and moderating variables. Theoretically, the father's role, along with that of the mother, is to provide the means and opportunities by which children achieve health and well-being, progress developmentally, and learn the skills to assume a meaningful place in society as adults. A cohesive model that delineates clearly and comprehensively the factors defining and influencing health and the criteria for achievement of well-being within the context of disability has been developed by Trieschmann (1987, 1988). With expansion, this model has far-reaching implications for understanding and defining health and adjustment in general. The Biological-Psychosocial-Environmental Model can provide the rationale and methodological factors needed to investigate the process and outcome of parenting by persons with disabilities.

In this model, health is a dynamic, ever-changing balance of biologic-organic, psychosocial, and environmental influences that enable a person to achieve well-being in "survival" (self-care) activities, relationships, and productivity (Trieschmann, 1987, 1988). Biologic factors are bodily and mental functions determined by genetic, congenital, environmental, and behavioral lifestyle factors that vary with age, disease status, and general physical status. Biologic factors include age, developmental status, sex, integrity of the body systems, nutritional status, strength, coordination, intelligence, and learning ability. Psychosocial factors are the characteristics generally called personality, which include stylistic ways of perceiving oneself and the world, behavioral tendencies and skills, and emotional patterns. Examples include cognitive styles, emotional responsiveness, behavior, self-image, independence, judgment, social skills, coping styles, values, gender role, cultural group, education, and work history. Environmental factors are those variables external to the person that affect the course of adaptation. Examples are social support system; socioeconomic status; access to and payment for health care resources; housing; transportation; educational, vocational, and recreational resources; geographical and environmental barriers; environmental diversity; and rural or urban residence.

A healthy biologic-psychosocial-environmental balance enables one to achieve well-being, defined by three general criteria: 1) performance of self-care and survival behaviors, such as avoidance of medical and psychosocial problems, activities of daily living, eating a nutritionally balanced diet, and using mobility, language, and perceptual-motor skills; 2) harmonious living and working relationships—those behaviors that contribute to a stable environment for living, working, and interacting in a meaningful way with others, including peers, colleagues, health-care providers, authorities, and to the ability to manage personal affairs; and 3) productivity, or activities that contribute to a sense of usefulness, satisfaction, and worth, such as employment, educational pursuits, family roles, community service, and avocations.

Treischmann's model of health (1988) provides a heuristic foundation for identifying essential factors in the family system, parent, child, and environment to consider in future investigations of physical disability in parenting. It specifies biologic, psychosocial, and environmental variables defining health and the criteria of well-being in parents and children. In addition, Table 1 summarizes other important variables to consider in designing research on the role of disability in a father.

Implications for Persons with Disabilities

Individuals who plan to or have families often express concerns about the impact of their disability on their children. Education and counseling must be based on empirical data about parental disability and knowledge of parent–child relations in general. Information should be provided sensitively, factually, and in a manner that does not promulgate unfounded negative opinions. Attention needs to be given to the individual concerns, problems, and strengths of a family, with the view of reinforcing family strengths and teaching constructive problem-solving and coping skills to manage problem

Table 1. Research on parental disability: Variables of importance

Cultural variables	Family variables
Race/ethnicity	Socioeconomic status
Rural/urban residence	Parent education
Religious context	Family size, structure
Social support network	Parent absence from home
Environmental diversity/opportunities	Divorce/stepparents
	Extended family support
Parent variables	**Child variables**
Sex of parent with disability	Age when parent disabled
Type of disability	Child sex
Effects of disability on abilities	Birth order
Acquired, genetic, or congenital disability	Developmental status
Severity of disability	Biologic and temperamental factors
Static versus progressive disability	Psychosocial variables
Chronicity of disability	
Onset (sudden or gradual)	
Brain-related cognitive/emotional deficits	
Time since onset (physical and psychosocial adjustment)	
Treatment status (hospitalized, frequency of medical problems)	
Social stigma of disability	
Parents' accommodations and style of coping with disability	
Child-rearing behaviors and values of parents	
Decision-making, discipline, and communication patterns	
Parents' biologic–psychosocial–environmental health status	

areas. Within these general guidelines, several specific recommendations are offered.

With the onset of a disability, counseling and education of families may have the following goals: 1) Ease the emotional distress that the disability and hospitalization of the parent may elicit by supportive counseling of both parents and children. 2) Assist parents and children to develop realistic expectations and understandings about the parent's abilities and limitations in general, as well as specific parenting and family issues. 3) Attend particularly to the mother, as many children in Buck's study (1980) noted difficulty not so much with their father's disability as with their mother's reactions. Data also suggested that mothers may attempt to compensate for what they misperceive to be problem areas. 4) Support the role of the father with a disability in decision-making and family functioning from the outset. Even during the initial hospitalization, avoid isolating him from the family because of beliefs that "it is too much stress for the newly injured" and that "being in the hospital is not good for children." The well-being of mothers, children, and fathers with disabilities benefits from including the father in usual family functions to the extent possible. Altering the mutuality of relationships and stripping the father of his role are helpful to no one. 5) Educate the father and mother on what are known to be the important factors in parenting. Effective communication and parenting skills can be learned. Focusing on the disability, which cannot be changed, only serves to promote undue guilt, anxiety, and attempts to compensate for a condition that cannot be changed. 6) Caution parents against inadvertently and inappropriately attributing difficulties to the disability. Buck (1980) found that families misattributed some perceived losses (e.g., "Dad couldn't engage in physical activities with me") and presumed differences (e.g., discipline style) to the disability, although fathers with SCI were behaving no differently than other fathers. When these mistaken beliefs and concerns are reinforced, there is the danger of developing a self-fulfilling prophecy that paternal disability is destructive to family life and engenders many losses. 7) When the disability does pose a barrier, urge parents to confront the issue directly, sensitively, and realistically rather than to avoid or compensate for the problem in other areas. For example, parents can acknowledge, "Yes, Dad is different because he is in a wheelchair. People may be uncomfortable and make fun of anything or anyone different. How can we help your friends learn being different is OK and feel comfortable with Dad? How can you respond to your friends' stereotypes?" 8) Professionals and parents alike need to remember that obstacles and stresses, even when they are traumatic and unpleasant, may not necessarily be harmful to the psychological well-being of children, but rather can serve as an impetus for personal growth, feelings of competence and mastery, and greater understanding. The job of parenting is not to enable children to avoid facing life's misfortunes when they occur, but to help them to learn the skills to confront them honestly, realistically, and gracefully.

On a personal note, many parents with disabilities and professionals across the country have spoken to me over the past 12 years since publishing the Buck (1980) study. The most gratifying aspect of having conducted this study has been the ability to allay the concerns of these parents with disabilities about their ability to parent effectively and to offer reassurance that they can succeed in one of life's most challenging yet rewarding goals—parenthood. Many of these parents have contacted me again as their children have grown up. They have expressed appreciation of having their fears reduced by objective data at a vulnerable point in their lives. They were proud of themselves and their children for their accomplishments, and their lives were more complete and meaningful for having pursued parenthood. With the many losses that disability entails, it is important that we professionals do not add to that list unnecessarily by undermining individuals' roles as parents.

In closing, given the often-found negativity among professionals, and the concerns of fathers with disabilities and their partners themselves, one young woman in Buck's study (1980) has a powerful message for us all:

> I feel I have learned a lot about myself, my family, and being prepared. I feel I am more capable of facing anything that may come up than my friends. I have benefitted greatly from watching and participating in the survival of a family where life depended on strength and courage. I have learned how to take care of myself and others. I know many secrets to the art of living as well as surviving in the face of many tragedies and disappointments. I have learned the tricks to success—not just survival— through my father and his series of trial and error. (p. 59)

REFERENCES

Anthony, E. (1970). The mutative impact of serious mental and physical illness in a parent on family life. In E. Anthony & C. Koupernik (Eds.), *The child in his family* (Vol. 1, pp. 131–136). New York: John Wiley & Sons.

Arnaud, S. (1959). Some psychological characteristics of children of multiple sclerotics. *Psychosomatic Medicine, 21,* 8–22.

Bem, S. (1974). The measurement of psychological androgyny. *Journal of Consulting and Clinical Psychology, 42,* 155–162.

Bem, S. (1977). On the utility of alternative procedures for assessing psychological androgyny. *Journal of Consulting and Clinical Psychology, 45,* 196–205.

Bene, A. (1977). The influence of deaf and dumb parents on a child's development. *Psychoanalytic Study of the Child, 32,* 175–194.

Biller, H. (1971). *Father, child, and sex role: Paternal determinants of personality development.* Lexington, MA: Lexington Books.

Bishop, D., & Epstein, N. (1980). Family problems and disability. In D. Bishop (Ed.), *Behavioral problems and the disabled* (pp. 337–363). Baltimore: Williams & Wilkins.

Bray, G. (1970). Rehabilitation of spinal cord injured: A family approach. *Journal of Applied Rehabilitation Counseling, 9,* 70–78.

Bruhn, J. (1977). Effects of chronic illness on the family. *Journal of Family Practice, 4,* 1057–1060.

Buck, F. (1980). *The influence of parental disability on children: An exploratory investigation of the adult children of spinal cord injured fathers.* Unpublished doctoral dissertation, University of Arizona, Tucson.

Buck, F., & Hohmann, G. (1981). Personality, behavior, values, and family relations of children of fathers with spinal cord injury. *Archives of Physical Medicine and Rehabilitation, 62,* 432–438.

Buck, F., & Hohmann, G. (1982). Child adjustment as related to severity of paternal disability. *Archives of Physical Medicine and Rehabilitation, 63,* 249–253.

Buck, F., & Hohmann, G. (1983). Parental disability and children's adjustment. In E. Pan, T. Backer, & C. Vash (Eds.), *Annual review of rehabilitation* (Vol. 3, pp. 203–241). New York: Springer-Verlag.

Buck, F., & Hohmann, G. (1984). Child adjustment as related to financial security and employment status of fathers with spinal cord injuries. *Archives of Physical Medicine and Rehabilitation, 65,* 327–333.

Burnett, M. (1973). Social work note: "On disabling the normal." *British Journal of Social Work, 3,* 504–507.

Cattell, R., Eber, H., & Tatsuoka, M. (1970). *Handbook for the Sixteen Personality Factor Questionnaire.* Champaign, IL: Institute for Personality and Ability Testing.

Christopherson, V. (1968). Role modifications of the disabled male. *American Journal of Nursing, 68,* 290–293.

Coates, D., Vietze, P., & Gray, D. (1985). Methodological issues in studying children of disabled parents. In S.K. Thurman (Ed.), *Children of handicapped parents: Research and clinical perspectives* (pp. 155– 180). Orlando: Academic Press.

Dahlstrom, W., Welsch, G., & Dahlstrom, L. (1972). *An MMPI handbook. Volume I: Clinical interpretation.* Minneapolis: University of Minnesota Press.

DiCaprio, N. (1971). Factors affecting the child's evaluation of the visually handicapped parent. *New Outlook for the Blind, 65,* 181–186.

Gibson, G., & Ludwig, E. (1968). Family structure in a disabled population. *Journal of Marriage and Family Living, 30,* 54–63.

Gilhool, T., & Gran, J. (1985). Legal rights of disabled parents. In S.K. Thurman (Ed.), *Children of handicapped parents: Research and clinical perspectives* (pp. 11–34). Orlando: Academic Press.

Glass, D. (1985). Onset of disability in a parent: Impact on child and family. In S.K. Thurman (Ed.), *Children of handicapped parents: Research and clinical perspectives* (pp. 145–154). Orlando: Academic Press.

Greer, G. (1985). Children of physically disabled parents: Some thoughts, facts, and hypotheses. In S.K. Thurman (Ed.), *Children of handicapped parents: Research and clinical perspectives* (pp. 131–144). Orlando: Academic Press.

Hamilton, M. (1977). *Father's influence on children.* Chicago: Nelson-Hall.

Hanna, D., & Edwards, P. (1988). Physically disabled parents and their normal children: Assessment, diagnosis, and intervention. *Holistic Nursing Practice, 2,* 38–47.

Heslinga, K., Schellen, A., & Verkuyl, A. (1974). *Not made of stone: The sexual problems of handicapped people.* Springfield, IL: Charles C Thomas.

Hilbourne, J. (1973). On disabling the normal: The implications of physical disability for other people. *British Journal of Social Work, 3,* 497–504.

Kennedy, K., & Bush, D. (1979). Counseling the children of handicapped parents. *Personnel and Guidance Journal, 58,* 267–270.

Kopala, B., & Egenes, K. (1984). The physically disabled parent: Assessment and intervention. *Topics in Clinical Nursing, 6,* 10–18.

Kossoris, P. (1970). Family therapy. *American Journal of Nursing, 70,* 1730–1733.

Lamb, M. (1975). Fathers: Forgotten contributors to child development. *Human Development, 18,* 245–266.

Nordquist, I. (1972). *Life together—The situation of the handicapped.* Stockholm: E. Olofssons Boktryckeri.

Olgas, M. (1974). The relationship between parents' health status and body image of their children. *Nursing Research, 23,* 169–174.

Olsen, E. (1970). The impact of serious illness on the family system. *Postgraduate Medicine, 47,* 169–174.

Power, P. (1980). The adolescent's reaction to chronic illness of a parent: Some implications for family counseling. *International Journal of Family Counseling, 5,* 70–78.

Roe, A., & Siegelman, M. (1963). A Parent–Child Relations Questionnaire. *Child Development, 34,* 355–369.

Rokeach, M. (1973). *The nature of human values.* New York: Free Press.

Romano, M. (1976). Preparing children for parental disability. *Social Work in Health Care, 1,* 309–315.

Romano, M. (1984). The impact of disability on family and society. In J.V. Basmajian (Ed.), *Foundations of medical rehabilitation* (pp. 273–276). Baltimore: Williams & Wilkins.

Secord, P., & Jourard, S. (1953). The appraisal of body-cathexis: Body-cathexis and the self. *Journal of Consulting Psychology, 17,* 343–347.

Strasberg, P. (1991). Clinical notes. *SCI Psychosocial Process, 4,* 22–24.

Thomason, B., & Clifford, K. (1972). The disabled person and family dynamics. *Accent on Living, 17,* 20–35.

Thurman, S.K. (Ed.). (1985). *Children of handicapped parents: Research and clinical perspectives.* Orlando: Academic Press.

Thurman, S., Whaley, A., & Weinraub, M. (1985). Studying families with handicapped parents: A rationale. In S.K. Thurman (Ed.), *Children of handicapped parents: Research and clinical perspectives* (pp. 1–10). Orlando: Academic Press.

Trieschmann, R. (1987). *Aging with a disability.* New York: Demos Publications.

Trieschmann, R. (1988). *Spinal cord injures: Psychological, social, and vocational rehabilitation* (2nd ed.). New York: Demos Publications.

16

Orgasmology
Relevance for Persons with Physical Disabilities

John Money

There are three phases of sexuality and eroticism. In reverse order they are: conception and pregnancy, acception and copulation, and proception and foreplay. They are listed in reverse order because, historically, this is the order in which they have become medically and scientifically respectable. The title *Reproductive Issues for Persons with Physical Disabilities* is itself an indication of how skittish the medical/scientific establishment is regarding a book that should address not only reproduction, but also copulation and erotic imagery. Professional avoidance of the phase of mutual acception and copulation is contingent on the fact that orgasm and its difficulties are still only barely a topic for polite medical and scientific discourse. Similarly, professional avoidance of the phase of proception and foreplay is contingent on the fact that both involve the imagery and ideation of sexuoerotic arousal, whether in dreaming, daydreaming, fantasizing, or actual practice. Erotic imagery and ideation are still stigmatized as being in the realm of pornography. Insofar as pornography is characterized as illicit and possibly criminal, it is rendered off-limits to science and medicine.

CIRCUMVENTING SOLIPSISM

We all work on the assumption that the experience of orgasm in others, if they have it, is similar to our own. We use the rule-of-thumb test that no matter how they name it, those who are not sure if they've had an orgasm almost certainly have not had one. We generally assume that, sooner or later, they will share our capacity. Nonetheless, we do not know whether there may be degrees of "orgasm blindness" (orgasm agnosia) analogous to degrees of color blindness.

One strategy for circumventing the dilemma of solipsism is to rely on information transmitted not as spoken or written language, but as instrumentally recorded physiologic changes in the person having an orgasm. It is a little known fact of history that John B. Watson, the Johns Hopkins professor of psychobiology world famous as the originator in 1913 of the theory of behaviorism, was also in 1919 the originator of the instrumental method of recording the physiology of orgasm (Magoun, 1981; Pauly, 1979). In the aftermath of litigation, his data were forever lost, and only a box containing the apparatus survived to bear mute witness.

Watson's orgasm research soon became no more than an unverified rumor. It was probably unknown to Alfred Kinsey when, in the late 1930s, he began his career in sex research. Thus, Kinsey began anew the accumulation of data on the bodily accompaniments of orgasm. Kinsey's data were derived from either the analysis of explicit films, or the direct observation of volunteer couples. Information on the anatomy and physiology of sexual response and orgasm is presented in *Sexual Behavior in the Human Female* (Kinsey, Pomeroy, Martin, & Gebhard, 1953).

Kinsey died in 1956 before having to confront the political and funding hazards of equipping a laboratory for orgasm research. That task fell to Masters and Johnson. The first major report of their work is well known as *Human Sexual Response* (1966). This book is important not only for its contents, but also because it was not censored. It reports the direct observation and recording of human sexual response and orgasm not only in individuals, but also in copulating couples.

ANIMAL MODELS

There are vogues in sex research. Victimology is presently in vogue, and words heard everywhere are "exploitation," "perpetrator," "sexual abuse," "survivor," and "victim." Being a sex therapist, educator, or researcher is no guarantee of invulnerability to false charges of abuse. The present, therefore, is a time when an animal model is a necessity for explicit orgasm research. The obstacle is, of course, that animals cannot talk to us and tell us whether they have an orgasm or not. We must rely on trying to decipher body language in synchrony with physiologic changes that are instrumentally recorded. Then we must make an inference as to whether something happened that may legitimately be called orgasm.

This dual method has, to the best of my knowledge, allowed the existence of female orgasm to be attributed unequivocally to only one subhuman species, namely, the stumptailed macaque monkey (Goldfoot, Westerborg-van Loon, Groeneveld, & Slob, 1980; Slob, Groeneveld, & Van der Werff Ten Bosch, 1986). The two animals in the initial photographic record are females. One is in the receptive role typical of the female, the other in the mounting role, typical of the male. In each, the body language of orgasm corresponds respectively to that observed in a female/male pairing. Thus, one may infer that both females are having an orgasm. The animal in the male role has no penis and no ejaculate but otherwise exhibits the body language of orgasm as if a male. Thus it is obvious that, as in human beings, orgasm in stumptailed monkeys is not contingent on ejaculation of semen.

One of the bonuses of the study of orgasm in subhuman primates is the possibility of scheduling statistically controlled experiments of an invasive type that in human beings are ethically forbidden. For example, surgical deconnection of the brain from the innervation of the pelvic genitalia may be experimentally scheduled in animals, whereas the human alternative is the unscheduled clinical experiment of spinal cord deconnection by disease, wound, or accident.

DECONNECTION OF BRAIN AND
PELVIC GENITALIA AND RELATION TO ORGASM

The 33 vertebrae of the spinal cord are numbered from the neck in five levels: cervical, 1–7; thoracic, 8–19; lumbar, 20–24; sacral, 25–29; and coccygeal, 30–33. In the case of a broken neck, severance of the spinal cord is at the cervical level. Insofar as innervation of all four limbs is completely deconnected from the brain, the condition is named quadriplegia. If severance is below the cervical level so that innervation of the arms and hands is spared, but that of the lower torso is deconnected from the brain, then the condition is paraplegia.

If the deconnection of the brain from the spinal cord is at or above the thoracic level, T11, then all of the neural reflex feedback loops between the pelvic genitalia and the spinal cord below T11 remain intact. These reflex loops are prerequisite to the release of ejaculation in the male (Szasz & Carpenter, 1989). In such cases, ejaculation may be induced by applying a vibrator to the penis or via the rectum to the region of the prostate gland. In this way it is possible to collect semen, if noncoital insemination of the spouse is needed to ensure pregnancy.

A definition of orgasm that accommodates all foregoing considerations is as follows:

> *Orgasm:* the zenith of sexuoerotic experience that men and women characterize subjectively as voluptuous rapture or ecstasy. It occurs simultaneously in the brain/mind and the pelvic genitalia. Irrespective of the locus of onset, the occurrence of orgasm is contingent upon reciprocal intercommunication between neural networks in the brain, above, and the pelvic genitalia, below. Phenomenologically it fails to survive mutual deconnection of the brain and the pelvic genitalia by severance of the spinal cord. However, it is able to survive even extensive trauma at either location.

Electroejaculation is not referred to as orgasm, for the man has not had the cognitional experience of orgasm. Nor has he had the cognitional experience of ejaculation, unless he was able to look and see what was happening, or to palpate his genitalia with his fingers and know what was happening through the sense of touch. If the spinal cord deconnection is below T11, erection may be retained in response to vibration, independently of ejaculation. Here again, cognition of the erection is only by sight or touch.

The paraplegic female experience of orgasm is similar to that of the paraplegic male, except that there is less visual evidence to be seen and less tactual evidence to be touched. Pregnancy is possible for the paraplegic woman without any experience that corresponds to ejaculation or orgasm. One young paraplegic woman characterized her genital region in its entirety as "numb." She couldn't be bothered with going through the motions of sexual intercourse, she said, even for the sake of her lover. Her vernacular term for coital reciprocity was "corresponding." Being numb, she had lost the capacity to correspond. She was sure, therefore, that no matter what her boyfriend said to the contrary, there would be nothing in it for him (Money, 1960).

Not all paraplegic men and women lose interest in sex. With practice and experience, some achieve an intensification of erotic sensuousness in the nipples and the upper part of the body, the neural innervation of which is not deconnected from the brain. They do not, however, have the experience of orgasm as they did when the spinal cord was intact. If they do experience an orgasm-like build-up of voluptuous rapture, it is not cognized as happening in the genital region.

PHANTOM ORGASM

In paraplegia, it is only while dreaming during sleep that the experience of orgasm as it was prior to the spinal cord injury may be again experienced (Money, 1960). This dream orgasm is properly characterized as a phantom orgasm, for it occurs only in the imagery and ideation of the dream, deconnected from the pelvic genitalia.

The phantom orgasm of the dream is not reported by all paraplegics. Among those who have reported the experience, its occurrence is infrequent until progressively it disappears within a maximum of 2 years after the spinal cord injury. Sexologically, it can be concluded that orgasm may exist retroactively as a mental representation in a brain that has been deconnected from orgasm in the pelvic genitalia. However, the long-term continuity of the existence of orgasm in the brain is contingent on the continuity of its synchronous existence in the pelvic genitalia. Synchrony itself is contingent on uninterrupted connectedness between the brain and the neural innervation of the pelvic genitalia, by way of the spinal cord. The orgasm is not exclusively a physiologic phenomenon, nor is it exclusively a disembodied psychological or transcendental phenomenon. It is, par excellence, a phenomenon of mind/body unity.

For the paraplegic, the orgasm becomes a memory and a penumbra of its former self. Like pain, the orgasm cannot be evoked and relived exactly as it was. It can be longed for, and its loss is a bitter loss, but one that the paraplegic appears to bear not frantically, but stoically. Lacking reciprocal communication between orgasm in the brain and orgasm in the genitalia, the paraplegic lacks also the post-traumatic desperation of the man who, with his orgasm otherwise intact, is the victim of irreversible traumatic loss of the penis (Money, 1961).

As is evident from cases of accidental or surgical peotomy or clitoridectomy, orgasm is not absolutely contingent on the intactness of the penis or clitoris. This comes as no surprise to those who have had the experience of orgasm induced simultaneously in the brain and in the genitals from nongenital parts of the intact body. Many lovers have discovered a uniquely personal "lover's spot" in some unlikely place on the torso. Adolescent lovers, not undressed, but already primed with excitement, may have an orgasm (with ejaculation also in the male) triggered by passionate tongue kissing, by being squeezed on the thigh, or by breast fondling.

Some men and women may have an orgasm, complete with genital manifestations, induced by having the nipples sucked, either without genital contact or as an adjunct to it. Some nursing mothers have an orgasm induced by the suckling of the baby at the breast. Many women are able to testify on the basis of personal experience regarding orgasm induced by penile penetration of the vagina without direct clitoral stimulation—as in the quadrupedal ("doggie") coital position, for example.

HORMONES AND ORGASM

In men, as in mammalian males in general, loss of the testicles is fairly rapidly followed by loss of the secretion and expulsion of the ejaculatory fluid. In a majority of castrates, the loss of ejaculation probably signifies the loss of orgasm. What may remain is the peak of sensation resembling that experienced by some prepubertal boys. The full orgasm with ejaculation can be restored by endocrine replacement therapy with the hormone testosterone.

It is possible for a prepubertal male to have a build-up of orgasm-like sensation toward a nonejaculatory peak. Before-and-after accounts, from hypogonadal patients who require testosterone replacement therapy in order to enter puberty and to mature, indicate that the peak attained with ejaculation after hormone therapy is not the same as the pretreatment peak without ejaculation. The peak of ejaculatory orgasm is reported as better and stronger (Money & Alexander, 1967).

Loss of ejaculation without the loss of orgasmic peak, the so-called dry orgasm, is a pharmacologically induced side effect associated chiefly with antihypertensive drugs and with some antipsychotic drugs (see review by Sitsen, 1988). The sexological effects of these drugs are unpredictable and individually variable. In men, they may suppress orgasm as well as ejaculation, and they may induce impotence. In women, they may also suppress orgasm, and in both sexes these drugs may induce sexual anergia.

The estrogenic and progestinic female hormones have an antiandrogenic effect in males. This effect includes suppression of ejaculation, although orgasm may be retained. Surgical castration is permanently antiandrogenic, since it removes the testicles, which are the source of the androgenic hormone, testosterone. The effects of hormonal antiandrogenic treatment resemble those of surgical deandrogenization, but with the extremely great advantage of being temporary and reversible, which is the rationale for the use of the progestinic antiandrogen, medroxyprogesterone acetate (Depo-Provera) in the treatment of male sex offenders (Money, 1970, 1987).

In the normal mature female, hormones secreted from the ovaries include a low level of testosterone. There is also a low level of androgenic steroids secreted by the adrenocortical glands. The relationship of ovarian and adrenocortical androgens to orgasm in females remains still to be elucidated.

DISABILITY AND INDIVIDUALS WITH GENITAL DISABILITIES

Among individuals with disabilities there is one group whose rehabilitation is consistently neglected and denied, namely, those with specifically genito-sexual disabilities, that is, disabilities involving the sex organs themselves. Such a disability may originate prenatally and be manifested as a birth defect of the sex organs, as in, for example, hermaphroditism of various diagnostic types, hypospadias, micropenis, penile aplasia, and vaginal atresia.

Sex organ disability may also originate postnatally as an accidental injury or traumatic mutilation. In boys, an extreme example is total loss of the penis in the wake of circumcision by cautery, not to mention less total mutilatory errors or side effects of male circumcision, worldwide.

In girls, postnatal trauma occurs routinely in ritual mutilation of the genitalia of which the most extreme type, Pharaonic circumcision or infibulation, is actually a complete vulvectomy. As many as 60 million females in the Nilotic and Sahelian cultures of Africa are estimated to have undergone some degree of ritual genital mutilation.

Genital trauma may originate postnatally also as a product of surgical intervention for the treatment of prostate cancer (prostatectomy) for example, or for cancer of the penis (penectomy) or the vulva (vulvectomy).

In the present national climate of antisexualism, it is virtually impossible to obtain sexological research or clinical service funding for those with genital disabilities. For example, birth defects of the sex organs are the only types of birth defect that are not recognized by the National Foundation/March of Dimes. In addition, it is also virtually impossible to obtain sexological research funding relevant to persons whose disability is not primarily genital, but which does affect their sex lives. Regrettably, it has also become almost impossible to publish case history material that pertains to the diagnosis, prognosis, or treatment of people with sexological problems, because it is classified by review committees as "too sensitive."

ORGASMOLOGY

Béjin (1985) wrote an essay on "The Decline of the Psycho-analyst and the Rise of the Sexologist." In a footnote (p. 183) he attributes to Wilhelm Reich the term *orgasmography*, and he himself coined the terms *orgasmotherapy* and *orgasmology*.

Orgasmology is a name for the science of orgasm that sounds respectable and user-friendly and promises to destigmatize the scientific study of human coition and give it legitimacy as a phenomenon of research. Scientifically, it gives prominence to the zenith of personal sexuoerotic experience, instead of relegating orgasm to an inconspicuous niche in the science of reproductive behavior. Orgasmology has many tangents and many avenues for experimental and clinical research and clinical application to the establishment of a joyful sex life for persons with all types of disabilities.

REFERENCES

Béjin, A. (1985). The decline of the psycho-analyst and the rise of the sexologist. In P. Aviés & A. Béjin (Eds.), *Western sexuality: Practice and precept in past and present time* (pp. 180–200). Oxford: Blackwell.

Goldfoot, D.A., Westerborg-van Loon, H., Groeneveld, W., & Slob, A.K. (1980). Behavioral and physiological evidence of sexual climax in the female stump-tailed macaque (*Macaca arctoides*). *Science, 208,* 1477–1479.

Kinsey, A.C., Pomeroy, W.B., Martin, C.E., & Gebhard, P.H. (1953). *Sexual behavior in the human female.* Philadelphia: W.B. Saunders.

Lightfoot-Klein, H. (1989). *Prisoners of ritual: An odyssey into female genital circumcision in Africa.* New York: Haworth Press.

Magoun, H.W. (1981). John B. Watson and the study of human sexual behavior. *Journal of Sex Research, 17,* 368–378.

Masters, W.H., & Johnson, V.E. (1966). *Human sexual response.* Boston: Little, Brown.

Money, J. (1960). Phantom orgasm in the dreams of paraplegic men and women. *Archives of General Psychiatry, 3,* 373–382.

Money, J. (1961). Components of eroticism in man: II. The orgasm and genital somesthesia. *Journal of Nervous and Mental Disease, 132,* 289–297.

Money, J. (1970). Use of an androgen depleting hormone in the treatment of male sex offenders. *Journal of Sex Research, 6,* 165–172.

Money, J. (1987). Treatment guidelines: Antiandrogen and counseling of paraphilic sex offenders. *Journal of Sex and Marital Therapy, 13,* 219–223.

Money, J., & Alexander, D. (1967). Eroticism and sexual function in developmental anorchia and hyporchia with pubertal failure. *Journal of Sex Research, 3,* 31–47.

Pauly, P.J. (1979). Psychology at Hopkins: Its rise and fall and rise and fall and . . . *Johns Hopkins Magazine, 30*(6), 36–41.

Sitsen, J.M.A. (1988). Prescription drugs and sexual function. In J. Money, H. Musaph, & J.M.A. Sitsen (Eds.), *Handbook of sexology: Vol. VI. The pharmacology and endocrinology of sexual function.* Amsterdam: Elsevier.

Slob, A.K., Groeneveld, W.H., & Van der Werff Ten Bosch, J.J. (1986). Physiological changes during copulation in male and female stumptail macaques (*Macaca arctoides*). *Physiology and Behavior, 38,* 891–895.

Szasz, G., & Carpenter, C. (1989). Clinical observations in vibratory stimulation of the penis of men with spinal cord injury. *Archives of Sexual Behavior, 18,* 461–474.

17

Current Research Trends in Spinal Cord Injuries

Beverly Whipple and Barry R. Komisaruk

This chapter reviews current research in the area of spinal cord injury, with a particular focus on sexual response. Little is known about the relationship between the level of spinal cord injury and the nature of sexual function and sexual response associated with it. Germane to the present context is the question of the relative contributions of periphery, spinal cord, and brain to sexual response. Specifically, what components of sexual response occur in relation to the level and type of spinal cord injury?

The current literature concerning sexuality and sexual response in individuals after a spinal cord injury (SCI) provides psychosexual data largely from anecdotal evidence or information from questionnaires and interviews. This type of data collection and dissemination has inherent biases as it is based on subjective reports. In addition, the literature that is available pertains mostly to male sexual function.

SEXUAL FUNCTION IN WOMEN AFTER SPINAL CORD INJURY

After reviewing the literature concerning female sexual function after SCI (Becker, 1978; Berard, 1989; Bregman, 1975; Bregman & Hadley, 1976; Campling, 1981; Comarr & Vigue, 1978a, 1978b; Griffith & Trieschmann, 1975; Hale-Harbaugh, Norman, Bogle, & Shaul, 1978), it can be concluded that women with spinal cord injuries are capable of menstruating, conceiving, and giving birth. Most of the current literature is not concerned with whether women with SCI have any sexual desire or sexual response (Whipple, 1990). For example, Billings and Stokes (1982) report that women with SCI, because their role can be passive, may enjoy intercourse and be perfectly capable of satisfying the male. They state that little is known about their capacity for orgasm.

However, Bregman and Hadley (1976) interviewed 31 women with spinal cord injury and report that most of the women's descriptions of orgasm since the injury were very similar to those of non-disabled women. Three of the women reported orgasms that were not different from the orgasms they experienced before their injuries.

Berard (1989) discusses physiological responses based on interviews of 15 women with SCI and reports a correlation between richness of fantasy and fulfillment of sexual life. Berard (1989) does address orgasm and states that pleasure may be heightened by concomitant stimulation of an erogenous zone either above or at the level of injury.

Laboratory studies need to be conducted to record objective data concerning sexual response and orgasm in both males and females who have experienced SCI. We have designed a project to fill this gap in the literature, which involves physiologic studies of sexual functioning after spinal cord injury. Before this study is discussed, it is important to review some of the recent research conducted in animals.

SOME CURRENT RESEARCH
ON PLASTICITY IN THE NERVOUS SYSTEM

New research developments have indicated that the nervous system is more plastic in adult mammals and humans than previously believed.

Preventive

An important concept that has developed recently is that of excitotoxicity, in which trauma to the central nervous system (CNS), such as that produced by ischemic hypoxia, which occurs during birth trauma, stroke, or traumatic ischemia, stimulates release in the CNS of excitatory amino acid neurotransmitters. These, particularly glutamate and aspartate, produce secondary damage to postsynaptic neurons. Another significant finding is that the action of these excitotoxins can be effectively blocked.

Persons with acute SCI who received the steroid methylprednisolone within 8 hours of injury showed significantly more improvement in motor, touch, and pinprick scores when they were
tested 6 weeks and 6 months post-injury than those receiving this
steroid *more* than 8 hours after injury, or those receiving naloxone or
a placebo. Benefit of early methylprednisolone treatment was evident even in patients whose injuries were initially evaluated as neu-
rologically complete, as well as in individuals believed to have incomplete lesions. According to the authors (Bracken et al., 1990), the
most likely explanation for the effect of methylprednisolone treatment is that, at the site of injury, it suppresses the hours-long process of breakdown of membranes by inhibiting lipid peroxidation,
which in turn improves the flow of blood at the injury site. The
blood flow is critical because ischemic hypoxia releases excitotoxic
amino acids locally in the CNS (Hagberg, Andersson, Kjellmer,
Thiringer, & Thordstein, 1987). The consequent CNS damage can be
significantly reduced by administration of receptor antagonists of
the excitatory amino acids (Andine et al., 1988).

Restorative

While the concept of excitotoxic neural activity is of applied significance, it involves primarily preventive measures. What is the current status of basic research on restoration of function? There has
been some progress in stimulating restoration of function in adult
mammals, but it has apparently not yet been applied to humans.
Some recent studies are reviewed that show that, in adult rats, corticospinal axons, transected at the thoracic level of the spinal cord,
can be stimulated to regrow more than 1 cm into the spinal cord
beyond their site of transection and that spinal motor neurons can
be stimulated to grow through implanted "bridges" into skeletal
muscles and form functional connections. In addition, based on
electron microscopic analysis, synapse formation has been demonstrated between regenerating axons passing through a nerve bridge
and neurons in the brain (Vidal-Sanz, Bray, Villegas-Perez, Thanos,
& Aguayo, 1987). Restoration of spinal reflexes has been demonstrated by implantation into the adult spinal cord of fetal neurons
that synthesize specific neurotransmitters. In other experiments to
be described, there is evidence that fetal neuron implants into an
adult spinal cord become innervated by neural pathways that descend from the brain to the spinal cord.

Schnell and Schwab (1990) utilized the hypothesis that the formation of myelin inhibits further neuronal plasticity. They devel-

oped a monoclonal antibody to myelin (named IN-1). After transect-
ing the spinal cord, including the corticospinal tract, they injected
the antibody-producing hybridoma cells into the frontal-parietal
cortex in young rats. They found that the transected fibers in the
spinal cord grew new projections that traveled around the spinal
cord cut, proceeding caudally 7–11 mm and probably farther, within
2–3 weeks. The animals receiving a control antibody showed re-
growth not farther than 1 mm. Thus, by neutralizing the myelin
chemical signals received by the cell bodies in the cortex, the axons
in the spinal cord of these same neurons can be disinhibited from
regenerating. Whether these regenerated corticospinal axons established functional connections has yet to be determined.

In addition to this regeneration of upper motor neurons, there is
also evidence of regeneration and functional reconnection of lower
motor neurons. As shown in adult rats (Horvat, Pecot-Dechavassine,
Mira, & Davarpanah, 1989), spinal motoneurons can evidently grow
new axons that travel through a transplanted nerve segment and
form functional connections with skeletal muscle. A neck muscle
was denervated and a 20–30 mm segment of peroneal nerve was
removed from the leg. One end of this nerve segment was inserted
into an incision in the dorsal spinal cord, and the other end was
inserted into an incision in the muscle. Within 5 weeks of the surgery, electrical stimulation of the nerve produced muscle contraction. Injection of markers and use of the neuromuscular cholinergic
receptor blocker, curare, and electron microscopy, provided evidence
that motor neurons, as far as 8 mm from the end of the nerve segment where it was implanted into the spinal cord at levels C3–C7,
sent functional processes into the nerve segment, traveled through
it, and terminated in functional cholinergic motor endplates in the
muscle, which is normally innervated by motoneurons from C1
and C2.

Restoration of reflex locomotor (Yakovleff et al., 1989) or reflex
ejaculatory (Privat, Mansour, Rajaofetra, & Geffard, 1989) function
has been produced by transplants of fetal neurons into adult rat
spinal cords. In the latter case, serotonin synthesizing raphe neurons
from fetal rats were implanted into the spinal cord below the (lower
thoracic) level of complete transection in adult male rats. After systemic administration of zimelidine, a specific inhibitor of serotonin
re-uptake, reflex ejaculation could be elicited in the raphe neuron-
grafted, but not the non-grafted, control rats (Privat et al., 1989).

While this is evidence of restoration of a local spinal reflex,
there is also evidence that grafts of fetal neurons into the adult
spinal cord can become innervated by descending axons from the

brain stem (Nothias, Horvat, Mira, Pecot-Dechavassine, & Peschanski, 1990).

Other properties of spinal cord function have been manipulated by pharmacologic agents. Specifically, androgen treatment has been shown to stimulate the growth of specific types of genital motor neurons in rats (Arnold & Breedlove, 1985). Local spinal androgen application facilitates penile reflexes in rats, and systemic estrogen facilitates sexual reflexes in spinal transected female cats and dogs (Hart, 1978). Amplification of responsiveness to tactile stimulation has been demonstrated by the application of receptor antagonists of the inhibitory amino acids, GABA and glycine, directly to the spinal cord (Beyer, Roberts, & Komisaruk, 1985; Roberts, Beyer, & Komisaruk, 1985). Amplification of sensory and/or motor responsiveness is of potential therapeutic value.

It must be emphasized that these studies, most published since 1985, are basic research in animals. They provide the basic paradigms that could guide the future direction of research in humans.

Vaginocervical Stimulation

We have analyzed the role of the spinal cord in mediating the effects of vaginal stimulation (VS). Vaginocervical afferent activity enters the spinal cord via the pelvic nerve (Komisaruk, Adler, & Hutchison, 1972) and hypogastric nerves (Peters, Kristal, & Komisaruk, 1987; Cunningham, Steinman, Whipple, Mayer, & Komisaruk, in press) and in the sacral region activates post-synaptic neurons in laminae 1, 2, 5, and 10 (Chinapen, Swann, Steinman, & Komisaruk, in press).

We are currently analyzing the afferent pathway by which vaginal sensory input continues to the brain. A powerful pain-blocking "gate" mechanism is activated in the spinal cord at the level of laminae 1 and 2 (Johnson, Pott, Siegel, Adler, & Komisaruk, 1987). This blocks ascending pain but not tactile input to the somatosensory thalamus in the brain and elevates pain thresholds in rats (Komisaruk & Wallman, 1977). Consistent with this, vaginal self-stimulation in women elevates pain thresholds but not tactile thresholds (Whipple & Komisaruk, 1985, 1988). It is possible that this mechanism could be activated in women who experience neurogenic pain in the sacral area, known in the vernacular as "burning butt," to help alleviate this form of pain. Additionally, the analgesic effect of VS is manifested throughout the body and could therefore have therapeutic value for the alleviation of other types of pain.

We have investigated alternative forms of orgasm and the effect of orgasm on pain thresholds and autonomic activity (Whipple,

Ogden, & Komisaruk, 1992). This study has demonstrated that it is possible to experience orgasm in the absence of any physical stimuli. Based on these data and the approaches used in animals, which may lead to pharmacologic methods of amplification of existing mechanisms, it may be possible to expand the types of orgasmic processes available to persons with SCI.

SENSORY RESPONSE IN THE ABSENCE OF GENITAL SENSORY INPUT

Orgasm has been reported to occur in response to imagery in the absence of any physical stimulation in nondisabled women (Ogden, 1981) and in people with spinal cord injury (Money, 1960). Whipple et al. (1992) undertook a study to ascertain whether the subjective report of imagery-induced orgasm is accompanied by physiologic and perceptual events that are characteristic of genitally stimulated orgasm. Based on previous studies, we hypothesized that arousing imagery that resulted in orgasm would produce a significant elevation in pain thresholds. We also hypothesized that the physiologic correlates of imagery-induced orgasm would not differ from those of orgasm produced by genital self-stimulation.

The subjects in this study ($N = 10$) were women who claimed that they could experience orgasm from imagery alone. The mean age of the subjects was 44.6 years (range, 32–67 years).

During each control and experimental condition (i.e., guided imagery via an audio tape, self-induced imagery, and genital self-stimulation), noninvasive physiologic measures of heart rate, blood pressure, and pupil diameter were recorded via a BioLab system, and thresholds to mechanically stimulated pain and touch were measured on the hand.

The relative effects of two types of imagery and genital self-stimulation were determined in each subject. One subject reported orgasm during the guided imagery condition, 10 during the genital self-stimulation condition, and seven during the self-induced imagery condition.

Orgasm from both self-induced imagery and genital self-stimulation was associated with significant increases in blood pressure, heart rate, pupil diameter, and pain thresholds over resting control conditions. These two orgasm conditions did not differ significantly from each other on any of the physiologic measures. No significant elevation over resting control levels (with the exception of pain tolerance thresholds) was observed in the guided imagery condition.

During genital self-stimulation orgasm, systolic blood pressure increased 126%, heart rate increased 44%, pupil diameter increased 52%, pain detection threshold increased 39%, and pain tolerance threshold increased 40%. During self-induced imagery orgasm, systolic blood pressure increased 94%, heart rate increased 32%, pupil diameter increased 33%, pain detection threshold increased 61%, and pain tolerance increased 42%. There were no significant differences in tactile thresholds between the groups for any of the measurements (see Whipple et al., 1992).

Based on these findings that orgasm from self-induced imagery and genital self-stimulation is associated with significant and substantial net sympathetic activation and concomitant significant increases in pain thresholds, it would seem appropriate to broaden the commonly accepted concept of orgasm. On the basis of these findings, it is evident that physical genital stimulation is not necessary to produce a state that is reported to be an orgasm.

An interesting question, based on these findings, is whether the perception of orgasm is generated directly within the central nervous system, and/or whether it is a consequence of the perception of muscular exertion and/or peripheral sympathetic activity. During this study, some of the subjects experienced vigorous muscular movement during genital and imagery-induced orgasms, while others appeared to be lying still. That is, there were instances in which orgasm was accompanied by sympathetic activation with no evident skeletal muscular activity. The proposed study of persons with SCI who show no skeletal muscular activity, and therefore no concomitant sensory input resulting from muscular activity, affords an opportunity to ascertain whether orgasm and concurrent sympathetic activation can occur in the absence of peripheral musculoskeletal and sensory activity. If such orgasm does occur, this will lead us to conclude that peripheral skeletal muscle activity and peripheral sensory input are not essential to orgasm. Furthermore, it will raise the question of whether afferent activity resulting from sympathetic activation contributes to orgasm.

STRUCTURE–FUNCTION RELATIONSHIP
IN PEOPLE AFTER SPINAL CORD INJURY

The purpose of our current study (conducted in collaboration with researchers from the Kessler Institute for Rehabilitation, West Orange, New Jersey) is to evaluate the sexual function of persons after a traumatic spinal cord injury and to develop a physiologic basis for prediction of sexual function based on residual neurologic function. This will allow more focused interventions for persons who have a spinal cord injury.

Based on studies with nondisabled individuals, several physiologic measurements (i.e., blood pressure, heart rate, respiratory rate, skeletal muscle contractions just above the level of injury and in the perineal area) and perceptual measurements (i.e., pain and tactile thresholds) are being monitored. The degree of erection and amount of anterograde or retrograde ejaculation in males and the quantity of lubrication in females are also being determined.

The subjects in this study (ages 21–50) include 12 males and 12 females with spinal cord injuries who report that they experience orgasm. Two males and two females from each group will be tested: complete quadriplegics or paraplegics above T6, incomplete quadriplegics or paraplegics above T6, complete paraplegics below T6, incomplete paraplegics below T6, complete cauda equina, incomplete cauda equina, and two nondisabled men and two nondisabled women.

Since it is not clear from previous studies what constitutes an orgasm in people with SCI, we will be determining: 1) where in the body the orgasm is experienced, 2) the nature of that experience, and 3) the most effective eliciting stimuli. The perceptual and physiologic properties of an orgasm elicited by stimulation of the skin above the level of injury may differ from an orgasm elicited by vaginal or other visceral stimulation below the level of injury. For example, in personal communication with three women with paraplegia, they have stated that they enjoy intercourse because they have orgasms during intercourse that they describe as being experienced "deep inside." Additionally, an orgasm produced by stimulation of multiple body regions may have concomitant physiologic and perceptual properties that are different from an orgasm produced by stimulation of a single body region.

The research protocol consists of an initial medical and psychological assessment, including the Minnesota Multiphasic Personality Inventory (MMPI) (Woychysln, McElheran, & Rommey, 1992) and the Derogatis Sexual Functioning Inventory (Derogatis & Melisaratos, 1979).

Each person will then participate in two laboratory sessions. During the first session, the individual will watch a nonstimulating videotape and then self-apply manual or vibratory stimulation to any body region they choose while watching a nonstimulating videotape. During the second session, the individual will view an erotic video and then will self-apply stimulation while viewing the erotic video. Physiologic and perceptual measurements will be taken during each condition, during orgasm, and after orgasm.

This study with people with SCI may provide further insight into the nature of the orgasmic process. It is possible that persons with spinal cord injuries may have been given misleading or inaccurate information regarding their potential for sexual response and fertility. The findings may help people with spinal cord injury improve the quality of their life, since sexual/intimate interaction and reproductive potential are important aspects of rehabilitation and daily living.

REFERENCES

Andine, P., Lehmann, A., Ellren, K., Wennberg, E., Kjellmer, I., Nielsn, T., & Hagberg, H. (1988). The excitatory amino acid antagonist kynurenic acid administered after hypoxic-ischemia in neonatal rats offers neuroprotection. *Neuroscience Letters, 90,* 208–212.

Arnold, A.P., & Breedlove, S.M. (1985). Organizational and activational effects of sex steroids on brain and behavior: A reanalysis. *Hormones and Behavior, 19,* 469–498.

Becker, E.F. (1978). *Female sexuality following spinal cord injury.* Bloomington, IL: Cheever.

Berard, E.J.J. (1989). The sexuality of spinal cord injured women: Physiology and pathophysiology: A review. *Paraplegia, 27,* 99–112.

Beyer, C., Roberts, L.A., & Komisaruk, B.R. (1985). Hyperalgesia induced by altered glycinergic activity at the spinal cord. *Life Science, 37,* 875–882.

Billings, D.M., & Stokes, L.G.: (1982). *Medical surgical nursing.* St. Louis: C.V. Mosby.

Bracken, M.B., Shepard, M.J., Collings, W.F., Holford, T.R., Young, W., Baskin, D.S., Eisenberg, H.M., Flamm, E., Leo-Summers, L., Maroon, J., Marsha, L.F., Perot, P.L., Piepmeir, J., Sonntage, V.K.H., Wagner, F.C., Wilberger, J.E., & Winn, H.R. (1990). A randomized, controlled trial of methylprednisolone or naloxone in the treatment of acute spinal-cord injury. *The New England Journal of Medicine, 322,* 1405–1411.

Bregman, S. (1975). *Sexuality and the spinal cord injured woman.* Minneapolis: Sister Kenny Institute.

Bregman, S., & Hadley, R.G. (1976). Sexual adjustment and feminine attractiveness among spinal cord injured women. *Archives of Physical Medicine and Rehabilitation, 57,* 448–450.

Campling, J. (1981). *Images of ourselves: Women with disabilities.* Boston: Routledge & Kegan Paul.

Chinapen, S., Swann, J.M., Steinman, J.L., & Komisaruk, B.R. (in press). Expression of C-fos protein in lumbosacral spinal cord in response to vaginocervical stimulation in rats. *Neuroscience Letters.*

Comarr, A.E., & Vigue, M. (1978a). Sexual counseling among male and female patients with spinal cord and/or cauda equina injury. *American Journal of Physical Medicine, 57,* 107–122.

Comarr, A.E., & Vigue, M. (1978b). Sexual counseling among male and female patients with spinal cord and/or cauda equina injury. *American Journal of Physical Medicine, 57*, 215–227.

Cunningham, S.T., Steinman, J.L., Whipple, B., Mayer, A.D., & Komisaruk, B.R. (1991). Differential roles of hypogastric and pelvic nerves in the analgesic and motoric effects of vaginocervical stimulation in rats. *Brain Research, 559*, 337–343.

Derogatis, L.R., & Melisaratos, N. (1979). The DSFI: A multidimensional measure of sexual functioning. *Journal of Sex and Marital Therapy, 5*, 244–280.

Griffith, E.R., & Trieschmann, R.B. (1975). Sexual functioning in women with spinal cord injury. *Archives of Physical Medicine and Rehabilitation 56*, 18–21.

Hagberg, H., Andersson, P., Kjellmer, I., Thiringer, K., & Thordstein, M. (1987). Extracellular overflow of glutamate, aspartate, GABA, and taurine in the cortex and basal ganglia of fetal lambs during hypoxia-ischemia. *Neuroscience Letters, 78*, 311–317.

Hale-Harbaugh, J., Norman, A.D., Bogle, J., & Shaul, S. (1978). *Within reach: Providing family planning services to physically disabled women.* New York: Human Sciences Press.

Hart, B.L. (1978). Hormones, spinal reflexes, and sexual behavior. In J.B. Hutchison (Ed.), *Biological determinants of sexual behavior* (pp. 320–347). New York: John Wiley & Sons.

Horvat, J.C., Pecot-Dechavassine, M., Mira, J.C., & Davarpanah, Y. (1989). Formation of functional endplates by spinal axons regenerating through a peripheral nerve graft: A study in the adult rat. *Brain Research Bulletin, 22*, 103–114.

Johnson, B.M., Pott, C., Siegel, A., Adler, N.T., & Komisaruk, B.R. (1987). Spinal antinociceptive action of vaginocervical stimulation: 2-DG autoradiographic evidence. *NIH Centennial MBRS-MARC Symposium Proceedings, 15*, 93.

Komisaruk, B.R., Adler, N.T., & Hutchison, J. (1972). Genital sensory field: Enlargement by estrogen treatment in female rats. *Science, 178*, 1295–1298.

Komisaruk, B.R., & Wallman, J. (1977). Antinociceptive effects of vaginal stimulation in rats: Neurophysiological and behavioral studies. *Brain Research, 137*, 85–107.

Money, J. (1960). Phantom orgasm in the dreams of paraplegic men and women. *Archives of General Psychiatry, 3*, 373–382.

Nothias, F., Horvat, J., Mira, J., Pecot-Dechavassine, M., & Peschanski, M. (1990). Double step neural transplants to replace degenerated motoneurons. In S.B. Dunnett & S.J. Richards (Eds.), *Progress in brain research, 82* (pp. 239–246). New York: Elsevier/North Holland.

Ogden, G. (1981). *Perception of touch in easily orgasmic women during peak sexual experiences.* Unpublished doctoral dissertation, Institute for Advanced Study of Human Sexuality, San Francisco.

Peters, L.C., Kristal, M.B., & Komisaruk, B.R. (1987). Sensory innervation of the external and internal genitalia of the female rat. *Brain Research, 408*, 199–204.

Privat, A., Mansour, H., Rajaofetra, N., & Geffard, M. (1989). Intraspinal transplants of serotonergic neurons in the adult rat. *Brain Research Bulletin, 22*, 123–129.

Roberts, L., Beyer, C., & Komisaruk, B.R. (1985). Strychnine antagonizes vaginal stimulation-produced analgesia at the spinal cord. *Life Science, 36,* 2017–2033.

Schnell, L., & Schwab, M.E. (1990). Axonal regeneration in the rat spinal cord produced by an antibody against myelin-associated neurite growth inhibitors. *Nature, 343,* 269–272.

Vidal-Sanz, M., Bray, G.M., Villegas-Perez, M.P., Thanos, S., & Aguayo, A.J. (1987). Axonal regeneration and synapse formation in the superior colliculus by retinal ganglion cells in the adult rat. *Journal of Neuroscience, 7,* 2894–2909.

Whipple, B. (1990). Female sexuality. In J.F.J. Leyson (Ed.), *Sexual rehabilitation of the spinal-cord-injured patient* (pp. 19–38). Clifton, NJ: Humana Press.

Whipple, B., & Komisaruk, B.R. (1985). Elevation of pain threshold by vaginal stimulation in women. *Pain, 21,* 357–367.

Whipple, B., & Komisaruk, B.R. (1988). Analgesia produced in women by genital self-stimulation. *Journal of Sex Research, 24,* 130–140.

Whipple, B., Ogden, G., & Komisaruk, B.R. (1992). Relative analgesic effect of imagery compared to genital self-stimulation. *Archives of Sexual Behavior 21,* 121–133.

Woychysln, C.A., McElheran, W.G., & Rommey, D.M. (1992). MMPI validity measures: A comparative study of original with alternative indices. *Journal of Personality Assessment, 58* (1), 138–148.

Yakovleff, A., Roby-Brami, A., Guezard, B., Mansour, H., Bussel, B., & Privat, A. (1989). Locomotion in rats transplanted with noradrenergic neurons. *Brain Research Bulletin, 22,* 115–121.

18

The Impact
of Spinal Cord Trauma
on Female Sexual Function

Marca L. Sipski

When an individual sustains a spinal cord injury (SCI), it is a tragic occurrence. In addition to the partial or complete paralysis associated with SCI, a myriad of physical changes occur, including loss of bladder and bowel control, spasticity, and neurogenic sexual dysfunction. Neurogenic sexual dysfunction is known to affect both males and females; however, the literature focuses primarily on male sexual dysfunction. One reason for this is that males have external genitalia with a much more visually apparent sexual response (e.g., erection) than females who have the internal response of lubrication. Thus, the male response is conducive to study via self-report, the traditional means of studying sexual function after SCI. Social biases that women are passive sexual partners concerned only with giving pleasure to males, combined with an emphasis on reproduction and childbirth, are additional reasons for the lack of information on female sexual dysfunction after SCI.

In this chapter, the available literature on female sexual dysfunction after spinal cord injury is reviewed. Studies pertaining to sexuality, the sexual response cycle, and menstruation as they relate to SCI are discussed, and recommendations are made for areas of future research.

SEX ACTS AND SEXUALITY

Early studies of sexual functioning after spinal cord injury painted a bleak picture. Money (1960) interviewed seven SCI females about their sexual capacity. He described one individual, a 32-year-old with sensory-incomplete quadriplegia, in detail. After her injury, she reported a complete loss of sexual desire with retention of pleasurable sensations above, but not below, her injury. She also reported erotic dreams with climaxes during the dreams and orgasm accompanied by voiding. The other women interviewed described intercourse, ranging from "terrible" to "just a waste of time" to "some pleasure but no genital sensation." They denied the feelings of sexual urge and gratification that they had experienced in the past. Money concluded that cognitional eroticism can be a variable of sex independent of genitopelvic sensation and action. He stated, "The brain, in other words, can work independently of the genitalia in the generation of erotic experience just as the genitalia of paraplegics can work reflexively and independently of the brain" (Money, 1960, p. 381).

Weiss and Diamond (1966) were the next to study sexual function after spinal cord damage, interviewing 26 males and 21 females with illness-related myelopathy. Fifty-two percent of these females had early onset of disability. Forty-eight percent of these women were married prior to disability. Following injury, 77% of these were still married, and 23% were divorced or separated. Fourteen percent of single females married after injury while 38% of the women never married.

Forty-eight percent of the female subjects in the Weiss and Diamond study (1966) reported conscious sexual desire pre-injury, in comparison to 62% post-injury. Fifty-two percent of women had engaged in some form of sexual activity pre-injury whereas 62% reported such activity post-injury. Twenty-four percent reported "undifferentiated" sexual sensations pre-injury compared to 33% post-injury. Thirty-eight percent reported "localized sexual sensations" pre-injury compared to 52% post-injury. Thirty-eight percent of the women said their partners were accepting in their attitudes toward sexual situations before the injury compared to 42% post-injury. Forty-three percent of women said that they themselves had been accepting in their attitudes before their injuries whereas 56% reported attitudes of acceptance post-injury. Eighty-six percent of women reported no sexual problems prior to disability whereas only 48% reported no difficulties post-disability. Subjects were given two sexual adjustment tests: the Wechsler Work Interest Inventory and the Weiss Sex Role Noun Test. Results indicated that women with myelopathy had less sex-role identification than comparison females without myelopathy on the Wechsler Work Interest Inventory and greater sex-role identification on the Weiss Sex Role Noun Test.

This study suffers from a lack of reported demographic information. Age at injury, current age, and etiology of the subjects' myelopathies are unknown. Without this information, results are difficult to interpret. Moreover, the terminology used in this report is vague (e.g., "undifferentiated sexual sensations"). Without more precise definitions, the significance of these results is questionable.

It was not until 1976 that SCI females were again studied via semi-structured interviews (Bregman & Hadley 1976). Sexual positions were described as were various means of psychological and physical stimulation. Only 2 of 31 subjects reported difficulty with bowel programs during intercourse while subjects with catheters preferred to leave them in during sexual activity. Orgasm, sexual positions, and means of stimulation were discussed as shown in Tables 1 and 2.

Sexual adjustment scores were derived from responses of subjects and their mates regarding their satisfaction with the frequency of their sexual encounters, their degree of sexual adjustment, and the degree of pleasure experienced in their sexual encounters. No significant correlations were noted between these scores and time

Table 1. Descriptions of orgasms by 31 subjects

Description	Number of subjects
Physical sensations	22
Pleasant sensation, release, relaxful, glowing tingling feeling	11
Strong, overwhelming, breathless, high intense excitement	8
High buildup of feelings, tension, and then a release and relaxation	3
Psychological sensations of good mental feelings and strong feelings of closeness and affection towards mate	4
Orgasm no different from before	3
Preferred not to discuss subject of orgasm with interviewer	1
No orgasms before or after injury	1
(total)	31

From Bregman, S., & Hadley, R.G. (1976). Sexual adjustment and feminine attractiveness among spinal cord injured women. *Archives of Physical Medicine and Rehabilitation, 57,* 449; reprinted by permission.

Table 2.   Method used for physical and social attractiveness by 31 subjects

Wear clothes that cover catheter leg bag, (long dresses, full skirts)	11
Wear slacks for style, comfort and transferring from the wheelchair	8
Transfer from wheelchair to couch or chair	3
Wear short jackets or ponchos instead of long coats	2
Wear clothes that draw attention to upper torso	2
Wear one-piece undergarments to support upper torso (hook and wire girdle)	2
Wear tight-fitting hose for support	2
Cross legs at ankles for back support and good appearance	2
Wear cut-off slacks that are easy to take off	1
Use attractive wheelchair (favorite color)	1
Dance sitting down	1

From Bregman, S., & Hadley, R.G. (1976). Sexual adjustment and feminine attractiveness among spinal cord injured women. *Archives of Physical Medicine and Rehabilitation, 57,* 450; reprinted by permission.

since injury; nor could any significant correlation be found between the scores and whether or not the subjects had received information regarding their potential for sexual function after injury.

Although this study is the largest to date, it failed to collect neurologic data and provided an inadequate description of the subjects' physical sensations associated with orgasm. Despite these shortcomings, the study appropriately concludes that women with SCI can adjust both socially and sexually. It was noted that sexual stimulation in areas where women had partial feeling might be enjoyable, that most women enjoyed breast stimulation, and that the psychological aspects of the relationship were the most meaningful for some women.

Two years after the Bregman and Hadley investigation, Fitting, Salisbury, Davies, and Mayclin (1978) studied 24 women with SCI between the ages of 20 and 40. Their ages at injury ranged from 11 to 34 with a mean of 20; time since injury varied from 2 to 20 years with a mean of 8. Over 80% were traumatically injured. Thirteen females had complete injuries, while 11 had incomplete injuries with levels ranging from C-4 to the lumbosacral junction. All were heterosexual pre-injury, however, post-injury, two were bisexual and one was homosexual. Twenty-two of the women had attended college and 11 had gone on to advanced degree programs. Fourteen women had been involved in sexual relations pre-injury, however, only two remained in these relationships post-injury. Fifty percent of the women believed the dissolution of their relationship was due to the injury. Twenty had been involved in sexual relationships since their injury, and 13 were currently in such a relationship. Fifty-four percent said sex was "very enjoyable" post-injury. Most women viewed themselves as "honest," "independent," and "intellectual." Moreover, they viewed themselves as more active sexual partners post-injury compared to pre-injury. Over half of the women viewed themselves as generally more independent after their injuries. Twenty-two of the women noted their self-image had changed since injury but thought the change was related to their maturing in general. Only 11 of these women had received sexual counseling after injury.

The report of Fitting et al. (1978) is notable because it provides more descriptive information than do previous studies; however, the extremely high educational level of the subjects may have significantly biased the results. Nevertheless, this study concludes that sexual interest can remain post-injury and that there may be an interrelationship between sexuality and self-concept in a woman's adaptation to acquired disability.

Sipski and Alexander (1991) studied 25 females with SCI using an 80-item multiple choice questionnaire. Subjects' ages ranged from 18 to 61 with a median of 34, and time since injury ranged from 6 to 220 months with a median of 50. Educational level ranged from 11 to 17 years with a median of 14. Five women exhibited complete quadriplegia, nine had incomplete quadriplegia, four had complete paraplegia, and seven had incomplete paraplegia.

The women were questioned about their sexual activities and preferences both pre- and post-injury. Twenty-four percent reported having no sexual experiences pre-injury, while 28% reported no sexual experiences post-injury. Forty percent, however, resumed sexual activity within 6 months of injury. The frequency of sexual activity pre-injury was at least weekly in 64%, while post-injury frequency was weekly in only 40%. Since injury, individuals had engaged in a variety of sex acts with 76% engaging in kissing and hugging, 68% penis-vagina intercourse, 68% touching, 56% oral sex, 40% manual stimulation, 24% vibratory stimulation, and 12% anal intercourse. Pre-injury, favorite activities included intercourse, kissing, and hugging. Post-injury, preferred activities were kissing, hugging, and touching.

Forty-four percent of these women reported they received information about sex after their spinal cord injuries. Twenty-eight percent of the women and 20% of their partners had undergone sexual counseling. Forty-four percent believed their spinal cord injuries negatively affected the quality of their relationships, and 32% believed their injuries negatively affected their ability to raise children. Twenty percent reported they had not adjusted well sexually, while 76% reported they had adjusted well sexually, and 4% were uncertain. Twenty-four percent reported their ability to become sexually aroused ranged from none to low, 40% reported it was appropriate, and 28% reported it was high. Desire for sexual activity and sexual satisfaction were noted to decrease after injury. Although this study suffers from a small sample size, it is notable because it provides detailed information on the sexual practices and satisfaction of SCI women.

SEXUAL RESPONSE CYCLE

In 1966, Masters and Johnson described four phases of the human sexual response cycle: excitement, plateau, orgasm, and resolution. Three pathways for the sexual response cycle are described by Masters and Johnson (1966) and are shown in Figure 1. Pathway A shows a woman who achieves multiple orgasms, pathway B describes a non-orgasmic woman, and pathway C describes a pathway in which the woman achieves a single orgasm.

The female excitement phase is characterized by clitoral enlargement in diameter, uterine elevation out of the deep pelvis, nipple erection and areolar enlargement, and vaginal lubrication, along with constriction of the lower third and dilation of the upper two thirds of the vagina. During the plateau phase, the clitoral shaft and glans retract along the pubic symphysis, the sex flush may appear, breast size continues to increase, and dilation of the upper portion of the vagina continues. Additionally, an orgasmic platform forms in

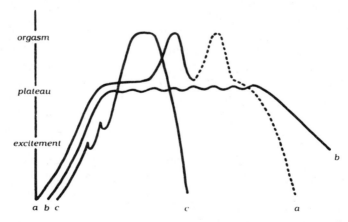

Figure 1.   The female sexual response cycle. (From Masters, W.H., & Johnson, V.E. [1966]. Human sexual response, p.5. Boston: Little, Brown; reprinted by permission of the authors.)

the vagina secondary to vasocongestion, and heart rate, respiratory rate, blood pressure, and muscle tone begin to increase. With orgasm, even greater elevation of heart rate, respiratory rate, and blood pressure occur along with 5–7 rhythmic contractions in the perineal musculature which last 0.7–1.0 seconds in length. Contraction of the fallopian tubes and uterus also occurs. One or a number of orgasms can occur, followed by the resolution phase involving slow reversal of the anatomic changes, along with generalized perspiration.

Little has been written regarding the effects of SCI on the sexual response cycle. Cole (1979) compared the sexual responses of females both before and after SCI and reported there were similarities in the responses of nipples, musculature, breasts, breathing, pulse, blood pressure, and skin changes, and that swelling remained in the labia and clitoris. However, he did not comment on vaginal and uterine changes (see Table 3) or the effect that variation in degree or level of injury would have on sexual response.

To determine the effects of specific types of SCI on sexual function, the normal physiology of sexual response must be clearly understood. If reflex lubrication is analogous to reflex erection, then it is probably mediated by sacral parasympathetic nerves, while psychogenic lubrication should be mediated by thoracolumbar sympathetic and sacral parasympathetic pathways. Griffith and Trieschmann (1975) described a female equivalent to ejaculation, including uterine, fallopian tube, and paraurethral smooth muscle contraction during the emission phase along with the contraction of striated

Table 3. Human sexuality—Female sexual response cycle: Comparison of sexual response cycles in able-bodied and spinal cord injured females

	Able-bodied female	Spinal cord injured female
Wall of vagina	Moistens	
Clitoris	Swells	Swells
Labia	Swells and opens	Swells
Uterus	Contracts	
Inner 2/3 of vagina	Expands	
Outer 1/3 of vagina	Contracts	
Nipples	Erect	Erect
Muscles	Tense, spasms	Tense, spasms
Breasts	Swell	Swell
Breathing	Increases	Increases
Pulse	Increases	Increases
Blood pressure	Increases	Increases
Skin of trunk, neck, face	Sex flush	Sex flush

From Cole, T.M. (1979). Sexuality and the spinal cord injured. In R. Green (Ed.), *Human sexuality: A health practitioner's text* (2nd ed., p. 164). Baltimore: Williams & Wilkins; copyright © 1979, The Williams & Wilkins Co., reprinted by permission.

pelvic musculature, perineal, and anal sphincter muscles during the ejaculation phase. If analogous to males, emission should be mediated by thoracolumbar sympathetic nerves, while ejaculation should be mediated by S2–S4 parasympathetic and somatic efferent nerves. It follows that, with this basis, examination of the type of SCI allows prediction of future effects on sexual function.

Unfortunately, specific types and degrees of SCI and their effects on female sexual responses such as lubrication, the equivalent of ejaculation, and orgasm have not been studied. One research study (Comarr & Vigue, 1978) examined some of these issues, reviewing the experiences of 21 females with SCI in addition to providing complete neurologic information. Although descriptions of sexual practices and orgasmic capability are coupled with excellent neurologic details, no mention is made of lubrication. Rather, it is simply stated that females could stimulate orgasm in various areas. Moreover, the major contribution of this study is the recommendation that similar counseling be used for both males and females with SCI with regard to potential sexual function. Comarr and Vigue reported that the ability of males to perceive sacral pain sensation indicated potential for psychogenic erection; similarly, in females, potential for psychogenic lubrication may be related to the preservation of sacral pain sensation.

The only direct observation of female sexual response post-SCI is that of Leyson (1983), who studied 10 women with SCI age 18 to 81 with an EMG anal probe inserted first into the vagina and then into the rectum while clitoral stimulation was performed to reach orgasm. Synchronous vaginal and rectal contractions were noted when orgasm was reported to occur, while without orgasm, neither of these occurred. Although Leyson's study is noteworthy, it lacks specific neurologic and procedural data that would have added to its significance and replicability.

The next published study that examined female sexual response post-SCI is that of Berard (1989), who interviewed 15 women with SCI about pleasant feelings, orgasm, dreams, lubrication, genital swelling, attractiveness, spasticity, and mobility. This study provided detailed neurologic information; however, responses to the interviews are noticeably absent. Rather, an anecdotal description of the alterations in sexual function that should occur after SCI is provided.

In women with upper motor neuron complete injuries, Berard (1989) predicts reflex lubrication will be maintained but not psychogenic lubrication. This is consistent with the site of neurologic damage and the literature on male physiology, where 70%–93% of men report reflex erections. Berard makes no mention, however, of the ejaculatory equivalent. Bors and Comarr (1960) reported that 4% of males with upper motor neuron complete injuries do have the capacity to ejaculate. Therefore, one can postulate that 4% of females with complete injuries also have the potential to experience this ejaculatory equivalent.

Women with upper motor neuron incomplete injuries are reported to have reflex lubrication and may also have psychogenic lubrication (Berard, 1989). According to Comarr and Vigue (1978), preservation of psychogenic lubrication may depend on the integrity of the spinothalamic tracts innervating the sacral cord. Considering the male counterpart, 80% are noted to experience isolated reflex erections while 19% have combination reflex and psychogenic erections, and 32% have ejaculations (Bors & Comarr, 1960). Thus, one can hypothesize that 99% of women with incomplete injuries should lubricate, and 32% of females with incomplete upper motor neuron injuries have potential for the ejaculatory equivalent. However, whether or not there is a relationship between sacral pain sensation and the ability to achieve psychogenic lubrication must still be tested in a laboratory.

Psychogenic lubrication is reported as "possible" with lower motor neuron complete injury affecting the sacral cord (Berard, 1989). This is consistent with the site of the neurologic damage and with self-report studies of males in which 25% were reported to attain psychogenic erections while none achieved reflex erections (Bors & Comarr, 1960). Of the 25% of males achieving psychogenic erections, 18% were noted to ejaculate (Bors & Comarr, 1960). Thus, if male and female sexual function are similar, 25% of women with complete lower motor neuron injuries in the sacral region can be expected to have psychogenic lubrication and 18% to have an ejaculatory equivalent. With lower motor neuron incomplete injury affecting the sacral cord, 95% of males were reported to have a combination of reflex and psychogenic erections, while ejaculation occurred in 70% (Bors & Comarr, 1960). Thus, one can hypothesize that 90%–95% of females with incomplete lower motor neuron damage should have combined psychogenic/reflex lubrication and the ejaculatory equivalent should occur in 70%.

Based on the neurologic pathways responsible for sexual functioning and Berard's descriptive information resulting from the questionnaire studies on SCI males, sexual function in women post-SCI can be predicted. In order to do this, it is important to know the level of injury, whether neurologic damage in the sacral spinal cord is complete or incomplete, and whether there is an upper or lower motor neuron injury affecting the sacral region. To date, no studies have attempted to examine this area in a laboratory setting and only one has done so by means of a questionnaire. Sipski and Alexander (1991) questioned women with varying degrees of SCI about lubrication, and results are shown in Table 4. Subjects with complete injuries reported they had only reflex or reflex combined with mental lubrication, while women with incomplete injuries reported the ability to achieve purely mental lubrication. It is notable that 16% reported they could not achieve lubrication at all, and, of those who could, 12% said it was insufficient for penetration.

ORGASM

In the same study, Sipski and Alexander (1991) examined the relationship between subjects' abilities to perceive orgasm and type of injury and noted no significant relationship. Perhaps this was partly because subjects defined their own orgasms and because orgasm is known to be, at least in part, a cerebral event. Furthermore, they noted that, to truly understand orgasm in the individual with SCI, laboratory analysis of the physiologic responses during the sexual response cycle must be performed. Although this study begins to examine, in greater detail, specific aspects of the female sexual response after SCI, it too is limited because of the reliance on self-report data. As stated previously, physiologic studies are necessary in women with varying types of SCI in order to understand whether reflex lubrication and/or psychogenic lubrication are maintained with different types of injuries. Moreover, the response described as orgasm in women with SCI must be examined in the laboratory to determine how physiologic responses such as blood pressure, heart rate, and respiratory rate compare to those in women without SCI, and what types of stimuli are most successful in allowing women to achieve orgasm.

MENSTRUATION

Spinal cord injury has long been known to affect the menstrual cycle. As early as 1952, Cooper and Hoen noted the absence of menses for 3–6 months post-SCI, with scanty flow when cycles resumed. Comarr (1966) reported on the menses of 25 women with SCI. No significant relation was found between level or type of injury and interruption of the menstrual cycle. Fifty percent of the women queried had amenorrhea following SCI with resumption of menstruation within 6 months. Comarr concluded that those women with regular cycles pre-injury would maintain regular cycles post-injury and that dysmenorrhea would cease post-injury.

Table 4. Lubrication

Response	Quadriplegic complete (n = 5)	Quadriplegic incomplete (n = 9)	Paraplegic complete (n = 4)	Paraplegic incomplete (n = 7)
Don't know	40	11	50	14
No	20	11	25	14
Yes, reflex only	20	22	25	0
Yes, mental only	0	22	0	14
Yes, combination	20	33	0	57

From Sipski, M.L., & Alexander, C.J. (in press). Sexual activities and satisfaction in females pre- and post-spinal cord injury. *Archives of Physical Medicine and Rehabilitation;* reprinted by permission.

In 1968, Durkan studied seven patients with high traumatic SCI noting that amenorrhea had persisted from 9 months to 14 years. Four patients spontaneously resumed their menses, two patients remained amenorrheic, and one responded to gonadotropins. No information was given on dysmenorrhea.

The most comprehensive study on menstruation was reported by Axel (1982), who interviewed 32 women with SCI. Fifty-eight percent noted an interruption of menses for an average of 5 months with a range of 1.25–12 months. The menstrual cycle was variable in 6% of women pre-SCI and 9% post-SCI. Eleven percent noted an increase in time between cycles, 11% noted a decrease, and 68% reported no change. Duration of flow was variable in 3% of women, increased in 14%, decreased in 23%, and remained the same in 60%. Amount of flow was increased in 9%, decreased in 15%, and unchanged in 76%. Unlike the results in Comarr's study, 22% of the subjects interviewed noted greater menstrual discomfort post-SCI. Fifty-six percent reported no change in the level of discomfort, and only 22% noted decreased discomfort post-SCI.

Although these studies provide basic information regarding the effects of SCI on the menses, all data collected are retrospective and, thus, its accuracy is questionable. Studies begun immediately post-injury are needed for more accurate detail regarding the changes in the menstrual cycle after SCI.

In conclusion, female sexual dysfunction after SCI has not been adequately studied. Questionnaire studies pertaining to the effects of SCI on sexuality must be accompanied by detailed neurologic data and, ideally, should begin immediately post-SCI so that previous sexual functioning can be accurately recalled. Future research must more accurately examine the female sexual response, including lubrication and orgasm with varying types of SCI. This will require physiologic, rather than self-report, studies. Only after such information is obtained can accurate prognostication of female sexual function after SCI be possible. With knowledge of the natural history of the condition, future development and evaluation of treatment interventions aimed at improvement of anorgasmia or loss of psychogenic lubrication will be facilitated.

REFERENCES

Axel, S.J. (1982). Spinal cord injured women's concerns: Menstruation and pregnancy. *Rehabilitation Nursing, 7,* 10–15.

Berard, E.J.J. (1989). The sexuality of spinal cord injured women: Physiology and pathophysiology. A review. *Paraplegia, 27,* 99–112.

Bors, E., & Comarr, A.E. (1960). Neurological disturbances of sexual function with special reference to 529 patients with spinal cord injury. *Urological Survey, 110,* 191.

Bregman, S., & Hadley, R.G. (1976). Sexual adjustment and feminine attractiveness among spinal cord injured women. *Archives of Physical Medicine and Rehabilitation, 57,* 448–450.

Cole, T.M. (1979). Sexuality and the spinal cord injured. In R. Green (Ed.), *Human sexuality: A health practitioner's text* (2nd ed., pp. 243–263). Baltimore: Williams & Wilkins.

Comarr, A.E. (1966). Observations on menstruation and pregnancy among female spinal cord injury patients. *Paraplegia, 3,* 263–272.

Comarr, A.E., & Vigue, M. (1978). Sexual counseling among male and female patients with spinal cord and/or cauda equina injury. *American Journal of Physical Medicine, 57,* 215–228.

Cooper, I.S., & Hoen, T.I. (1952). Metabolic disorders in paraplegics. *Neurology, 2,* 332–340.

Durkan, J.P. (1968). Menstruation after high spinal cord transection. *American Journal of Obstetrics and Gynecology, 100,* 521–524.

Fitting, M.D., Salisbury, S., Davies, N.H., & Mayclin, K. (1978). Self-concept and sexuality of spinal cord injured women. *Archives of Sexual Behavior, 7,* 143–156.

Griffith, E.R., & Trieschmann, R.B. (1975). Sexual functioning in women with spinal cord injury. *Archives of Physical Medicine and Rehabilitation, 56,* 18–21.

Leyson, J.F. (1983). Electromyographic (EMG) urodynamic anal probe as a diagnostic tool in the management of sexual dysfunctions in female spinal cord injured patients. *Journal of the American Paraplegia Society, 6,* 79–80.

Masters, W.H., & Johnson, V.E. (1966). *Human sexual response.* Boston: Little, Brown.

Money, J. (1960). Phantom orgasm in the dreams of paraplegic men and women. *Archives of General Psychiatry, 3,* 372–383.

Sipski, M.L. (1991). Spinal cord injury: What is the effect on sexual response? *Journal of the American Paraplegia Society, 14,* 40–43.

Sipski, M.L., & Alexander, C.J. (in press). Sexual activities and satisfaction in females pre- and post-spinal cord injury. *Archives of Physical Medicine and Rehabilitation.*

Weiss, A.J., & Diamond, M.D. (1966). Sexual adjustment, identification, and attitudes of patients with myelopathy. *Archives of Physical Medicine and Rehabilitation, 47,* 245–250.

19

A Summary of Normal Female Reproductive Physiology

Sandra Ann Carson

The female reproductive system functions through the integration and complex interaction of many systems (Figure 1). Each level of this systematic hierarchy stimulates its successor and receives hormonal feedback, which both facilitates and inhibits its own function. These complex interactions are designed with one goal: the propagation of the human species. This important obligation requires the female reproductive system to be ready each month to nurture a fertilized ovum and, in the absence of such opportunity, to reprogram and ready itself quickly in the following month for another possible pregnancy. Each level of the system has important functions in meeting this goal.

The central nervous system synthesizes a host of chemicals that influence the hypothalamus. The neurotransmitters norepinephrine and serotonin facilitate gonadotropin-releasing hormone (GnRH) pulses secreted by the hypothalamus. Dopamine inhibits GnRH release; opiates also influence the hypothalamus and decrease GnRH. The neurotransmitters influence the function of the hypothalamus at all levels, but reproductive function is directly influenced in the arcuate nucleus. The hypothalamic response to the neurotransmitters varies at different times of the menstrual cycle, reflecting effects of the ovarian steroid milieu. These compounds are altered in times of stress, by extremes of weight, and by administration of certain drugs, particularly antihypertensives, an-

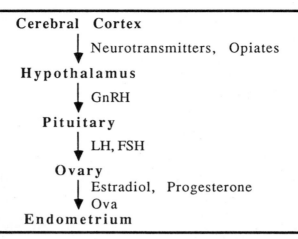

Figure 1. Systematic hierarchy of the female reproductive system.

tidepressants, and tranquilizers. The compounds are also altered acutely in acquired disability from an accident.

CONTROL OF GnRH

The hypothalamic neurons synthesize gonadotropin-releasing hormone in the cell bodies that lie in the arcuate nucleus. The neuronal axons extend down the pituitary stalk to synapse on blood vessels comprising the pituitary portal system. GnRH, packaged in small vessels, is transmitted down the long axons and released in the blood vessels of the portal system.

A small decapeptide, GnRH has a half-life of about 4 minutes. After secretion into the portal vessels, GnRH travels to the pituitary where it binds to specific receptors and is degraded. Very little GnRH is secreted into the peripheral circulation.

GnRH secretion is also unusual by its pulsatile pattern. GnRH pulses lasting approximately 6 minutes occur every 60–90 minutes in the human. This pulse frequency has a very narrow range before normal function is altered: Pulses more frequent than every 30 minutes or less than every 2 hours stop pituitary function and, consequently, gonadal function. GnRH pulse amplitude and frequency are influenced by neurotransmitters. Conditions altering the neurotransmitter balance sensed by the hypothalamus will ultimately interfere with GnRH pulse frequency with subsequent pituitary effects.

GONADOTROPINS

The role of GnRH in the pituitary is to stimulate both the synthesis and release of the gonadotropins, follicle-stimulating hormone (FSH), and luteinizing hormone (LH). Both gonadotropins consist of 2 polypeptides, one α and one β chain. The α chains are almost identical in LH, FSH, thyroid-stimulating hormone (TSH), and human chorionic gonadotropin (hCG). It is the β chain of all of these hormones that confers molecular specificity and individual biologic function to each. It is also through binding sites on the β chains that serum concentrations of these gonadotropins are measured by radio-immuno assays (RIAs).

Both LH and FSH are synthesized in the pituitary gonadotroph. These cells respond to stimulation by GnRH pulses differently during different times of the menstrual cycle, depending on the concentrations of ovarian steroids. For example, GnRH pulses in a low-estradiol environment stimulate high FSH release, whereas the same GnRH pulses in a high-estradiol environment stimulate low FSH release (Figure 2). This feedback is important in modulating gonadotropin release, particularly the midcycle LH and FSH surge.

During the first days of the menstrual cycle, LH is at its nadir; FSH is at its highest follicular phase concentration until the midcycle surge (Figure 3). As ovarian follicles develop and secrete increasing concentrations of estradiol during the follicular phase, the pituitary increases its secretion of LH but decreases its secretion of FSH.

OVARY

When the ovary develops a single dominant follicle, estradiol is produced at its follicular phase maximum, and progesterone secretion begins when the follicle is ready to release its ovum. It is the simultaneous rise in progesterone in the presence of the elevated estradiol concentration that the pituitary interprets as ovarian "readiness" for ovulation, and releases the midcycle surge of LH and FSH. Although the pituitary surge is the trigger for ovum release, it is actually the ovary that signals the pituitary of its readiness. This process is termed the "ovarian clock" and suggests that defective follicular development interferes with ovulation as easily as do pituitary disorders.

Gonadotropin function and ovarian follicular development are clearly interrelated at several levels. Ovarian follicular development

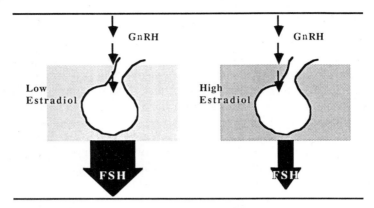

Figure 2. Pituitary release of FSH is modulated by the estradiol environment.

depends on the gonadotropins. Early in the cycle, 7–10 follicles are recruited for stimulation by a gonadotropin-independent process about which little is known. Once recruited, these follicles are stimulated by FSH to grow and produce estradiol.

Receptors for FSH and LH progressively increase in the follicles. The follicle that develops the highest estradiol environment develops more FSH receptors and becomes more sensitive to the dropping follicular phase concentrations of FSH (see Figure 3). The other follicles develop a more androgen-dominant environment, fail to develop receptors that would allow them to respond to lower levels of FSH, and thus become atretic. Eventually, one ovarian follicle becomes dominant and destined for ovulation. Approximately 36 hours after the initiation of the midcycle LH surge, the dominant follicle ovu-

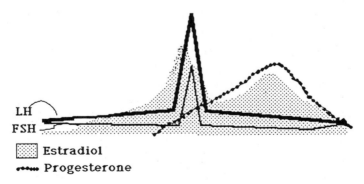

Figure 3. Schematic diagram of hormonal changes throughout the menstrual cycle.

lates. The follicle then is invaded by blood vessels and hormone production is increased dramatically. Cholesterol is concentrated in the follicle in order to have steroid precursors readily available. The cholesterol storage gives the follicle its yellow color and has led to the term corpus luteum, or "yellow body." The corpus luteum produces both estradiol and progesterone, both of which peak approximately 7 days after ovulation (Figure 3). It is the progesterone production during the luteal phase that results in physical changes that provide most presumptive evidence that ovulation has taken place (Table 1).

Progesterone has a thermogenic effect and is responsible for the 0.6° F rise in basal body temperature that occurs in the luteal phase. This hormone also reverts the thin, elastic cervical mucus, classic of the follicular phase, to a thick and sticky gel. If monitored daily, changes in cervical mucus lend presumptive evidence that ovulation occurred. Progesterone also results in secretory changes in the endometrium, which may be documented through an endometrial biopsy.

In addition to hormone production, the ovary is, of course, the source of oocytes. The oocytes reach their maximum number when the woman herself is a fetus at 20 weeks gestation. At this time, the oocytes have entered meiosis I, which is not completed until ovulation. Meiosis II is completed only upon fertilization. Oocyte numbers decline steadily throughout life until only 600,000 remain at the time of puberty. Nonetheless, this number is well in excess of the 400–500 oocytes released during a woman's reproductive years. When ovulated, the oocyte sits on a mound of granulosa cells atop the dominant follicle. The fimbria of the fallopian tube freely traverse the surface of the ovary to sweep the oocyte from its granulosa pedestal.

Table 1.   Definite and presumptive evidence of ovulation

Definite evidence of ovulation
   Pregnancy
   Laparoscopic visualization of oocyte release

Presumptive evidence of ovulation
   LH surge
   Progesterone concentration > 4 ng/ml
   Secretory endometrium
   Cervical mucus thickening
   0.6° F rise in base body temperature

FERTILIZATION AND EMBRYONIC DEVELOPMENT

The oocyte is fertilized in the fallopian tube. If intercourse has occurred recently, sperm reside throughout the entire reproductive tract. Those present in the ampulla of the tube bind to the ovum's outer covering, the zona pellucida. Once a sperm penetrates the zona, biochemical changes in the zona pellucida help prevent more sperm from penetrating. The sperm then binds to the plasma membrane and enters the ovum. After penetration, the oocyte undergoes a "cortical reaction" in which small granules appear just below the cell membrane and prevent any further penetration in the unlikely event that other sperm have traversed the zona pellucida.

Fertilization in the human requires up to 18 hours, and the first cell division occurs approximately 24 hours after fertilization. The second cell division also takes about 24 hours. Thereafter, cell divisions occur much more rapidly. These initial human cell divisions take place in the fallopian tube, where the embryo resides for about 3 days. The tubal fluid provides the nutrients necessary for continued cell division. Approximately 4 days after fertilization, the embryo enters the uterus, where it remains freely floating for another 3 days. During the 6–7 days between ovulation and implantation, the embryo develops into a 200–300 cell blastocyst. The blastocyst has begun to differentiate: The trophectoderm layer of cells is destined to become the placenta, and the inner cell mass becomes the fetus. Despite the increased number of cells, the embryo has not grown in size and remains within the walls of the zona pellucida. In addition to preventing polyspermy as discussed above, the zona pellucida also serves to keep the early embryonic cells in contact with each other. This cell contact seems important for cell differentiation. Immediately prior to implantation, the embryo hatches from its zona. Implantation occurs on Day 21 of the menstrual cycle in an endometrium that is lush, full of engorged blood vessels, and glycogen-laden secretory glands.

ENDOMETRIAL DEVELOPMENT

The endometrial development to prepare for implantation takes approximately 3 weeks, a phenomenon made possible by the hormonal milieu provided by the ovarian follicle. In the early follicular phase, estrogen levels begin to rise and stabilize the shedding menstrual flow. Rising levels of estradiol stimulate mitosis of the endometrial stroma and glandular development begins. In the follicular phase, glands proliferate; however, they show no secretions and remain long and straight. Blood vessels in the endometrium are also straight during the follicular phase. Stromal cells proliferate, but the cellular stroma contains little edema. After ovulation, progesterone stops the stimulation of endometrium by estradiol. Although the endometrium thickens a little during the luteal phase, the main influence of progesterone is to stimulate glandular secretions that are glycogen-rich and to stimulate blood vessels to grow, coil, and become engorged. In addition, the vessels of the endometrium become porous and the endometrial stroma, edematous. An implanting blastocyst is able to invade the vessel walls and gain access to the maternal vascular system. Decidualization of the endometrial stroma during pregnancy, predominantly a progesterone effect, serves to limit the invading trophoblast from progressing into the myometrium. This protects the maternal organism and provides a layer of cleavage at which the placenta will later separate.

In the absence of an implanting blastocyst, the corpus luteum no longer delivers the abundance of steroid hormones to the endometrium after mid-luteal phase. The lower steroid levels can no longer support the thick endometrium, leading to disruption of vessels and glands. Cells release lytic enzyme that lyse and necrose the upper layers of endometrium. The lining then sloughs as a menstrual period, and the entire cycle begins again.

CERVICAL MUCUS

The female reproductive system must also host the male gametes and lead them to the site of fertilization. This is one major function of the cervical mucus. As mentioned earlier, the cervical mucus also reflects changes in the hormonal milieu of the menstrual cycle. During the early follicular phase, the cervical mucus is almost absent. In the 5 days prior to ovulation, increasing estradiol concentrations stimulate the production of mucus by the cervical glands. The mucus is clear and "stretchable" at this time. Presumably, the mucus serves to introduce sperm to the upper reproductive tract after intercourse. In addition, the alkaline nature of the mucus serves to protect the sperm from the acidity of the vagina, to feed and to store them in order to provide a continued source of sperm in search of an ovum. After ovulation, progesterone causes the cervical mucus to thicken, making it sticky and "hostile" to sperm. However, the mucus may also prevent bacteria from entering the upper reproductive tract during the time when a fertilized ovum may be present.

Clearly, the integrated function of the many aspects of the female reproductive system have been designed with the ultimate goal of reproduction. The many checks and balances not only serve to prevent the system from going awry, but also provide opportunities for external control. In these ways, we have been able to control female reproduction far more consistently, reversibly, and with fewer undesirable side effects than ever before.

SUGGESTED ADDITIONAL READINGS

Mishell, D.R., & Davajan, V. (1989). *Reproductive endocrinology, infertility and contraception* (2nd ed.). Philadelphia: F.A. Davis.
Speroff, L., Glass, R.H., & Kase, N.G. (1989). *Clinical gynecologic endocrinology and infertility* (4th ed.). Baltimore: Williams & Wilkins.
Yen, A.A.S., & Jaffe, R.B. (1986). *Reproductive endocrinology* (2nd ed.). Philadelphia: W.B. Saunders.

20

Sexuality Issues after Traumatic Brain Injury
Clinical and Research Perspectives

Nathan D. Zasler

Brain injury may adversely affect the expression of sexuality secondary to alterations of both genital and nongenital function. Before the functional ramifications of such injuries on sexual function can be discussed and understood, it is critical to have an understanding of the basic neuroanatomic pathways and neurophysiologic mechanisms involved in the mediation of sexual function. Appropriate neuromedical and rehabilitative intervention should be available to individuals with traumatic brain injury to allow maximal reintegration into pre-injury sexual lifestyles at the community, personal, and family level.

REVIEW OF RELEVANT RESEARCH LITERATURE

There is a significant dearth of clinical research studies examining specific issues related to sexual dysfunction following traumatic brain injury. Most of the more methodologically sound studies examining sexuality issues from a holistic perspective have been performed since 1980. Bond (1976) was one of the first researchers to examine issues of psychosocial changes arising from severe brain

This work was partly supported by Grant No. G0087C0219 from the National Institute on Disability and Rehabilitation Research, United States Department of Education.

injury via interview assessments. He found that there was not a relationship between post-traumatic amnesia, level of physical disability, the level of cognitive impairment, and level of sexual activity. Specific sexual function patterns were not examined in Bond's study.

Rosenbaum and Najenson (1976) interviewed wives of wartime neurotrauma patients, with both brain and spinal cord injuries. Reduced sexual function and emotional distress were more often present in the group with brain injury relative to a group of controls with no injuries. They also reported the greatest level of mood disturbance for the wives of persons with brain injury, relative to the group with spinal cord injury and the control group. No clear-cut relationship was found between the locus of injury and the specific sexual dysfunction reported. In a secondary analysis by the same authors, a 22-item mood inventory was utilized to assess the relationship between mood disturbance and sexual activity level. Data analysis revealed that greater levels of mood disturbance were associated with decreased levels of sexual activity. Additionally, negative attitudes toward perceived sexual changes were associated with a lower mood level.

Oddy and colleagues studied 50 adults with TBI who were at least 6 months post-injury and who had a minimum of 24 hours of post-traumatic amnesia (Oddy, Humphrey, & Uttley, 1978). Half of the 12 married patients reported an increase in sexual intercourse and half reported a decrease. In a subsequent study, Oddy and Humphrey (1980) investigated alterations in sexual behavior 1 year post-injury. Just under 50% of spouses reported that they were significantly less affectionate toward their injured spouses. Oddy and colleagues in 1985 followed up their original group of patients at 7 years post-injury, but data regarding sexual activity were not included (Oddy, Coughlan, Tyerman, & Jenkins, 1985).

In 1978, Lezak reported that many patients suffered from completely absent libido and some from increased sexual drive (Lezak, 1978). Alterations in sexual interest, as well as behavior problems, reportedly contributed to family and marital difficulties. Lezak theorized that spouses were sexually frustrated, in part due to their spouses' poor interpersonal skills and diminished capacity for empathy.

Social adjustment 2 years after severe TBI was assessed by Weddell and colleagues who interviewed relatives of a group of patients who had completed a rehabilitation program (Weddell, Oddy, & Jenkins, 1980). Although no direct inquiries were made regarding sexuality issues, personality changes were examined. Irritability was listed as the most frequent alteration from a behavioral standpoint, followed by alterations in expression of affection. Other common behavioral sequelae included childishness, disinhibition, and increased talkativeness.

One of the best early studies on sexual function alterations following brain injury was done by Kosteljanetz and colleagues on a group of 19 post-concussional male patients. They found that a majority of patients (53%) reported reduced libido and that a lesser but still significant percentage (42%) reported erectile dysfunction. A positive correlation was noted between reports of sexual dysfunction and intellectual impairment (Kosteljanetz, Jensen, Norgard, Lunde, Jenson, & Johnsen, 1981).

A survey of wives and mothers of male patients with brain injury, not necessarily post-traumatic, by Mauss-Clum and Ryan (1981) found that a large proportion of the respondents reported that the survivor was either disinterested in sex or preoccupied with it. Forty-two percent of wives reported that they had no sexual outlet.

Kreutzer and Zasler administered the PAQ (Psychosexual Assessment Questionnaire) to 21 sexually active (post-injury) male patients following TBI (Kreutzer & Zasler, 1989). They found that the majority reported negative changes in sexual behavior including decreased libido, erectile dysfunction, and decreased frequency of intercourse. Common personality changes included depression and reduced self-esteem and sex appeal. There did not seem to be any relationship between the level of affectual change and alterations, negative or positive, in sexual behavior. Interestingly, despite these negative changes, there was evidence that the marital relationship quality was preserved relative to pre-injury.

Garden, Bontke, and Hoffman (1990) studied the status of 11 men and 4 women post-traumatic brain injury at least 2 months prior to evaluation. Both the spouses and the patients completed a sexual history and function questionnaire. Although a variety of factors were assessed including libido; intercourse frequency; time spent in foreplay; sexual attractiveness; erectile, ejaculatory, and orgasmic capabilities, and marital adjustment, only a few strong correlations were found. Intercourse frequency decreased for 75% of female patients, while 55% of the male patients reported a decline. Interestingly, although male genital sexual dysfunction rarely was reported, female spouses reported a significant decline in their ability to achieve orgasm after their partner was injured (Garden, Bontke, & Hoffman, 1990).

In a recent article, O'Carroll, Woodrow, and Maroun (1991) examined the psychosexual and psychosocial sequelae of TBI in a series of 36 patients followed for up to 4 years post-injury. Using several previously validated scales, they assessed both patients and partners. Approximately one half of all male patients scored within the dysfunctional range on the psychosexual profiles. The major psychosexual complaint was decreased frequency of sexual intimacy. A large number of patients demonstrated significant emotional distress, and/or anxiety, and/or depression (61%, 25%, and 22%, respectively). Of the partners evaluated, the percentages were 41%, 18%, and 6%, respectively. Findings did not seem to correlate with severity of neurologic insult; however, age and time post-injury were related to degree of psychosexual dysfunction.

In summary, it becomes readily apparent to even the novice researcher that the literature in the area of traumatic brain injury and sexuality and sexual function is significantly lacking. Few studies have focused specifically on sexual behavior, and the results have been somewhat disparate in the few that have. Many of the commonly quoted studies are at best anecdotal reports and do not provide any empirical evidence to guide clinical decision-making or to relate to patients and families. Given the multiplicity of sequelae of TBI, including physical, emotional, cognitive, and behavioral, it is not surprising that alterations occur in sexuality as well as sexual function. As of now, we have only a sense of the magnitude of this area of functional deficit, which is unfortunate given the importance of sexuality to most persons, single or married.

PHYSIATRIC ASSESSMENT OF SEXUALITY ISSUES

Traumatic brain injury can result in sexual problems due to a number of factors including nongenital and genital dysfunction. Genital dysfunction may result in erectile dysfunction, ejaculatory problems, orgasmic dysfunction, vaginal lubrication problems, and vaginismus. Nongenital problems that may adversely affect sexual intimacy include sensorimotor deficits, linguistic-pragmatic deficits, perceptual deficits, limited joint range of motion, neurogenic bowel/bladder dysfunction, dysphagia with or without problems controlling secretions, motor dyspraxias, post-traumatic behavioral deficits, as well as alterations in self-image and self-esteem (Zasler & Horn, 1990).

There is not much literature available that might assist neurorehabilitationists in gaining an appreciation for the clinical assessment of sexual function in an individual following a traumatic brain injury. Professionals working with this patient population must have an appreciation for the appropriate neuromedical assessment and management of this class of functional deficits. One protocol that has been proposed is the GRASP (General Rehabilitation Assessment Sexuality Profile), which divides assessment into sexual history, sexual physical exam, and clinical diagnostic testing (Zasler & Horn, 1990).

Sexual History

A complete sexual history defines needs, expectations, and behavior. Additionally, it identifies problems, misconceptions, and areas for education, counseling, and reassurance in relation to sexuality issues. Interviews should be conducted with both the patient and the sexual partner where applicable and possible. The assessment should include demographic and personal information. The patient's medical history is essential to clarify any and all medical disorders that could potentially affect sexual function. Premorbid sexual functioning, practices, and relationships should be explored. Both sexes should be questioned about their specific genital function. Patients and couples should be questioned regarding their specific concerns (e.g., birth control, fertility, genital dysfunction, libidinal alterations). Sexuality issues may not be important for all professionals. Key points when interviewing include providing a private atmosphere, not rushing the interview, being frank yet empathetic, using nondirective techniques, and using vocabulary appropriate to the patient. Professionals should avoid putting the patient in a position that conflicts with his or her moral or ethical beliefs. Lastly, the status of an individual's sexual preference should never be assumed and should always be discussed. Ultimately, the interview can serve as a foundation for demonstrating to the patient that he or she has a right to be sexual just like anyone else and that sexual expression resulting in intimacy, not necessarily vaginal intercourse, is the goal of the process (Zasler, 1991).

Sexual Physical Exam

The sexual physical exam really begins when the clinician first sees the patient. Mobility deficits may give clues to physical limitations that may adversely affect sexuality and sexual function. The flexibility of the hips and degree of adductor spasticity are of particular importance. During the examination, the clinician should note the patient's general hygiene status and use of adaptive equipment. The genitals should be examined from both a neurologic and non-neurologic standpoint. In the female, the genitalia should first be inspected, followed by a bimanual examination. If the primary physician does not feel comfortable performing a bimanual exam then a referral should be made to a qualified physician. The vaginal walls should be evaluated for tone and mucosal alterations. In the male, the penis should be palpated for presence of plaques, as are found in Peyronie's disease. Testicular presence in the scrotal sacs should be assessed as should size and consistency. In both males and females, the clinician should check hair distribution in the genital region and in locations of secondary sexual hair growth to rule out possible endocrinopathies that could be either primary or secondary in nature. The neurologic assessment of the genitalia should include a rectal exam, sensory testing, and assessment of lumbosacral reflex integrity. The skilled clinician can utilize the information from bedside testing to guide recommendations as well as to prognosticate genital sexual function relative to the neurologic insult in question (Zasler, 1991; Zasler & Horn, 1990).

Clinical Sexual Diagnostic Testing

Urodynamics may assist the neurorehabilitationist in gaining a better understanding of the integrity of sexual organ innervation. Afferent neurologic assessment can be accomplished with penile biothesiometry and/or dorsal nerve somatosensory evoked potentials. Efferent neurologic assessment, whether motor or autonomic, can be accomplished in a gross manner via nocturnal penile tumescence (NPT) and/or response to intracavernosal pharmacotherapy (ICP). Female clinical assessment is less sophisticated; however, photoplethysmography and heat electrode techniques have been utilized to assess vaginal hemodynamics and can be employed to treat orgasmic and arousal deficits via biofeedback training (Zasler, 1991; Zasler & Horn, 1990).

PHYSIATRIC MANAGEMENT OF SEXUAL DYSFUNCTION

The physiatric management of sexual dysfunction must take into consideration the many issues that may directly or indirectly contribute to alterations in sexual function following traumatic brain injury. Neuroendocrine dysfunction may occur following TBI; however, the general clinical experience has been that this phenomenon is relatively rare in the TBI population. Initial laboratory evaluation should include assessment of FSH, LH, PRL, and free testosterone in males. In females, the same hormones should be assessed, in addition to estradiol and dehydroepiandrosterone. Clinicians should keep in mind that other factors may contribute to neuroendocrine abnormalities, the most common in this patient population being medications and, in the acute care setting, physiologic stress factors.

In postpubertal females, cyclic administration of oral estrogen-progesterone preparations will restore the menstrual cycle, maintain secondary sexual characteristics, and reduce the risk for osteoporosis. In the postpubertal male, hypogonadism may be treated with intramuscular testosterone replacement, typically given every 2–4 weeks. In cases of delayed puberty, treatment should begin during adolescence; males are typically treated with hCG for 1–2 years followed by maintenance testosterone therapy and in females, cyclic estrogen and progesterone therapy is instituted to establish menses and secondary sexual characteristics (Zasler & Horn, 1990).

The skilled neurorehabilitationist should also examine other areas of nongenital neurologic impairment to assess potential treatment, whether pharmacologic, surgical, or compensatory, for these specific deficits. Sensorimotor deficits, cognitive-behavioral deficits, language-based alterations, changes in libido, as well as neurogenic bowel and bladder dysfunction, can all be addressed by the clinician as they affect the ability for sexual expression. (See Zasler & Horn, 1990, for more in-depth discussion on management strategies.)

Genital sexual dysfunction after TBI may take a number of forms. Males may present with erectile, ejaculatory, and/or orgasmic dysfunction. The present state-of-the-art in neurourologic management of erectile dysfunction focuses on one of three main treatment categories: penile prostheses, intracavernosal pharmacotherapy, and external management. Enteral agents have been used, including dopamine agonists and noradrenergic agonists such as yohimbine; however, research is ongoing relative to their efficacy in this patient population. Problems with premature ejaculation should first be addressed behaviorally to assess how much of the problem is functionally based. Methods such as the "squeeze" technique can be taught to the patient and partner. On occasion, medication might be considered for the male patient suffering from premature ejaculation; this might include topical anesthestic applied to the penile shaft or anticholinergic medication administered enterally. Orgasmic dysfunction is generally approached from a behavioral standpoint in both men and women. Females may complain of alterations in vaginal lubrication and/or orgasmic dysfunction. Inadequate vaginal lubrication can generally be addressed by artificial lubrication with water-soluble products. Behavioral therapy, including imagery and body exploration/sensitization training, may benefit some females who have arousal or orgasmic dysfunction (Zasler, 1991).

Patients as well as family members should be counseled regarding dealing with sexuality issues in the home and community

(Zasler & Kreutzer, 1991). All patients should be instructed relative to safer sex practices, issues regarding sexually transmitted disease, and appropriate birth control (Zasler & Horn, 1990).

CONCLUSIONS

Professionals are just beginning to examine the neurologic and functional ramifications of traumatic brain injury on sexual function. Currently, there is a relative dearth of information on which clinicians can base prognostication, assessment, or treatment; however, our knowledge base is expanding slowly but surely. Better acknowledgment of the importance of sexuality and sexual function to the quality of life may stimulate researchers and clinicians to allocate more resources to answering many of the questions that remain. In the interim, clinicians and researchers should be aware of the importance of sexual expression to other areas of human function following TBI. Awareness, in and of itself, will provide an impetus for further critical examination of this important area of psychological and physiologic function.

REFERENCES

Bond, M.R. (1976). Assessment of psychosocial outcome of severe head injury. *Acta Neurochirurgica, 34,* 57–70.

Garden, F.H., Bontke, C.F., & Hoffman, M. (1990). Sexual functioning and marital adjustment after traumatic brain injury. *Journal of Head Trauma Rehabilitation, 5*(2), 52–59.

Herzog, A. (1984). Endocrinological aspects of epilepsy. *Neurology and Neurosurgery Update Series, 5*(11).

Horn, L.J., & Zasler, N.D. (1990). Neuroanatomy and neurophysiology of sexual function. *Journal of Head Trauma Rehabilitation, 5*(2), 1–13.

Kosteljanetz, M., Jensen, T.S., Norgard, B., Lunde, I., Jensen, P.B., & Johnsen, S.G. (1981). Sexual and hypothalamic dysfunction in postconcussional syndrome. *Acta Neurologica Scandinavica, 63,* 169–180.

Kreutzer, J.S., & Zasler, N.D. (1989). Psychosexual consequences of traumatic brain injury: Methodology and preliminary findings. *Brain Injury, 3*(2), 177–186.

Lezak, M.L. (1978). Living with the characterologically altered brain injured patient. *Journal of Clinical Psychiatry, 39,* 592–598.

Mauss-Clum, N., & Ryan, M. (1981). Brain injury and the family. *Journal of Neurosurgical Nursing, 13,* 165–169.

O'Carroll, R.E., Woodrow, J., & Maroun, F. (1991). Psychosexual and psychosocial sequelae of closed head injury. *Brain Injury, 5*(3), 303–313.

Oddy, M., Coughlan, T., Tyerman, A., & Jenkins, D. (1985). Social adjustment after closed head injury: A further follow-up seven years later. *Journal of Neurology, Neurosurgery, and Psychiatry, 48,* 564–568.

Oddy, M., & Humphrey, M. (1980). Social recovery during the first year following severe head injury. *Journal of Neurology, Neurosurgery, and Psychiatry, 43*, 798–802.

Oddy, M., Humphrey, M., & Uttley, D. (1978). Subjective impairment and social recovery after closed head injury. *Journal of Neurology, Neurosurgery, and Psychiatry, 41*, 611–616.

Rosenbaum, M., & Najenson, T. (1976). Changes in life patterns and symptoms of low mood as reported by wives of severely brain-injured soldiers. *Journal of Consulting and Clinical Psychology, 44*, 881–888.

Weddell, R., Oddy, M., & Jenkins, D. (1980). Social adjustment after rehabilitation: A two year follow-up of patients with severe head injury. *Psychological Medicine, 10*, 257–263.

Zasler, N.D. (1991). Sexuality in neurologic disability: An overview. *Sexuality and Disability, 9*(1), 11–27.

Zasler, N.D., & Horn, L.J. (1990). Rehabilitative management of sexual dysfunction. *Journal of Head Trauma Rehabilitation, 5*(2), 14–24.

Zasler, N.D., & Kreutzer, J.S. (1991). Family and sexuality after traumatic brain injury. In J. Williams & T. Kay (Eds.), *Head injury: A family matter* (pp. 253–270). Baltimore: Paul H. Brookes Publishing Co.

21

Spinal Cord Injured Women, Pregnancy, and Delivery

Walter H. Verduyn

The author's interest in pregnancy and delivery involving spinal cord injured women was sparked by his involvement with two of the spinal cord injured women in his hospital unit. As a result of the lack of significant information in the literature, an effort was made to collect information about a larger number of pregnancies and deliveries. The collected information was classified in different groupings in order to deal with a number of important issues related to the spinal cord injury.

CASE REPORTS

With the improvement of acute care and effective rehabilitation, pregnancy and delivery involving spinal cord injured women will occur more frequently. Our staff from the spinal cord injury reha-

---

This chapter is adapted from an article of the same title, originally published in 1986 in *Paraplegia, 24,* 231–240 and is reprinted and adapted by permission, copyright © 1986 International Medical Society of Paraplegia, Churchill Livingstone, Edinburgh.

Author's note: The problem of autonomic hyperreflexia during childbirth is a major threat to survival during childbirth to the woman with a spinal cord injury with a level of paralysis of thoracic 6 and above.

The paper, "Pregnancy and delivery of spinal cord women," published in *Paraplegia,* 1986, needs to be read by all physicians performing deliveries who might be involved in the pregnancies of women with spinal cord injuries. Publication of this paper in this volume is important because of the wider audience of health professionals who will read this.

bilitation unit felt fortunate when we had two tetraplegic patients who were pregnant. Staff members were involved in prenatal care, were present during delivery, and were involved with postnatal care. Potential problems were identified as: 1) early labor, 2) hyperreflexia, 3) urinary tract infection, and 4) spinal cord injury care.

Active early labor was stopped effectively with terbutaline. Hyperreflexia was controlled with amyl nitrate, Arfonad if needed, and if the hyperreflexia was uncontrollable, a cesarean section (c-section) would be performed with epidural anesthesia. Urinary tract infection was treated with long-term antibiotics such as ampicillin or Keflex, and related yeast vaginitis was treated with Mycostatin.

A case study was written on both of the pregnant women. Case number 1 was a C5–C6 tetraplegic who delivered a 2,339-gram baby girl with an Apgar score of 9–10. Case 2 was a C2–C7 subtotal resection ependymoma tetraplegic (incomplete) who delivered a 2,637-gram baby girl with an Apgar score of 8–10. Both babies were considered mature, with a gestational age of 38 weeks. Both babies were delivered with outlet forceps and did not need episiotomy. Babies were kept in reverse isolation in the newborn nursery. Mothers went back to the spinal cord injury unit after a few hours observation in the delivery room. A mail survey and literature review continues. So far, 33 spinal cord injured women were identified who delivered a total of 50 babies (2 sets of twins and 1 intrauterine death). In 22 of the 27 deliveries in women with injuries at T6 level and above, hyperreflexia occurred (Rossier, Ruffieux, & Ziegler, 1969, 1970) (7 c-sections, 1 after hyperreflexia developed). Twelve women were below T6 and delivered 23 babies (12 c-sections).

PATIENT SURVEY AND LITERATURE REVIEW

The separation of patients with a neurologic level of T6 and above from those with a level below T6 was primarily to separate out the women who were likely to have hyperreflexia. Of the 27 deliveries in the category of T6 and above, 22 had hyperreflexia. Seven had cesarean sections (one patient reported hyperreflexia as indication for cesarean section).

Of the total of 50 deliveries, there were 19 c-sections, certainly a high incidence. These were in 11 patients: 1 patient had 4 c-sections, 1 had 3 c-sections, 3 patients had 2 c-sections, and 6 patients each had 1. The indications given were hyperreflexia, ruptured membranes, and fear of bladder damage. The incidence of the use of forceps is 15, which is fairly high. There was one breech delivery.

Prematurity

There were only four premature births, one at 5 weeks, two at $6^{1}/_{2}$ weeks, and a pair of twins at 8 weeks. One was treated with terbutaline successfully and delivered 5 weeks early. One, a pair of twins, was born at 8 weeks, post c-section, because of presenting cord. There were some deliveries from 2 to 4 weeks prior to the expected due dates but not really premature. Post-maturity did not appear to be a real problem. The time varied from $1^{1}/_{2}$ weeks to 4 weeks.

With regard to birth control, pills were used by 9 women, either alone or in combination with IUD, condoms, or foam. The rhythm method was used by one patient, who had 5 pregnancies. One woman had artificial insemination.

Birth Weight

There were nine babies under 2,500 grams (1,361 g; 1,531 g; 1,616 g; 1,701 g; 1,871 g; 2,013 g; 2,098 g; 2,296 g; 2,325 g).

Anesthesia

Most of these babies were delivered without anesthesia. Some of the patients who had a cesarean section had general anesthesia. Epidural anesthesia (Watson & Downey, 1980) was used for six deliveries because of hyperreflexia.

Delivery complications were minor except for hyperreflexia. One patient induced with Pitocin sustained a cerebral intraventricular bleed and coma. There were two patients with prolapsed cord and one patient with ruptured membranes.

Postpartum Complications

The dehiscence of the episiotomy in two patients is probably significant for spinal cord injured women. Thrombophlebitis and pulmonary emboli should also be considered to be a risk of pregnancy in spinal cord injured women.

The problems related to pregnancy and delivery show a significant number of women with urinary tract infections (Greenland & Young, 1984; Young, Katz, & Klein, 1983). This is most likely related to the large number of women who had Foley catheters. Two women had bladder stones, and five had decubitus ulcers.

It is interesting to note that two women found that they had difficulties with their transfers toward the end of their pregnancies because of weight gain.

The treatment of hyperreflexia shows significant variation from epidural anesthesia (Watson & Downey, 1980), to general anesthesia, to the use of drugs, varying from amyl nitrate (Spector, 1983) to magnesium sulphate and Demerol. This most likely reflects the experience and practice of the physician managing the deliveries. It is noted that only two deliveries were managed by a spinal cord injury specialist. In four deliveries, the spinal cord injury specialist was a consultant. The great majority of the deliveries was done by an obstetrician (38), while four were done by a family practitioner/ general practitioner. One delivery was done by the father on the ranch because they just managed to reach the hospital for the previous delivery. They are expecting a third child.

One T4 paraplegic and one T12 paraplegic each had twins.

The congenital abnormality rate was not a special feature in these spinal cord injured women, but the sample is too small for any definite impressions. (Goller & Paeslack, 1980).

Problems of child following delivery: one anoxia, one Valium withdrawal, one possible Valium withdrawal.

It was noted that four women were pregnant at the time of their paralysis and three of them delivered normal babies. (Goller & Paeslack, 1972, 1980). The fourth patient had an intrauterine death with induction at 20 weeks.

Urinary bladder management varied widely from ileo conduit to intermittent catheterization. Controlled voiding was present in women with a cord lesion below T6. One was an incomplete tetraplegic at C5–C6. Many of the controlled-voiding women had required a catheter for a short time after delivery.

There were 5 inductions in this group. One was for intrauterine death, two were for recurring hyperreflexia, and two were done on the due date. In one of these, the induction was directly responsible for hyperreflexia and cerebral intraventricular bleed and coma. Only three blood pressures were taken over a 4-hour period (124/80, 140/90, 210/100; prenatal 106/60, 98/60, 110/54, 110/64). (McGregor & Meeuwsen, 1985). (Abouleish [1980] reported death 2 days postparum due to cerebral hemorrhage as a result of autonomic hyperreflexia.)

Comments by women were: "Problems with labor and delivery room staff," and, "I knew more than the docs." One woman reported that she called a nurse from the neighboring spinal cord injury hospital to come and manage her hyperreflexia. Several of the women felt that they were either overtreated or they were not believed about what they felt was necessary for their care.

One individual was severely overtreated at the time of delivery: She had an arterial line, CVP line, an epidural catheter, an intra-uterine catheter, a fetal scalp electrode, and a Foley catheter. She delivered a 2,013-gram baby approximately 5 weeks prior to due date. It was delivered vaginally by outlet forceps, after amniotomy and oxytocin. The indication for induction was hyperreflexia. Fortunately this patient did not have any iatrogenic complications after her delivery.

CONCLUSION

In reviewing the figures, I feel very strongly that those of us who treat spinal cord injured patients should take the initiative to be involved with their pregnancies and deliveries; possibly not actually doing the deliveries but certainly maintaining good communications with the obstetricians so that these patients are managed properly. Autonomic hyperreflexia, or dysreflexia, is a severe threat to SCI women with neurologic involvement at T6 and above.

I also feel it is essential for the staff of the spinal cord injury center to be involved in the postpartum care in order to teach quadriplegic women to care for their babies in the immediate postpartum period. I feel that the additional hospitalization necessary to accomplish this is certainly worthwhile.

RECOMMENDATIONS

1. Most spinal cord injured women know their disability well. Listen to the patient, ask questions about skin care, bowel care, and bladder care. Review patients' independence skills.
2. Instruct office staff and labor and delivery room staffs to be sensitive to the patient's special needs. She is the final authority with regard to her special needs in skin, bowel, and bladder care.
3. If the level of paralysis is T6 and above, the patient will probably have autonomic hyperreflexia or dysreflexia during her contractions while in labor. Ask if she has ever had hyperreflexia (this can occur with a full bladder, due to a plugged catheter or a spastic sphincter; it may occur during a bowel program or indeed from any prominent stimulus below the level of paralysis); and ask her how she manages such a complication. Many spinal cord injury centers give patients printed outlines concerning hyperreflexia.

4. Early labor is common in spinal cord injured women. Weekly checks after 32 weeks are prudent. If dilation occurs, bed rest in the hospital is advised (proper bowel, bladder, and skin care is needed). Brethine (terbutaline) is an effective drug to stop or prevent early labor, and other drugs have been developed.

5. Induction can be difficult in patients with a neurologic level of T6 and above because of the risk of hyperreflexia. In my opinion, induction is contraindicated in these women because of the complications of hyperreflexia, unless the physician and the delivery room staff understand hyperreflexia and are capable of monitoring and managing hyperreflexia.

6. If the physician accepting the obstetrical care of a spinal cord injured woman is not familiar with such patients, a consultation with a spinal cord injury center physician is recommended.

7. The spinal cord injured woman has a disability but is otherwise healthy. She needs proper medical care and close supervision by medical staff alerted to special problems when needed for her and her child.

8. Treat when needed, do not overtreat.

9. Most spinal cord injured women can deliver normal babies vaginally.

10. Always be aware of the threat of decubitus ulcers. Patients need to be turned and padded, especially if on a delivery table for a long time (leg straps could cause problems, especially if the patient is very spastic). The easiest place of delivery for a spinal cord injured woman is in bed.

REFERENCES

Abouleish, E. (1980). Hypertension in a paraplegic parturient. *Anesthesiology, 53*(4), 348–349.

Daw, E. (1973). Pregnancy problems in a paraplegic patient with an ileal conduit bladder. *Practitioner, 211,* 781–784.

Dickinson, F.T. (1977). Paraplegia in pregnancy and labor: Report of case and review of literature. *Journal of the American Osteopathic Association, 76,* 537–539.

Goller, H., & Paeslack, V. (1972). Pregnancy damage and birth complications in the children of paraplegic women. *Paraplegia, 10,* 213–217.

Goller, H., & Paeslack, V. (1980). Our experiences about pregnancy and delivery of the paraplegic woman. *Paraplegia, 8,* 161–166.

Greenland, V.C., & Young, B.K. (1984). When the mother is a paraplegic. *Contemporary Ob/Gyn, 24,* 201–210.

McGregor, J.A., & Meeuwsen, J. (1985). Autonomic hyperreflexia: A mortal danger for spinal cord-damaged women in labor. *American Journal of Obstetrics and Gynecology, 151,* 330–333.

Nath, M., Vivian, J., & Cherny, W. (1979). Autonomic hyperreflexia in pregnancy and labor: A case report. *American Journal of Obstetrics and Gynecology, 134,* 390–392.

Oppenheimer, W. (1971). Pregnancy in paraplegic patients: Two case reports. *American Journal of Obstetrics and Gynecology, 110,* 784–786.

Ravindran, R.S., Cummins, D.E., & Smith, I.E. (1981). Experience with the use of nitroprusside and subsequent epidural analgesia in a pregnant quadriplegic patient. *Anesthesia and Analgesia, 60*(1), 61–63.

Rossier, A., Ruffieux, M., & Ziegler, W. (1970). Faits cliniques [Clinical facts]. *Gynecologie et Obstetrique [Gynecology and Obstetrics]* 69, 537–543.

Rossier, A., Ruffieux, M., & Ziegler, W. (1969). Pregnancy and labour in high traumatic spinal cord lesions. *Paraplegia, 7,* 210–215.

Spector, R. (1983). Intravenous nitroglycerin: New uses for an old drug. *Journal of Iowa Medical Society, 73*(3), 96.

Tabsh, K.M.A., Brinkman, C.R., & Reff, R.A. (1982). Autonomic dysreflexia in pregnancy. *Obstetrics and Gynecology, 60*(1), 119–121.

Watson, D.W., & Downey, J.O. (1980). Epidural anesthesia for labor and delivery of twins of a paraplegic mother. *Anesthesiology, 52*(3), 259–261.

Young, R.K., Katz, M., & Klein, S.A. (1983). Pregnancy after spinal cord injuries: Altered maternal and fetal response to labor. *Obstetrics and Gynecology, 62*(1), 59–63.

22

Male Reproduction
Fertility

Richard V. Clark

Male infertility is defined as the inability to induce a pregnancy with unprotected intercourse with a presumably fertile female partner for a minimum period of 1 year (Sherins & Howards, 1986). Infertility involves a couple and, therefore, can be based on male factors, female factors, or both. A variety of clinical settings can be associated with infertility, and often patients are unaware of any existing abnormality. A male factor is suspected when the female partner shows a normal menstrual cycle with ovulation, adequate duration of the luteal phase, patency of the oviducts, and lack of pelvic pathology, especially endometriosis or tubal adhesions.

When evaluating a patient with spinal cord injury, as with any male with infertility, a directed history and physical examination with assessment of reproductive hormone levels and semen characteristics form the basis of evaluation (Table 1). Male factor infertility is suggested if the male has an abnormal semen analysis, with a low sperm count, poor motility, or abnormal morphology (Clark & Sherins, 1986). As is discussed, it is difficult to select minimal criteria for any of these values below which fertility is impossible, unless considering azoospermia or necrospermia (Silber & Rodriguez-Rigau, 1981). Evidence of hormonal abnormalities may indicate testicular failure, although most infertile men have normal reproductive hormone levels. Paraplegia or quadriplegia are associated with an increased incidence of prostatitis and elevated testicular temperature, and these factors should be especially considered during screening evaluations.

Table 1. Causes of male infertility

Potentially reversible	Usually irreversible
Gonadotropin deficiency	Chromosomal abnormality
Vas or epididymal occlusion	Androgen resistance
Retrograde ejaculation	Nonmotile sperm
Prostatitis, epididymitis	Mumps orchitis
Varicocele	Cryptorchidism
Drugs/toxins	Young syndrome
Heat exposure	Epididymal dysfunction
Sexual dysfunction	Absent vas deferens
Immune process	Radiation exposure
Systemic illness	

BACKGROUND: NORMAL PHYSIOLOGY

Differentiation of the male reproductive tract begins early in fetal life, between 6 and 12 weeks. It is dependent on secretion of two products from the fetal testes: 1) Mullerian inhibiting factor from Sertoli cells, which causes regression of the embryonic female tract and allows development of the male ducts—the epididymis, vas deferens, seminal vesicle, and ejaculatory duct; and 2) testosterone from Leydig cells, which induces differentiation of the Wolffian structures and formation of the male external genitalia (by intracellular conversion to dihydrotestosterone by 5 alpha-reductase). In addition, a testes-determining factor derived from a locus in the short arm of the Y chromosome is necessary for fetal testes formation. This factor appears distinct from the cell surface antigen, H-Y antigen, which had been previously proposed as the critical determinant for testicular differentiation. Testicular descent is dependent on normal testicular function and hormonal milieu as well as adequate intra-abdominal pressure. Puberty begins with nocturnal secretion of LH- and FSH-stimulating testosterone secretion and growth of the seminiferous epithelium.

Normal male reproductive function is dependent upon normal stimulatory signals from the hypothalamus in the form of pulsatile bursts of gonadotropin-releasing hormone (GnRH). GnRH, in turn, stimulates the pituitary gland to secrete both luteinizing hormone (LH) and follicle-stimulating hormone (FSH). LH and FSH, in turn, stimulate the testes to make both testosterone and sperm. Normal testicular function is dependent upon LH stimulation of Leydig cells to produce testosterone. Normal seminiferous tubular function and sperm production are dependent upon both elevated intra-testicular levels of testosterone as well as adequate stimulation by FSH. Interruption of any phase of this axis can lead to disruption of testicular function, causing either hypogonadism or infertility. Evaluation of the male includes measurement of reproductive hormones as well as evaluation of testicular size and semen analysis (Mortimer, Templeton, Linton, & Coleman, 1982). The following section covers the major disorders causing testicular dysfunction and the methods for evaluation.

OVERVIEW: MALE REPRODUCTIVE DYSFUNCTION

Disorders of the male reproductive system can be grouped into three broad categories. First is primary testicular failure—hypergonadotropic hypogonadism. These disorders are caused by primary testicular processes, resulting in failure of testicular function at either the level of Leydig cells or the seminiferous tubule. These disorders are characterized by low sex steroids but elevated gonadotropins, since negative feedback on the hypothalamus by testicular steroids and/or inhibin is lost. Clinically, patients with acquired testicular failure show evidence of hypogonadism with loss of libido, impotence, decreased muscle mass, and gradual loss of sex-dependent hair. Patients may also present with delayed puberty, and a eunuchoid habitus.

A second major category covers disorders characterized by impairment of hypothalamic or pituitary dysfunction, secondary testicular failure—hypogonadotropic hypogonadism—in which there is inadequate stimulation of the testes leading to inadequate levels of testosterone or impaired sperm production. These disorders are characterized by low gonadotropins and low sex steroids. The clinical presentation is also hypogonadism.

The third category, eugonadal testicular failure, which is the most common disorder of the male reproductive system, is characterized by male infertility with low sperm counts, but otherwise normal virilization and sexual function as well as normal testicular size and normal hormonal concentrations. This disorder is often called idiopathic male infertility, or idiopathic oligospermic infertility. The cause of impaired sperm production is not understood, but is likely multifactorial.

HYPERGONADOTROPIC SYNDROMES (TESTICULAR FAILURE)

Testicular Injury

A variety of factors can cause primary testicular injury. These include infectious agents, toxic agents, and direct radiation injury. A common condition in males is mumps orchitis, which can lead to acute inflammation of the testes with severe seminiferous tubule damage. In addition to the acute phase, there can be a gradual progression of residual inflammatory lesions, leading to some recovery after an acute injury, followed by a gradual failure of testicular function over several years. Mumps orchitis does not appear to occur before puberty.

Radiation causes direct injury to the spermatogonial cells producing the sperm. At doses of 400 rads–600 rads, recovery of testicular function is unlikely. Various chemical toxins, including pesticides, can cause injury to the seminiferous tubules. Elevated temperature, either in the form of a prolonged high fever or chronic exposure to very hot baths, can also lead to seminiferous tubule damage. Drugs used for cancer chemotherapy, especially procarbazine, chlorambucil, and cyclophosphamide, can severely damage the germinal epithelium. These patients are infertile and often have an elevated FSH as inhibin secretion from Sertoli cells is lost. In these conditions with pure germ cell injury, virilization and potency are usually maintained, and LH and testosterone are normal or near normal.

Klinefelter Syndrome

This is the most common primary testicular disorder that has a genetic basis. It is caused by an extra X chromosome, giving a karyotype of 47,XXY instead of the normal male karyotype of 46,XY. This disorder causes failure of development of seminiferous tubules, leading to azoospermia and gradual failure of Leydig cells, leading to inadequate testosterone levels. Seminiferous tubules in these patients rarely develop to any significant degree, and these patients are characterized by small testes—less than 6 mL in volume. Leydig cell function can persist in these patients for variable amounts of time, and many patients show normal puberty and virilization before overt Leydig cell failure begins in later decades. Definitive diagnosis is made by karyotype.

The classic presentation is delayed puberty with a eunuchoid habitus, gynecomastia, and small, firm testes. However, an increasing number of patients are now being identified on the basis of infertility and azoospermia, with or without evidence of late onset testicular failure, that is, impotence.

Reifenstein Syndrome

Androgen insensitivity is a broad condition that can range from very mild disorders, characterized only by hypospadias (the mildest developmental abnormality, reflecting incomplete fusion of the urethral

folds) to complete androgen insensitivity causing testicular feminiz-
ation with a normal female phenotype. These patients often present
with ambiguous genitalia, hypospadias, a bifid scrotum, diminished
virilization, and possibly gynecomastia. Diagnosis is difficult, rely-
ing heavily on clinical presentation. Evaluation of androgen binding
to the patient's genital skin fibroblasts provides the definitive diagnosis, but this technique is not readily available.

HYPOGONADOTROPIC SYNDROMES
(PITUITARY OR HYPOTHALAMIC FAILURE)

Hypogonadotropic Hypogonadism

Hypogonadotropic hypogonadism appears to be caused by an isolated impairment of the hypothalamus, leading to inadequate GnRH
stimulation of the pituitary gland. These patients fail to go through
puberty and are typically diagnosed between the ages of 16 and 20
for this reason. Individuals with this condition are characterized by
small testes, low gonadotropin levels, and low testosterone levels.
These patients typically fail to increase LH and FSH on initial
GnRH stimulation, but they can be primed with repetitive exposure. Many of these patients show anosmia as well. Anosmic patients studied at autopsy showed absence of olfactory tracts.

Delayed Puberty

Boys show evidence of entry to puberty by development of pubic and
axillary hair, phallus growth, testicular growth, and thinning of the
scrotal skin with the development of scrotal folds. This occurs on
the average at age 12, and the 95% confidence limits extend between
the ages of 10 and 14. After the age of 15, puberty is clearly delayed,
and consideration must be given to organic causes. Boys with "con-
stitutional" delay of puberty have no permanent organic lesion but
simply have late onset. There will often be a positive family history,
particularly in previous generations as opposed to siblings. Distinguishing between hypogonadotropic hypogonadism and delayed puberty is difficult. Careful measurement of testicular size can allow
documentation of testicular growth over a several month interval,
which is strongly suggestive of delayed puberty. Nocturnal rises in
testosterone, or a positive response of LH/FSH to GnRH stimulation, are early signs of pubertal onset. Stimulatory tests to see if
prolactin rises after an injection of either chlorpromazine or meto-
clopramide can be useful. A trial of therapy with low-dose testosterone enanthate or testosterone cypionate for 4–6 months may

stimulate the onset of puberty, and have obvious psychosocial benefits. However, vigorous androgen administration can lead to premature epiphyseal closure and loss of adult height.

Pituitary Insufficiency

Impairment of pituitary secretion of both LH and FSH can be caused
by a variety of factors. Local pituitary tumors can cause this, as well
as other mass lesions, by injury to the gonadotrophs. Granulomatous diseases, such as sarcoid and suprasellar tumors, can impair
pituitary or hypothalamic function.

Hyperprolactinemia

Elevated prolactin levels, caused either by a pituitary adenoma that
secretes prolactin or by the induction of prolactin with certain drugs
(i.e., tricyclic antidepressants or major tranquilizers), will impair
male reproductive function. The cause of this is multifactorial and
involves not only impairment of pulsatile secretion of GnRH, but of
testicular steroidogenesis as well.

EUHORMONAL MALE INFERTILITY (IDIOPATHIC OLIGOSPERMIA)

Infertile males usually present with an abnormal semen analysis
showing a reduced sperm count (< 20 million sperm/mL ejaculate
or < 60 million total sperm) and/or a reduced sperm motility
(< 40% with rapid forward progression) (Table 2). A growing number
of couples are being found in which an overt factor cannot be demonstrated in either the man or woman. In the absence of an identifia-
ble cause of impaired testicular function, the men are considered to
have "idiopathic infertility." They nearly always have normal virilization and potency, and hormonal levels are normal (with the exception of a mild elevation of FSH in less than 5% of cases). The
basis of infertility is unclear and likely involves some aspect of
sperm–egg interaction, as low counts of normal sperm can still

Table 2. Semen analysis

Semen characteristics	Good	Equivocal	Poor
Total sperm/ejaculate	$> 60 \times 10^6$	$40–59 \times 16^6$	$< 40 \times 10^6$
Sperm density (per mL)	$> 20 \times 10^6$	$10–19 \times 10^6$	$< 10 \times 10^6$
Volume	> 2.0 mL	1.0–1.9 mL	< 1.0 mL
Motility	> 60%	40–59%	< 40%
Motility grade	> 3.0	2.5–2.9	< 2.5
Oval forms	> 60%	40–59%	< 40%

achieve fertility without great difficulty. Treatment is frustrating and no medical therapy has been shown effective (Clark & Sherins, 1989; Sokol, Steiner, Bastillo, Petersen, & Swerdloff, 1988). The most consistent responses are found with repair of varicocele if present, intrauterine insemination with specially treated sperm, or in vitro fertilization.

Infections in the male reproductive tract can cause infertility. Clinically apparent infections of the testis, epididymis, or prostate can lead to reduced sperm count or motility. Epididymitis is considered secondary to urethritis or cystitis, and the ipsilateral testis is usually involved. Occult infections can be suggested by the presence of leukocytes in the semen or post-prostatic massage urine sample.

Sperm antibodies can arise in either the male or female and can bind to the sperm surface, blocking molecules important in capacitation or oocyte binding (Bronson, Cooper, & Rosenfield, 1984). Sperm are sequestered cells that possess several cell-surface antigens that are recognized as foreign and can incite an immune response and antibody formation in the male when exposed, for example, by vasectomy or trauma. Sperm antigens can be found in the circulation bound to immune complexes, and sperm-specific antibodies have been demonstrated against several sperm-surface antigens on ejaculated sperm. Development of sperm antibodies also has been associated with testicular biopsy, cryptorchism, varicocele, testicular cancer, and testicular inflammation (mumps orchitis).

Demonstration of sperm-surface antibodies is most frequently done using antihuman immunoglobulins bound to polyacrylamide beads or fluorescent isotopes. While the specificity of the probe depends on the anti-Ig antibody developed (most are polyclonal, the sensitivity depends on the particular probe), tests are regarded as positive if more than 10% of sperm show binding. However, binding levels of 10%–20% are considered borderline, while levels over 20% have a strong correlation with infertility.

The role that sperm antibodies play in infertility is not clear. Studies in which sperm-surface antibodies have been removed by specific proteases or by absorbent columns have shown recovery of heterologous ova penetration. This suggests that the surface antibodies are responsible for impaired sperm–egg interaction.

TREATMENT OF HORMONAL INSUFFICIENCY

Testosterone Replacement

Testosterone replacement is standard therapy for all forms of male hypogonadism. It is easily given by an injection of testosterone enanthate or testosterone cypionate, 100 mg intramuscularly once a week or 200 mg intramuscularly every 2 weeks. Most treatment facilities usually use the latter dose for convenience. Dosing intervals of longer than 2 weeks generally result in periods of inadequate levels of testosterone, despite an increased dose. These recommendations are based on elevations of gonadotropins prior to the next injection of testosterone at intervals of 3 or 4 weeks, indicating inadequate negative feedback.

Gonadotropin Replacement

Replacement with testosterone allows normal virilization and normal male sexual function. It does not promote stimulation of seminiferous tubules to produce sperm. This requires replacement with gonadotropins, which is done using human chorionic gonadotropin (hCG) alone or with human menopausal gonadotropin that is enriched in FSH. More recently, mechanical pumps giving pulsatile injections of GnRH have been used (Whitcomb & Crowley, 1990). All these treatment regimens can achieve good results, depending upon the stage of testicular development at the time therapy is initiated. Patients whose testes have evidence of some stimulation by endogenous gonadotropins, based on a testicular size greater than 4 mL, can show an excellent response to this therapy, with over 80% developing sperm production and fertility.

REFERENCES

Bronson, R.A., Cooper, G.W., & Rosenfield, D. (1984). Sperm antibodies: Their role in infertility. *Fertility and Sterility, 42,* 171–183.

Clark, R.V., & Sherins, R.J. (1986). Use of semen analysis in the evaluation of the infertile couple. In R.J. Santen & R.S. Swerdloff (Eds.), *Male reproductive dysfunction* (pp. 255–266). New York: Marcel Dekker.

Clark, R.V., & Sherins, R.J. (1989). Treatment of men with idiopathic oligospermic infertility using the aromatase inhibitor, testolactone: Results of a double blinded, randomized placebo controlled trial with crossover. *Journal of Andrology, 10,* 240–247.

Mortimer, D., Templeton, A.A., Linton, E.A., & Coleman, R.A. (1982). Influence of abstinence and ejaculation-to-analysis delay on semen analysis parameters of suspected infertile men. *Archives of Andrology, 8,* 251–256.

Sherins, R.J., & Howards, S.S. (1986). Male infertility. In P.C. Walsh, R.F. Gittes, A.D. Permitter, & T.A. Stamey (Eds.), *Campbell's urology* (5th ed., pp. 640–697). Philadelphia: W. B. Saunders.

Silber, S.J., & Rodriguez-Rigau, L.J. (1981). Quantitative analysis of testicle biopsy: Determination of partial obstruction and prediction of sperm count after surgery for obstruction. *Fertility and Sterility, 36,* 480–485.

Sokol, R.Z., Steiner, B., Bastillo, M., Petersen, G., & Swerdloff, R.S. (1988). Controlled comparison of the efficacy of clomiphene citrate in male infertility. *Fertility and Sterility, 49,* 865–870.

Whitcomb, R.W., & Crowley, W.F. (1990). Diagnosis and treatment of isolated gonadotropin-releasing hormone deficiency in men. *Journal of Clinical Endocrinology and Metabolism, 70,* 3–7.

23

Infertility

Alan B. Copperman and Alan H. DeCherney

Almost 2.4 million American couples, nearly 15%, are presently infertile, or unable to achieve pregnancy after 1 year of trying. The psychological and emotional burdens on the infertile couple as they attempt to understand and participate in technologically complicated treatment and evaluation can be overwhelming. The gynecologist is therefore challenged to perform the roles of educator and counselor, and then of healer.

The number of couples seeking a fertility workup is increasing each year (Jalfe & Jewelewicz, 1991). This increase is attributable to delayed childbearing, an increasing rate of pelvic infection, incomplete treatment, and the reduced availability of adoptive babies. Following an initial assessment of known risk factors for infertility, including age of partners, coital frequency, duration of infertility, and the compensatory balance of relative fertility between partners, the workup begins. In recent years, this has included semen analyses, postcoital testing, basal body temperature charting, endometrial biopsy, hysterosalpingography, and laparoscopy. Technologic advances have added new depth to this evaluation. New areas of infertility are being defined, and areas explored in the past are being reevaluated with increased sophistication.

In approximately 30%–50% of couples presenting for infertility workup, the male is found to be at least partly responsible. Historically, initial evaluation, following a detailed history of exposure to environmental toxins, sexually transmitted diseases, and absence of sexual dysfunction, involves a semen analysis. Following abstinence from ejaculation for 24–48 hours, a specimen is collected in a sterile, body-temperature container and evaluated within 1 hour of collection. Average values for a specimen include 2–5mL of semen with 20–150 million sperm of >50% motility, and >50% normal morphology with a mean velocity of >25 μm/s.

New technology has markedly improved the physician's ability to evaluate the "male factor." Multi-exposure photography (MEP) has allowed for finer differentiation in the quantification of sperm movement. The hamster test involves the penetration of hamster eggs following the removal of their outer zona pellucida. Sperm from men with proven fertility almost consistently penetrate over 10% of the ova. Some believe that failure to penetrate at least 10% of the ova suggests an impairment of male fertility (Rogers, 1985). In fact, some have shown a strong correlation between this test and subsequent ova fertilization in actual in vitro fertilization attempts (Kremer & Jager, 1990). There are detractors, however, who believe that this test just measures motility and the random interaction of motile sperm with the hamster oocytes. New biochemical markers such as sperm creatine kinase may serve as an objective indicator of the sperm's functional integrity and may thus predict fertilizing potential (Huszar, Corrales, Vigue, Quinn, & Androl, 1990).

An exciting area in the field of male infertility is the role of immunologic factors. Antibodies to sperm have been detected in serum, semen, and cervical mucus. Older tests for the presence of sperm antibodies, including the Franklin-Dukes and Isojima, were not terribly precise in their delineation. Today, the immunobead binding test provides the most reliable marker for immunologic infertility.

In cases of male-factor infertility, new treatments seem to be on the horizon. Surgical treatments are aimed at correcting specific physical defects. Varicocele correction, for example, may improve sperm parameters in some men (Dubin & Amelar, 1977). Correction of medical problems, especially endocrinological problems, may also improve the quality of sperm. Recently, attempts have been made to optimize sperm concentration and motility prior to insemination. These methods include pellet preparation, multiple tube swim-up techniques, and a two-layer Percoll density gradient technique (McClure, Nunes, & Tom, 1984). Each involves centrifugation and separation of the most motile sperm and subsequent direct intrauterine insemination.

The interaction of males and females is measured with the postcoital test. The test is performed on the anticipated day of ovulation, at which time the cervical mucus should be most hospitable. Within 8 hours of intercourse, the cervical mucus is removed using a forceps. Evaluation consists first of assessment of mucus adequacy, including amount, thinness, and stretchability (spinnbarkeit), which should be >8cm. The presence of 20 motile sperm per high-power field, swimming forward, is a good indicator of adequate coital technique and sperm count. In cases where there are no sperm or non-motile sperm, and especially in cases in which the sperm are found shaking in place, a complete immunologic workup, including a search for sperm antibodies, should be performed.

Female infertility evaluation begins with attempted documentation of ovulation. A history of regular menses with monthly complaints of premenstrual syndrome and dysmenorrhea is highly suggestive of ovulatory cycles. Documentation can be achieved with basal body temperature charts (and their characteristic ovulatory biphasic pattern), endometrial biopsy, and recently with new over the counter tests for the LH surge. In addition to their ability to suggest the occurrence of ovulation, these have greatly augmented the ability to appropriately time events such as artificial insemination, postcoital tests, and endometrial biopsy.

Transvaginal ultrasound, with its refined transducers, has enabled the study of the follicle in genesis. Transvaginal ultrasound has enabled us to know the number of follicles present, their size, health, and maturity. It has also allowed us to measure whether ovulation occurs and is probably the best way to detect luteinized unruptured follicle syndrome. In the near future, with finer discrimination on the part of the ultrasound, a cumulus will be identified, and other normal events of follicular physiology and growth will be elucidated. Transvaginal ultrasound has also been vital in the evaluation of other etiologies of infertility including critically placed myomas, endometriosis, and pelvic inflammatory disease.

The hysterosalpingogram has taken on new life as a diagnostic tool, and may actually be therapeutic as well (DeCherney, Kort, Barner, & DeVore, 1980). It gives information about the natural contour of the uterus, occasionally suggesting the presence of scar tissue, fibroids, and polyps, and about the patency of the fallopian tube. The reported but still debatable therapeutic effect of performing a hysterosalpingogram is possibly a result of oil-based dye mechanically lavaging tubes (perhaps dislodging mucus plugs or breaking adhesions) or stimulating cilia. If a hysterosalpingogram reveals proximal tubal obstruction, a patient may be offered the option of transcervical balloon tuboplasty or tubal recanalization (Confino et al., 1990). Prior to the availability of this outpatient procedure, only less cost-effective options such as in vitro fertilization (IVF) or tubal reconstructive surgery existed. Recent advances in hysteroscopy also allow for a better view of the uterine cavity and permit performance of a variety of surgical procedures, such as resection of endometrial polyps, submucus myomas, uterine septa, and synechiae.

Inspection of the tubal lumen can provide critical information as to the anatomic and functional capacity of the tube (Shapiro, Diamond, & DeCherney, 1988). The architecture of the tubal mucosa determines to a large extent its functional ability. Using a small caliber endoscope, direct examination of the tubal lumen can be carried out. The procedure can be performed at the time of diagnostic laparoscopy or at laparotomy. Preliminary data confirm the fact that a significant discrepancy exists between the external appearance of the tube and the findings at tuboscopy. This examination may allow one to identify the subgroups of patients with tubal disease who may not benefit from tubal surgery.

Laparoscopy has emerged as a routine and vital part of infertility evaluation and treatment. Adhesions and endometriosis can be identified and treated with laser technology, cautery, and microsurgical techniques. Second look laparoscopy, in fact, is often being advocated either in the immediate post-operative period or within 4 months of surgery (DeCherney & Mezer, 1984). This procedure allows for the relatively benign evaluation and correction of recurrent disease.

Historically, infections have been suspected as causes of infertility but have been difficult to document. Mycoplasma, for example, has long been implicated as a possible cause of habitual abortion and salpingitis in females and may also play a role in male factor infertility (Fowlkes, MacLead, & O'Leary, 1975). Recent advances in testing for chlamydia, specifically the utilization of a DNA probe (Gen-Probe), has allowed for rapid and easy diagnosis of this easily treated pathogen.

New endocrinologic and immunologic tests are emerging as possible adjuncts to infertility evaluation. Specific beta-pregnancy testing in conjunction with transvaginal ultrasound is well recognized in the management of ectopic pregnancy. New endocrine tests are continually becoming available. GnRH testing, if only to establish a specific diagnosis such as hypothalamic amenorrhea, might become routine office procedure. Ca 125, a membrane antigen expressed by nonmucinous epithelial ovarian carcinoma, may have promise with regard to detection and monitoring following treatment of endometriosis in infertile women presenting with chronic pelvic pain (Pittaway & Douglas, 1989).

Psychologic factors involved in infertility are becoming more important as the prevalence of infertility continues to increase and its evaluation and treatment becomes more invasive and complex.

Alteration in the neuropeptide beta-endorphin, for example, may contribute in some to reproductive dysfunction (Seifer & Collins, 1990). Adjunctive psychological testing and therapy may play significant roles as investigation into neurotransmitters and neuroendocrinology further defines their roles in the etiology of infertility.

Once the workup is complete, assessment of collected data is performed, and a treatment course initiated. If the patient is anovulatory, for example, ovulation can be medically induced with clomiphene citrate, human menopausal gonadotropin, gonadotropin-releasing hormone analogs, dexamethasone, bromocriptine, and other agents. Once initiated, these directed therapies can be effective in inducing ovulation in nearly 80% of cases (Whitelaw, & Kalmant, & Grams, 1970).

Artificial insemination may be an effective treatment in an appropriate patient population. The use of concentrated sperm preparations (often accomplished by taking the first part of a split ejaculate) or centrifugation has been found by some to be successful as treatment of oligospermia. This homologous artificial insemination, however, is usually reserved for the treatment of anatomic or local problems such as hypospadias, retrograde ejaculation, psychological impotence, or vaginismus.

Therapeutic donor insemination has been used to treat patients with male-factor infertility, antisperm antibodies, and unexplained infertility. The mechanism usually used is insertion of a cervical cup containing donor sperm; often the couple performs the insemination themselves. Alternatively, intrauterine insemination can be performed. This involves the direct transfer of washed, prepared sperm into the uterine cavity.

In-vitro fertilization and embryo transfer (IVF-ET) was initially used for women with severe tubal disease. Currently, however, indications include infertility secondary to immunologic reasons, male-factor infertility, endometriosis, cervical-factor infertility, exposure to diethylstilbesterol, and unexplained infertility. The first step in IVF-ET involves the stimulation of multiple follicle development by the use of clomiphene citrate (Clomid), exogenous gonadotropins (LH and FSH in combination or FSH alone), or gonadotropin-releasing hormone (GnRH) analogs. The timing of oocyte recovery is determined by serial ultrasounds and estradiol levels, and 36 hours after a dose of human chorionic gonadotropin (hCG), the recovery itself is performed via transvaginal aspiration under transvaginal ultrasonographic visualization. The oocytes are incubated for 48 hours with washed, concentrated sperm, and following the formation and division of a zygote, optimally 4 four-cell embryos are transplanted back into the uterine cavity.

Gamete intrafallopian transfer (GIFT) has been popularized since the mid-1980s. The initial stages are identical to IVF; however, in GIFT, the oocytes and prepared sperm are placed into a transfer catheter and injected directly into the fallopian tube. This procedure is only performed in patients with minimal tuboperitoneal disease. Theoretic advantages over IVF include fertilization occurring in its natural milieu and implantation occurring 5–6 days after ovulation, its "natural" time of entry (Diamond & DeCherney, 1987).

Collins's monumental work (Collins, Wrixon, Janes, & Wilson, 1983) in the *New England Journal of Medicine* discussing treatment and the success and failure of present "therapeutic" interventions has resulted in the reevaluation of treatment modalities. This work must be repeated and critically assessed to determine whether or not present interventions have a therapeutic impact.

In conclusion, there are many new ways to help the infertile couple. Many entities have been newly defined, and there is a greater sophistication and understanding of older disease processes. Success rates have not significantly increased since the late 1980s. With continued technological progress, however, combined with a greater understanding of human reproductive physiology, effective diagnosis and therapy for infertility should be possible.

REFERENCES

Collins, J.A., Wrixon, W., Janes, L.B., & Wilson, E.H. (1983). Treatment-independent pregnancy among infertile couples. *New England Journal of Medicine, 309,* 1201.

Confino, E., Tur-Kaspa, I. DeCherney, A.H., Corfman, R., Coulam, R., Coulam, C., Robinson, E., Haas, G., Katz, E., Vermesh, M., & Gleicher, N. (1990). Transcervical balloon tuboplasty: A multicenter study. *Journal of the American Medical Association, 264,* 2079.

DeCherney, A.H., Kort, H., Barner, J.B., & DeVore, G.R. (1980). Increased pregnancy rate with oil soluble hysterosalpingography dye. *Fertility and Sterility, 34,* 407.

DeCherney, A.H., & Mezer, H.C. (1984). The nature of posttuboplasty pelvic adhesions as determined by early and late luteal laparoscopy. *Fertility and Sterility, 41,* 643.

Diamond, M.P., & DeCherney, A.H. (1987). In-vitro fertilization (IVF) and gamete intrafallopian transfer (GIFT). *Obstetrics and Gynecology Clinics of North America, 14*(4).

Dubin, L., & Amelar, R.D. (1977). Varicocelectomy: 986 cases in a twelve year study. *Urology, 10*(5), 446.

Fowlkes, D.M., MacLeod, J., & O'Leary, W.M. (1975). T-mycoplasmas and human infertility: Correlation of infection with alterations in seminal parameters. *Fertility and Sterility, 26*(12), 1212.

Huszar, G. Corrales, M., Vigue, L., & Quinn, P. (1990). *Journal of Andrology.*

Jaffe, S.B., & Jewelwicz, R. (1991). The basic infertility investigation. *Fertility and Sterility, 56*(4), 599.

Kremer, J., & Jager, S. (1990). The significance of the zona-free hamster oocyte test for the evaluation of male infertility. *Fertility and Sterility, 54*(3), 509.

McClure, R.D., Nunes, L., & Tom, R. (1989). Semen manipulation: Improved sperm recovery and function with a two-layer Percoll gradient. *Fertility and Sterility, 51*(5), 874.

Pittaway, D.E., & Douglas, J.W. (1989). Serum CA-125 in women with endometriosis ad chronic pelvic pain. *Fertility and Sterility, 51,* 68.

Rogers, B.J. (1985). The sperm penetration assay: Its usefulness reevaluated. *Fertility and Sterility, 43*(6), 821.

Seifer, D.B., & Collins, R.L. (1990). Current concepts of beta-endorphin physiology in female reproductive dysfunction. *Fertility and Sterility, 54*(5), 757.

Shapiro, B.S., Diamond, M.P., & DeCherney, A.H. (1988). Salpingoscopy: An adjunctive technique for evaluation of the fallopian tube. *Fertility and Sterility, 49,* 1076.

Whitelaw, M.J. Kalman, L.G., & Grams, L.R. (1970). The significance of the high ovulation rate versus the low pregnancy rate with Clomid. *American Journal of Obstetrics and Gynecology, 107,* 865.

24

Effects of Medications on Fertility in Males with Physical Disabilities with Sexually Transmitted Disease

Jean L. Fourcroy

Until recently, the reproductive function of men with physical disabilities was not considered important; now, sexual counseling is an integral part of successful rehabilitation. It is thought that early intervention with males with physical disabilities improves overall results. Over 22 fertility programs across the country address issues related to disabling injuries and methods most appropriate to the injured man and his mate (U. Yarif, personal communication, March 22, 1991; Sims, 1991). A high percentage of men with physical disabilities have spinal cord injuries (SCI) and are between the ages of 18 and 35, which are the prime reproductive years. All need reassurance for successful parenting. Since all of these individuals have higher rates of spermatogenic abnormalities than men without physical disabilities (Hirsch, McCue, Allen, Lee, & Staas, 1991), the possible effects of medications, specifically those used for treatment of sexually transmitted diseases, on fertility potential are very important. Together with erectile and ejaculatory dysfunctions, these may increase fertility problems.

Many other factors alter the fertility potential in addition to the treatment of sexually transmitted diseases (STDs). These factors include immobility of the male with a disability and any neurologic changes. The immobility may create little-understood changes affecting not only the vascular system but also the bioavailability of medications. Similar changes have been seen in bed-rest models simulating microgravity and demonstrating the same hemodynamic shifts (Nicogossian, Huntoon, & Pool, 1989). The neurologic changes may alter the production and the emission of spermatozoa. It is well-known that a high incidence of men with spinal cord injuries (SCI) are infertile, either due to poor sperm production or ejaculatory failure. The technology of electroejaculation has greatly improved the outlook for these men (Bennett, Seager, & McQuire, 1987).

INFECTIONS IN MALES WITH DISABILITIES

Infections of the male genital system have long been thought to be a possible cause of infertility. The three sexually transmitted organisms that perhaps most affect fertility in both males and females are gonorrhea, chlamydia, and myocoplasmata (including *Ureaplasma urealyticum* and *Mycoplasma hominis*). These organisms have been recognized in both male and female reproductive tracts, with the suggestion that the infection rate by such organisms is higher among couples with idiopathic infertility (Fowler, 1981; Sherins & Howards, 1986). However, data on STDs and their effects on fertility are not consistent.

What are the genital infections common in men with disabilities? There are few data to suggest that incidence is any different than that in men without disabilities. The most common etiology of urinary tract infection in men younger than 35 years of age is *Chlamydia trachomatis*. Although rarely isolated from the urethral cultures of normal males, chlamydia has been thought to be a major cause of nongonococcal urethritis and epididymitis (Fowler, 1981). Until recently, this has been difficult to substantiate. Both Fowler (1981) and Megory, Zuckerman, Shoham, and Lunnenfeld (1987) have written excellent reviews of the normal colonization of the male urethra and accessory glands.

The risk factors for transmission of STDs for all men include sexual behavior such as multiple partners, as well as drug abuse and poor health care. Condom use, especially with the addition of spermacides, is thought to help prevent transmission of STDs, but, clearly, it also prevents conception. There are no data that suggest that a person with a disability has an increased incidence of STDs. Immobility increases the risk of urinary tract infections, but health habits clearly affect this problem. Treatment of infections that are known causes of infertility (e.g., syphilis, HIV, and HPV) are not discussed. Infertility by these agents is caused secondarily by obstruction and dysfunction of the genital system.

DIAGNOSTIC MARKERS

What are the diagnostic markers used to determine *when* to treat for a sexually transmitted urogenital tract disease, and what is the current understanding of the effects of these medications on fertility? Do any of these medications affect spermatogenesis or sperm function? Fertility potential can be altered at any site of development of sperm or sperm transport by infection or medication (see excellent reviews by Megory et al., 1987; Schlegel, Chang, & Marshall, 1991). Sexually transmitted diseases can alter the normal maturation and development of spermatozoa at many points in the genital anatomy. Spermatogenesis within the seminiferous tubules, the excretory system beginning with the rete, and the epididymis leading to the prostate and seminal vesicle, ejaculatory duct, and posterior urethra are all important sites where infection and medication as well as neurologic damage may alter the final product (Graney & Krieger, 1990). In the older man, the prostate is a prime site for chronic prostatitis of bacterial origin, while in the younger man of reproductive age, the infection is more likely to be chlamydia. There are few data of the role of instrumentation or indwelling catheters in males with disabilities in the prevalence of infections. Epididymitis in the young man (<35) is usually secondary to *C. trachomitis* and *N. gonorrhoeae* (Krieger, 1990), even without history of urethral discharge. Clean intermittent catheterization continues to be an important method to reduce infection rate because it reduces bacterial growth and permanent bladder overdistention.

The relation of infection to infertility is controversial for several reasons. Favorable reports have been published showing benefit from antibiotic therapy, although laboratory evidence of infection is often lacking (Fowler, 1981; Megory, Zuckerman, Shoham, & Lunnenfeld; Toth & Leser, 1987). Second, it is difficult to distinguish commensal growth from pathologic growth, and some of the organisms that may be incriminated (e.g., *Ureaplasma urealyticum* and *Chlamydia trachomitis*) are difficult to culture. On routine semen analysis in most laboratories, it is difficult to distinguish immature sperm cells from white cells (World Health Organization, 1987).

Eliasson (1976) reported that 40% of infertile men in Sweden have cytologic or bacteriologic evidence of inflammation of the accessory sex glands and that treatment should be given if two or more of the following criteria are present:

1. There is an excess of pus cells in the expressed prostatic fluid.
2. Palpation has revealed a clearly swollen and tender prostate and/or seminal vesicles.
3. A man has subjective symptoms indicating urethritis, cystitis, or prostatitis.
4. The semen contains more than occasional white blood cells.
5. The bacteriologic culture shows pathogenic bacteria or a massive growth of potentially pathogenic bacteria.
6. There is a rapid decline in motility and viability of spermatozoa resulting in less than 40% live, motile spermatozoa 2 hours after ejaculation.
7. There is decreased secretory function of the accessory genital glands.
8. The wife has a urogenital infection.

It is helpful to use segmented urine cultures before and after expressed prostatic secretions (EPSs) to document the infection and to identify the site. Many treatments for STDs are, unfortunately, not based on documented infection (Fowler, 1981).

Most of the medications used to treat STDs are presumably secreted into the genital fluids, thus affecting both sperm production and function, and they present, therefore, an additional hazard to a man's potential fertility. Reviews of the available data on known drugs used to treat sexually transmitted diseases are sparse and probably not representative of the population with diabilities.

ANTIBIOTICS COMMONLY USED TO TREAT STDs

Zovirax (Acyclovir)

Zovirax, used for the treatment for recurrent herpes simplex, is an excellent example of a drug whose effect on the male genital tract has been studied. This drug is a synthetic purine nucleoside analog that inhibits the growth of the herpes virus. The secretory pattern of this medication was studied because of its important use in the 18–35-year-old age group. The effect of herpes infections on maternal and fetal outcomes is not discussed here, but they are clearly important health risks that must be treated appropriately. Although secreted in high levels in the genital duct, this oral drug does not appear to alter spermatogenesis or mortality and appears not to alter fertility in the male (Douglas, 1988).

Nitrofurantoin

An antibiotic well-known for its use in treating urinary tract infections (UTIs) is nitrofurantoin (e.g., Macrodantin). The nitrofurantoins are highly concentrated in urine, which is a benefit in treating urinary tract infections. These antibiotics were first developed in 1944 and used for healing wounds (e.g., furacin) and are frequently used in association with chronic catheter care. Spermatozoa immobilization has been well-demonstrated by in vitro studies. Additionally, Nelson and Bunge (1957) demonstrated the effects on sperm production in an interesting study of 35 patients, 25 of whom were men with pre- and post-treatment testicular biopsies as well as semen analysis, while the other 10 had only semen analysis at the beginning and end of nitrofurantoin dosing. The dose used was 10 mg/kg for 2 weeks. Today, the generally accepted doses are much lower, usually 50–100 mg per day, in divided doses. Spermatozoa immobilization appeared to be fully reversible with recovery 9–32 weeks after cessation of treatment. Depression of total sperm counts was noted between 5 and 8 weeks after beginning treatment. In seven cases there was histologic evidence of drug effect and a "tendency toward arrest," possibly at the primary spermatocyte level (Nelson & Bunge, 1957). However, there are no studies on chronic use of nitrofurantoins at lower, more appropriate, doses. Urologists today very often take advantage of the spermicidal activity and use nitrofurantoin to flush the working end of the vas deferens at the time of vasectomy. Nitrofurantoin should be discontinued if fertility is desired, although more research is needed on this drug using current doses.

Macrolides: Erythromycin

There is evidence that suggests that erythromycin is capable of spermicidal activity and of producing impaired motility. The levels in prostatic fluids are approximately 40% of serum levels, which is the reason that erythromycin is so effective in the treatment of urinary tract infections (e.g., prostatitis, White, 1954). It is possible that this class of drugs can impair fertility, but the effects may be reversible. More information is needed on this aspect (Holmes, 1990).

Aminoglycsides: Gentamicin and Kanamycin

It was demonstrated in 1974 that gentamicin can arrest spermatogenesis at the level of the primary spermatocytes but has little, if any, effect on mature spermatozoa (Timmermans, 1974). These drugs are not used for treatment of STDs but for treatment of nonresponding UTIs. The patient desiring fertility should be cautioned about using these drugs.

Tetracyclines: Including Doxycycline

Tetracyclines and derivatives such as doxycycline are often first-line treatments for STDs. Doxycycline, the most widely used, has been used in an effort to improve fertility when infection has not been demonstrated clinically. Toth and Leser (1987) suggest that the use of a tetracycline—in particular doxycycline—improves fertility. A 79%–81% improvement in quantity and quality of motility was seen in a review of the treatment of 243 men given doxycycline for 2–4 weeks for ureaplasma (Toth & Leser, 1987). To date, there is no evidence that the use of tetracyclines inhibits the normal maturation or function of the reproductive tract. Tetracyclines are secreted by the kidneys and, therefore, high concentrations in the genital system probably also occur. There is a need for more data on the use of tetracycline in the treatment of STDs.

Sulfonamides

Sulfasalazine was first used in the 1940s for inflammatory bowel disease, but it was not until the 1970s that decreased sperm motility was noted. This effect on motility appears to be reversible and may be an effect that occurs late in the maturation of the sperm, since the reversibility is noted approximately 75 days after medication is stopped. Perhaps the sperm acrosomal membrane enzymes are the site of alteration in late-stage development. (Cosentino, Chey, Takihara, & Cockett, 1984; O'Morain, Smethurst, Dore, & Levi, 1985; Toovey, Hudson, Hendry, & Levi, 1981).

Combination Sulfa Drugs

Sulfamethoxazole and trimethoprim (Bactrim or Septra) are combined in medications used frequently for long periods of time for urinary tract infections. There are few data on use in patients of prime fertility years; however, the trimethoprim may deprive active dividing cells from folate by inhibiting dihydrofolate reductase. Evidence has been suggested that there is either a 37% decrease or a 42% improvement in semen analysis (Schlegel, 1991). Again, more studies are needed to define this drug effect on fertility potential. There may be evidence of altered pharmacokinetics in immobile patients.

Penicillin

There are no current human data. The apparent safety of penicillin has led to widespread acceptance as an extender in preparation of semen (Schlegel et al., 1991).

Quinolones

Nalidixic Acid Nalidixic acid was the first of the quinolones to be used for chronic UTI. It is clearly secreted into the genital ducts. When ejaculate samples are divided, there appears to be an equal amount in each sample. This suggests that nalidixic acid is secreted not only in the prostate and seminal vesicle, but perhaps in the epididymis as well. This has been an important drug for the treatment of chronic urinary tract infections.

Ofloxacin One study using single oral doses of 400 and 500 milligrams ofloxacin in 20 men did not address semen motility but confirmed the important excretory potential of this drug. The amount in semen exceeded inhibitory dose (Minimal Inhibitory Concentration) (MIC) of the medication (Berger, Yavetz, Paz, Gorrea, & Homonnai, 1990). The drug is effective for both chlamydia and mycoplasma species. (Tartaglione & Russo, 1990). Other quinolones that have not been reviewed but are commonly used for the treatment of STDs are norfloxacin and ciprofloxacin.

OTHER CONSIDERATIONS

There are very few data evaluating the drug availability and pharmacokinetics of drugs in the immobile man. There is reason to believe from existing studies on the pharmacokinetics of drugs that there are important changes with obesity, age, and immobility. Bedrest models of space microgravity have pointed out some of these differences that could affect availability of drugs within the genital tract milieu (Nicogossian et al., 1989). These facts should be considered in future research.

Any study of medications to be used in males with disabilities must include not only the drugs used to treat urinary tract infections, but also those used for other therapies that may affect fertility potential of these men. Examples of such drugs are alpha methyl dopamine (Aldomet), which may alter the normal nerve conduction through the adrenergic nervous system causing impotence, and cimetidine (Tagamet), which may enhance the secretion of prolactin and block the androgen effect. Autonomic dysfunction in a man with a physical disability may alter ejaculation by interfering with the innervation of the vas deferens and bladder neck. Phenoxybenzamine hydrochloride is an alpha adrenergic antagonist that has been used to control the manifestations of autonomic hyperreflexia in patients with spinal cord transection. This drug alters the closing of the bladder neck causing retrograde ejaculation. Ephedrine, an adrenergic agonist, is often used to increase the sympathetic tone at the bladder neck and prevent retrograde ejaculation. Phenytoin, used for seizure prevention, interferes with metabolism of 17-ketosteroids and 17-hydroxysteroids by suppressing androgen production. It also reduces semen quality and the percentage of motile sperm. (See Dixon, 1988, for a complete list of other agents that may affect the male reproductive system.)

Clearly, future research needs to identify the genito-urinary secretory patterns of medications in males with disabilities. Every drug used for the treatment of STDs in males with disabilities needs more data on the milieu in the genital tract. The concomitant medications used by the individuals must also be considered.

REFERENCES

Bennett, C.J., Seager, S.W.J., & McQuire, E.J. (1987). Electroejaculation for recovery of retrograde ejaculation. *Journal of Urology, 137,* 513–515.

Berger, S.A., Yavetz, H., Paz, G., Gorrea, A., & Homonnai, Z. (1990). Concentration of ofloxacin and ciprofloxacin in human semen following a single oral dose. *Journal of Urology, 144,* 683–684.

Bruce, A.W., & Reig, G. (1989). Prostatitis associated with chlamydia trachomatis in 6 patients. *Journal of Urology, 142,* 1006–1007.

Cosentino, M.J., Chey, W.Y., Takihara, H., & Cockett, A.T.K. (1984). The effects of sulfasalazine on human male fertility and seminal prostaglandins. *Journal of Urology, 132,* 682–686.

Dixon, R. (1988). Toxic responses of the reproductive system. In E.S.E. Hafez Klaassen, C.D., Amdur, M.O., & Doull, J. (Eds.). *Casarett and Doull's toxicology* (3rd ed., pp. 453–454). New York: Macmillan.

Douglas, J.M. (1988). A double-blind, placebo-controlled trial of the effect of chronically administered oral acyclovir on sperm production in men with frequently recurrent genital herpes. *Journal of Infections Disease, 157*(3), 588–593.

Eliasson, R. (1976). Clinical examination of infertile men. In E.S.E. Hafez (Ed.), *Human semen and fertility regulation* (pp. 321–331). St. Louis: Mosby.

Fowler, J.E. (1981). Infections of the male reproductive tract and infertility: A selected review. *Journal of Andrology, 3,* 121–131.

Graney, D.O., & Krieger, J.N. (1990). Anatomy and physical examination of the male genital tract. In K.K. Holmes, P. Mardh, P.F. Sparling, P.J. Wener, W. Cates, S.M. Lemon, & W.E. Stamm (Eds.), *Sexually transmitted diseases* (2nd ed., pp. 95–103.). New York: McGraw-Hill.

Hirsch, I.H., McCue, P., Allen, J., Lee, J., & Staas, W. (1991). Quantitative testicular biopsy in spinal cord injured men: Comparison to fertile controls. *Journal of Urology, 145*(73), 73–76.

Krieger, J.N. (1989). Prostatitis, epididymitits and orchitis. In G.L. Mandell, R.G. Douglass, & J.G. Bennett (Eds.), *Principles and practice of infectious disease* (3rd ed., pp. 971–976). New York: Churchill Livingstone.

Megory, E., Zuckerman, H., Shoham, Z., & Lunnenfeld, B. (1987). Infections and male infertility. *Obstetrical and Gynecological Survey, 42*(5), 283–290.

Nelson, W.O., & Bunge, R.G. (1957). The effect of therapeutic dosages of nitrofurantoin (furadantin) upon spermatogenesis in man. *Journal of Urology, 77,* 275–285.

Nicogossian, A.E., Huntoon, C.L., & Pool, S.L. (1989). *Space physiology and medicine* (2nd ed.). Philadelphia: Lea and Febriger.

O'Morain, C.O., Smethurst, P., Dore, C.J., & Levi, A.J. (1985). Reversible male infertility due to sulfasalazine: Studies in man and rat. *Gut, 25,* 1078–1084.

Osenkop, R., & MacLeod, J. (1947). Sulfadiazine: Its effect on spermatogenesis and its ecretion in the ejaculate. *Journal of Urology, 58,* 80–84.

Schlegel, P.N., Chang, T.S.K., & Marshall, F.F. (1991). Antibiotics: Potential hazards to male fertility. *Fertility and Sterility, 55,* 235–242.

Sherins, R.J., & Howards, S.S. (1986). Male infertility. In R.F. Walsh, G. Theis, A.D. Perlmutter, & T.A. Stamey (Eds.), *Campbell's urology* (5th ed.) (pp. 640–697). Philadelphia: W.B. Saunders.

Sims, B. (1991, March). What consumers are teaching us about sexuality. *Paraplegia News,* 4–26.

Tartaglione, T., & Russo, M.E. (1990). Pharmacology of drugs used in venereology. In Holmes, K.K., Mardh, P., Sparling, P.F., Wener, P.J., Cates, W., Lemon, S.M., & Stamm, W.E. (Eds.). *Sexually transmitted diseases* (2nd ed. pp. 993–1019). New York: McGraw Hill.

Timmermans, L. (1974). Influence of antibiotics on spermatogenesis. *Journal of Urology, 112,* 348–349.

Toovey, S., Hudson, E., Hendry, W.F., & Levi, A.J. (1981). Sulfasalazine and male infertility: Reversibility and possible mechanism. *Gut, 22,* 445–451.

Toth, A., & Leser, M.L. (1987). Ureaplasma urealyticum and infertility: The effect of different antibiotic regimens on the semen quality. *Journal of Urology, 128,* 705–707.

White, I.G. (1954). The toxocitiy of some antibacterials for bull, ram, rabbit and human spermatozoa. *Australian Journal of Experimental Biology and Medical Science, 32,* 41–48.

World Health Organization. (1987). *Laboratory manual for the examination of human semen and semen-cervical mucus interaction.* Oxford: Cambridge University Press.

25

Management Approaches to Sexually Transmitted Diseases in Women with Disabilities

Sandra L. Welner

Among the most common neurologic syndromes affecting spinal cord function are: external compression syndromes, autoimmune/ hereditary degenerative diseases, idiopathic/acquired and infectious diseases, and central cord syndromes (sacral sparing) (Aminoff, 1989; Beeson, McDermott, & Wyngaarden, 1979).

NEUROLOGIC SYNDROMES AFFECTING SPINAL CORD FUNCTION

External Compression Syndromes

Probably the most common neurologic syndrome is the class of lesions characterized as external compression syndromes. Benign and malignant tumors responsible for external compression of the spinal cord include meningiomas, neurofibroma, epidural hematoma, teratoma, and lipomas. Depending on the level of the compression, different deficits are manifest. If the compression is above the level of T10–T12, all sensation below the umbilicus is lost. Depending on which part of the cord is damaged, manifestations of impairment are variable. Most commonly the cord is only partially compressed. Ipsilaterally (same side as partial compression), there

Without the help of Dr. Mary Groesch, this chapter would not have been possible.

are spastic weakness, abnormal reflexes, and joint position sense and vibration sense impairment (dorsal columns). Contralaterally (opposite side of the partial compression), pain and temperature impairment are present due to the crossing of the spinothalamic pathways. In a woman affected in this way, the self-diagnosis of pelvic inflammatory disease (PID) would be extremely difficult because of obvious lack of sensation in the affected areas. Unfortunately, the organs are *not different* in their ability to become severely damaged by rampant, undiagnosed infection. T12–L1 levels of injury are associated with loss of sensory and motor function at and below the level of the inguinal ligament. Uterus and ovaries are innervated through nerves originating at the level of L1–L2. Peritoneal surfaces covering ovaries and uterus probably originate approximately at the T12 level. Thus, as can be observed, most spinal cord compression syndromes have a significant deleterious effect on sensory and motor function of the lower trunk and pelvis.

Hereditary and acquired causes of spinal cord compression include, among others, achondroplasia, Paget's disease, and congenital spinal stenosis. Deformities of the bony structure of the spinal cord may also result in compression syndrome manifestations. These include, among others, cervical or lumbar spondylosis.

Idiopathic/Acquired Diseases

Idiopathic/acquired diseases affecting the spinal cord include multiple sclerosis (MS) and, less commonly, amyotrophic lateral sclerosis (ALS), transverse myelitis, and sarcoidosis.

Multiple Sclerosis MS is associated with demyelinating plaques distributed widely throughout the white matter of the spinal cord. MS is sometimes divided into clinical types, depending upon which portion of the neuraxis is most involved (e.g., spinal, cerebral, brain stem-cerebellar, or mixed). The most common form is spinal with prominent features of spastic paraparesis, lower extremity paresthesias, and urinary complaints.

Amyotrophic Lateral Sclerosis ALS is an idiopathic syndrome associated with sporadic areas of nerve damage with associated muscle weakness and wasting in the areas of the affected nerves. Course may be rapid decompensation or gradual deterioration over many years.

Transverse Myelitis or Myelopathy Transverse myelitis refers to a clinical syndrome in which there is evidence of complete or partial loss of neurologic functions below a lesion that pathologically usually has a limited longitudinal dimension in the spinal cord. Thoracic and cervical segments are most frequently involved.

Demyelination, neuronal injury, and incomplete or complete necrosis of neural tissue have been described and may at times be associated with inflammatory cells, macrophages, or proliferation of astroglia. The onset is usually abrupt, with the neurologic deficit evolving from the initial symptoms to maximal disability within hours to a few days or occasionally a few weeks. A premonitory history of an upper respiratory or other infection or minor trauma is reported in ~25% of cases.

The earliest symptoms are muscle weakness, usually involving the lower limbs, sensory aberrations, back discomfort, or root pain, all occurring with about equal frequency. Signs may be asymmetrical, but bilateral involvement of the spinal cord is invariable at some time in the course of the disease. Bladder and bowel dysfunction are nearly universal as paresis of the limbs and sensory disturbances progress.

Sarcoidosis Neurosarcoidosis affects central and peripheral nerves with central nervous system (CNS) impairments predominating.

Central Cord Syndrome (Sacral Sparing)

Nerve fibers in the spinal cord are arranged with the outer fibers innervating lower portions of the body, and the inner fibers governing more proximal areas. There are a number of categories of central cord lesions that have the same sacral sparing properties (i.e., due to the central location of the lesion, the sacral area remains sensitive to stimuli). The first main grouping of central cord syndromes includes benign and malignant spinal cord tumors such as ependymomas and gliomas. Lesions that cause expansion from within the spinal cord include, among others, syrinx and hemorrhage inside the spinal cord due to trauma.

Autoimmune/Hereditary Degenerative Diseases

Autoimmune/hereditary degenerative diseases are a group of complex disorders that have in common progressive nerve degeneration in which ataxia and dysmetria (inability to control range of muscle action), resulting from predominant involvement of the cerebellum and its pathways, are combined to greater or lesser degrees, with impairment of other sensory and motor systems. All represent system degenerations, and many of the specific entities have a well-established genetic basis. Although clinical signs of cerebellar involvement predominate, the extension of the disorders to involve other regions of the nervous system can produce more complex neurologic symptoms. The important and common inherited spinocerebellar degenerations include: Friedreich ataxia, Roussey-Levy syndrome, Bassen-Kornzweig syndrome, Refsum's syndrome, olivo-pontocerebellar degeneration, Marie's ataxia, and dyssynergia cere-bellar myoclonica.

Infectious Diseases of the Nervous System

Among the more common infectious etiologies of spinal cord dam-age are neurosyphilis, herpes zoster, Lyme disease, tuberculosis, paralytic poliomyelitis, and chronic inflammatory demyelinating polyneuropathy. Depending on the level of damage due to the infec-tion, resultant impairments are variable.

Neurosyphilis All forms of neurosyphilis begin as meningitis, and some believe that all the subsequent damage to the nervous system is due to the chronic meningitis and its effects on the ves-sels. The meningitis is usually asymptomatic but can result in symptoms similar to those of other subacute meningitides, for ex-ample, headache, stiff neck, and cranial nerve palsies. With tertiary parenchymal neurosyphilis there is infection of the brain with spirochetes, and it seems probable that this infiltration by organ-isms and the subsequent inflammation leads to impaired function.

Herpes Zoster Pathologic studies of herpes zoster have shown an acute ganglionitis with an intense inflammatory response, cell necrosis, and occasionally hemorrhages within the ganglia. In addi-tion, there is inflammation in the adjacent segments of the cord or brain stem, which is predominantly unilateral, more prominent in gray matter, and involves the posterior more than the anterior horns.

Lyme Disease Lyme disease is caused by a spirochete that is carried by ticks. A distinctive primary skin lesion, erythema chron-icum migrans (ECM), characterizes this multisystem inflammatory disease. Many patients also show signs of arthritis and arthralgia, as well as neurologic and cardiac manifestations. Although it can be contracted by people of all ages, children and young adults are par-ticularly susceptible to Lyme disease because they generally spend more time outdoors and thus have more opportunities for exposure to ticks.

Tuberculosis Tuberculous meningitis is invariably fatal when untreated and often produces incapacitating neurologic damage. In-volvement is usually most marked at the base of the brain and may produce a grossly thickened, space-occupying exudate, causing pres-sure injury to adjacent cranial nerves and long tracts.

Paralytic Poliomyelitis Paralysis in paralytic poliomyelitis may develop with overwhelming rapidity, proceeding from barely detect-able weakness to tetraplegia in but a few hours, or it may pursue a more indolent course in which additional weaknesses appear over a

4- or 5-day period. Rarely, this indolent progression may last for as long as 10–12 days. In general, the more rapid the early progression, the more severe the eventual involvement.

The virus has a predilection for large motor neurons, with weakness about large joints usually being noted first. Spread of the disease shows no consistent pattern. Although there is a tendency for adjacent spinal and brain stem segments to be involved together, paralysis is nearly always asymmetric and at times widely scattered in its distribution. The lower extremities and lower trunk are involved most frequently, whereas upper extremities and cranial nerves are less often seriously paralyzed.

Chronic Inflammatory Polyradiculoneuropathy   In chronic inflammatory polyradiculoneuropathy, the neurologic deficit tends to develop slowly over months or years and persists for years. Some patients have a stepwise progression to their maximal deficit and then slowly improve. Others have a recurrent course with ultimate worsening or ultimate improvement. A few patients progress slowly to death several years later. As in the acute inflammatory polyradiculoneuropathies, the process tends to involve symmetrical proximal body structures and to affect motor, autonomic, and sensory peripheral neurons in varying proportions.

Miscellaneous Spinal Cord Dysfunctions

The list of miscellaneous spinal cord dysfunctions is quite long. Two more common dysfunctions are spinal trauma and vitamin B_{12} deficiency. As opposed to cord compression, spinal trauma can, in unfortunate cases, result in total spinal cord section with resultant severe impairment and total lack of function of any kind below the level of the lesion.

Vitamin B_{12} Deficiency   Insufficient absorption of vitamin B_{12} from the gastrointestinal tract can result in subacute degeneration of the spinal cord, optic nerves, cerebral white matter, and peripheral nerves. Among the more common causes of B_{12} deficiency are status post-GI surgery and extreme vegetarianism.

SEXUALLY TRANSMITTED DISEASES

Pelvic Inflammatory Disease (PID)

One hypothesis regarding the pathogenesis of acute PID suggests that it usually starts as a cervical infection with *Neisseria gonorrhoeae* and/or *Chlamydia trachomatis* with subsequent alteration in the cervical-vaginal microenvironment as a result of the consumption of nutrients and the production of metabolic waste products. These changes cause others, including alterations in vaginal pH and the availability of oxygen, which results in overgrowth of endogenous and anaerobic flora. The original cervical pathogens and/or endogenous organisms then ascend into the upper genital tract. This hypothesis would explain the polymicrobial nature of PID. Alternative theories assume that polymicrobial PID can be initiated without *N. gonorrhoeae* or *C. trachomatis*. Organisms isolated from women with polymicrobial PID have generally fallen into four broad categories: *N. gonorrhoeae* alone, *C. trachomatis* alone, *N. gonorrhoeae* and *C. trachomatis*, and anaerobic and/or facultative bacteria. As seen in Table 1, not every case of PID is caused by a sexually transmitted organism (Audio-Digest, 1990b; Glass, 1988). From a diagnostic standpoint, the presence of a pathogen in the endocervix does not always indicate that this is the organism causing infection in the endometrium, the fallopian tubes, or the peritoneal cavity. Further, infectious agents can be recovered from endometrial cultures even when cervical cultures for the same agents are negative. In their classic studies, Jacobsen and Westrom (1969) found that the clinical diagnosis of PID was erroneous in one third of cases where laparoscopy was used as the diagnostic criterion.

Table 1. Characteristics of pelvic inflammatory disease (PID)

Statistics

        1,000,000 cases in U.S. per year
        80% of cases are 15–29 years old
        By age 21, 1 out of 5 women have had ≥1 episode of PID
        U.S. health care cost: $3.5 billion per year

Nongonococcal, non-chlamydial causes of PID

Anaerobic bacteria	Aerobic bacteria
Bacteroides species	Nonhemolytic streptococci
Peptococci	Coagulase negative staphylococci
Peptostreptococci	Lactobacilli
Vilonella parvula	Gardnerella vaginalis
Others	Others

Long-term consequences if treatment of PID is delayed

	Infertility (closure of fallopian tubes)	Ectopic pregnancy
1st episode	15%–20%	6–10-fold increase
2nd episode	50%	6–10-fold increase
3rd episode	75%	6–10-fold increase

Because *C. trachomatis* infection of both the cervix and upper genital tract is often asymptomatic, diagnosis is difficult, especially when laparoscopy is not performed. *C. trachomatis* often causes substantial tissue destruction even in asymptomatic cases, and such destruction is a major factor in subsequent infertility. Clinical evidence of improvement therefore may not correlate well with resolution of primary pathology. Because symptoms may improve during antibiotic treatment despite continuing mucosal and soft tissue infection with *C. trachomatis*, clinical cure may be a poor measure of outcome (Glass, 1988).

The search for a single agent effective in the treatment of PID has led to several comparative studies of ciprofloxacin, a new quinolone, versus clindamycin plus an aminoglycoside. Although clinical cure rates with ciprofloxacin have been high, only small numbers of patients have been treated and the results of treatment of mucosal *C. trachomatis* infections appear inadequate. As seen in Table 2, effective treatment for chlamydia is limited to doxycycline, erythromycin, ampicillin, norfloxacin, clindamycin, and amoxicillin (Centers for Disease Control, 1990b). With these alternative medication regimens, test of cure is even more crucial than after a 10-day course of doxycycline, because failure to eradicate the organism is seen more commonly in these regimens. A new macrolide, azithromycin, shows promise as an alternative effective treatment

Table 2. Outpatient treatments for PID

Standard treatments	Effectiveness
ceftriaxone, 250 mg intramuscular	95% +
cefotaxime, 500 mg intramuscular	95% +
ceftizoxime, 500 mg intramuscular	95% +
and	
doxycycline, 100 mg, 2 times per day, 7–10 days	95% +
Alternative treatments for chlamydia (less effective, may need retreatment)	
erythromycin	70%
ampicillin	70%
clindamycin	70%
amoxicillin	70%
norfloxacin (quinolone), 400 mg, 2 times per day, 7–10 days	90% +
azithromycin (macrolide), 500 mg, 4 times per day, 1 day dosage	90% +
Alternative treatment for gonorrhea (greatly limited, because of prevalence of antibiotic-resistant strains)	
doxycycline, 100 mg b.i.d., 7 days	90%–95%
norfloxacin, 400 mg b.i.d., 7–10 days	85%–90%

for *C. trachomatis*. One of the most significant benefits of azithromycin is the 1-day dosing regimen that eliminates the need for compliance with a 7- to 10-day course of medication. As compliance to treatment is so crucial in the eradication of chlamydia, this could be a very important contribution.

Doxycycline is included in inpatient and outpatient regimens because *C. trachomatis* is increasingly being recognized as an initiating factor for PID and presumably requires treatment once PID is established. Treatment failures are more likely with low doses or short courses. Treatment for *C. trachomatis* with doxycycline probably requires more than the standard 7-day course of treatment.

N. gonorrhoeae strains that are resistant to tetracycline are becoming more of a problem. For gonorrhea treatment, ceftriaxone, cefotaxime, and ceftizoxime are still the treatments of choice. Emerging strains of ceftriaxone-resistant gonorrhea are now being seen in Southeast Asian patients and possibly could give rise to spread of these strains into the general population (Centers for Disease Control, 1987, 1990a, 1990b, 1990d).

Compliance with examinations for and treatment of PID can present major obstacles for women with physical disabilities, and not all outpatient facilities are able or want to examine disabled women. Therefore, treatment centers are not as available as would be optimal. Women with disabilities who have had previous negative experiences with logistic difficulties of the gynecologic exam may unfortunately be quite reluctant to seek attention until many of the more serious sequelae have occurred. In addition, the lack of painful sensations may result in lack of awareness of needing attention in the first place.

Compliance with medication regimens may also present obstacles. Women with hand coordination difficulties may be frustrated by pill bottle caps that make it impossible to comply with any medication regimens. This seems like such an easy problem to solve, but many women with disabilities are hindered by unaware pharmacists who need to be educated. One way to avoid this problem is for the prescribing physician to specify that the cap must be easy to open. This puts the responsibility on both the pharmacist and the physician.

A number of conditions, such as multiple sclerosis, amyotrophic lateral sclerosis, and traumatic brain injury, may result in dysphagia (swallowing difficulties). It is really up to the physician to know the patient and to locate a pharmacy or medical center that is able to provide the patient with liquid unit-dose medication. As can be imagined, more of the contents of large bottles of liquid antibiotic ends up on the counter and on the floor than in the patient.

A final point in assessing efficacy of a medication regimen in eradicating PID is the reduction of pain and fever. Obviously, if pain is not assessable, identification of elevated temperature is of major importance. Some women may already be taking anti-inflammatory medication, which could suppress temperature elevations and blunt a febrile response. In addition, patients who like to take charge of their own monitoring may be thwarted by not being able to read the small numbers on a thermometer. These problems are specifically seen in multiple sclerosis and traumatic brain injury. New innovations have enabled color temperature monitoring to solve this problem.

New information has uncovered some disturbing facts pertaining to HIV transmission and women. Men are more likely to transmit HIV to women (than vice versa) because there is more HIV in semen than in vaginal secretions. The anatomy of sexual intercourse places women at greater risk. Therefore, women with disabilities should definitely be included in HIV counseling sessions.

Herpes Simplex Virus (HSV)

Genital herpes can be transmitted when lesions are absent or unrecognized. Therefore, abstinence from intercourse when lesions are present may not completely protect the sexual partner, and use of condoms in all sexual encounters may be the only way to possibly prevent transmission of the virus. No tests are commercially available to identify asymptomatic shedders of HSV. Herpes is not curable, but outbreaks can be palliated by treatment with antiviral therapy (acyclovir). Acyclovir has been shown to decrease the length of viral outbreaks to some degree, but it does not eliminate the virus. Treatment for the first episode of HSV consists of acyclovir, 200 mg 5 times per day for 2 weeks. For recurrent episodes (<6 per year) the standard treatment is acyclovir, 200 mg 5 times per day for 5 days. Testing is underway to evaluate safety and efficacy of a regimen of 800 mg 2 times per day for 5 days. In patients with very frequent herpetic outbreaks (>6 per year), chronic suppressive therapy may be indicated. This regimen is acyclovir, 200 mg 5 times per day for 3–4 months. This regimen significantly reduces recurrences for all cases and completely eliminates recurrences in 73%–94% of cases (Audio-Digest, 1989a; American College of Obstetricians and Gynecologists Update, 1990a).

One of the important issues surrounding HSV in women with physical disabilities is lack of ability to promptly respond to a prodrome. A prodrome of HSV is characterized by subtle tingling or burning or itching in the area of the upcoming outbreak. In women with neuropathies that impair cutaneous sensation, this prodrome is impossible to identify. Obviously, women with spinal cord lesions below T10 are also prevented from identifying herpetic infection independently. Here we get into social issues. As can be seen in Table 3, HSV is quite rampant in the U.S. and in many cases is quite asymptomatic. Unlike gonorrhea, chlamydia, and syphilis, herpes, being a virus, is not curable. Outbreaks can be treated or suppressed on a long-term basis. However, the inability to identify the painful lesions could have dire consequences for a woman's health. Untreated primary herpes can result in massive perineal ulceration, urethral obstruction, hepatitis, and, rarely, encephalitis as well. The treating health care professional needs to educate women with physical disabilities on alternative identifying measures to avoid such dire consequences. The patient will need to learn to recognize changes such as markedly increased or decreased tone, malaise, low-grade fever, and more subtle, subjective clues. Counseling should be routine in women who may be shy about requesting information on birth control and safer sex. Do not wait until she asks; it might be too late.

Table 3.   Statistics and diagnostic issues in the management of genital herpes (HSV)

Statistics

300,000 new cases of herpes annually in the U.S.

30%–60% of PID patients have serologic evidence of previous exposure to herpes and are therefore possibly infectious to others.

HSV is most prevalent in the mid-to upper socioeconomic groups.

In two thirds of cases, partner transmitting infection has visible herpetic lesions.

In one third of cases, partner is an asymptomatic shedder.

Diagnosis primary infection (first episode)

Six-day incubation period

Vaginitis with itching and burning

Severely painful ulcerative lesions

Untreated cases can progress for 3–6 weeks with worsening symptoms

Herpetic lesions are usually seen on the vulva, vagina, and perineum. In severe cases, the meningeal tissues, and the urethral and rectal mucosa can be involved. In these cases fever is often noted.

Recurrent episodes (in first year after primary infection)

HSV type 2: 80% incidence of recurrence; HSV type 1: 40% incidence of recurrence.

After clearing of the first infectious episode, affected patients can expect 3–5 recurrences per year.

In two thirds of recurrent episodes, patient will experience a prodrome 24–72 hours prior to the onset of a lesion: pain, pins and needles, and itching in the vicinity of the primary lesion.

Ulcerative lesions with herpetic appearance should always be cultured for confirmation.

Syphilis

Syphilis is a complex infection that has many confusing symptoms (Beeson et al., 1979) (Table 4). It is usually described as having three stages of progressive debilitating sequelae (Beeson et al., 1979). In the primary stage of syphilis, patients may be seronegative immediately after exposure to a lesion, but darkfield examination of scrapings from a lesion will show spirochetes although the VDRL will not be positive. A new test, florescence treponemal antibody Igm test,

Table 4. Syphilis diagnosis and treatment

Primary stage
  30% chance of infection after first exposure to syphilis
  10- to 90- day incubation (21 days mean)
  Painless chancre develops at point of exposure
  Chancre heals in 3–9 weeks, even if untreated
  Florescence treponemal antibody IgM test

Secondary stage
  Skin rash
  Swollen glands
  Mucus patches
  Condyloma latum

Tertiary stage
  Spinal cord damage (tabes dorsalis)
  Joint, muscle pain; robot-like gait

Latent stage
  No lesions
  No symptoms

Standard treatment of syphillis
Primary, secondary, latent (<1 year)
  Benzathine penicillin G with probenecid: 2.4 million U IM
  Alternative therapy
    Tetracycline: 500 mg 4 times per day for 15 days; erythromycin: 500 mg 4 times per day for 15 days
    Check efficacy of treatment by monitoring VDRL titer every 3 months for 1 year. Titer should fall to 1/4, if it doesn't, retreat. If titer quadruples, retreat.
Seropositivity of unknown duration (>1 year presumed) or HIV-positive
  Benzathine penicillin G with probenecid: 7.2 million U total (2.4 million U IM for 3 successive weeks)
  If HIV-positive, lumbar puncture should be obtained. Some recommend treating with penicillin: 24 million U IV for 10 days
  Alternative treatment as above
  Check efficacy by VDRL titer as above at 18 and 24 months post-therapy. Lumbar puncture may be recommended (see text).
Neurosyphilis:
  Various penicillin regimens: IV, IM, PO

allows for faster and more accurate diagnosis of syphilis in its early stages. Primary stage lesions resolve without treatment in 3–9 weeks. There is clearly a neurosyphilis that occurs as part of primary infection in HIV-infected people that is more severe than that which occurs in people without HIV. It is therefore controversial as to whether a lumbar puncture is necessary in cases of primary syphilis in HIV-positive patients. Secondary stage syphilis is consistently associated with very high titers and is more symptomatic: Fever and malaise, condyloma latum, and palmar and plantar rash as well as other skin rashes are seen. Secondary syphilis lesions resolve within 2–3 weeks without treatment. Following the secondary stage, a latent stage is seen. There are usually no symptoms and no lesions. In addition, spirochetemia decreases after the first year, even if untreated.

In tertiary syphilis, appearance of gumma can be seen in lungs, brain, and other organs. The disease is still treatable in this stage. Infectious damage of major vessels such as the aorta (syphilitic aortitis) is seen, as well as infection of coronary vessels and cardiac valves. Late or tertiary syphilis is the destructive stage of the disease and can be crippling. It has affected many prominent figures in history, and, until the advent of penicillin, it was a dreaded complication of this infection. Late syphilitic complications are still important medical problems, but newly recognized cases of late syphilis have been declining steadily in the U.S. since the second world war.

Late syphilis is usually very slowly progressive, although certain neurologic syndromes may have sudden onset due to endarteritis and thrombosis in the CNS. Late syphilis is noninfectious. Any organ of the body may be involved, but three main types of disease may be distinguished: late benign (gummatous), cardiovascular, and neurosyphilis.

Tertiary Benign Syphilis (Late) Late benign syphilis or gumma has often been cited as the most common complication of late syphilis. In the penicillin era, gummas are quite rare. They typically develop from 1 to 10 years after the initial infection and may involve any part of the body. Although they may be very destructive, they respond very rapidly to treatment and therefore are clinically relatively benign. Histologically, the gumma is a granuloma. The histology is nonspecific and may be associated with central necrosis surrounded by epithelioid and fibroblastic cells and occasionally giant cells. There is sometimes vasculitis.

Gummas may start as a superficial nodule or as a deeper lesion that breaks down to form punched-out ulcers. They are indurated on palpation. There often is central healing with an atrophic scar surrounded by hyperpigmented borders. Cutaneous gummas may resemble other chronic granulomatous ulcerative lesions caused by tuberculosis, sarcoidosis, leprosy, and other deep fungal infections. Gummas may also involve deep visceral organs, of which the most common are the respiratory tract, the gastrointestinal tract, and bones. Precise histologic diagnosis may not be possible. However, the syphilitic gumma is the only such lesion to heal dramatically with penicillin therapy.

Cardiovascular Syphilis The primary cardiovascular complications of syphilis are aortic insufficiency and aortic aneurysm, usually of the ascending aorta. Less commonly, other large arteries may be involved, and, rarely, involvement of the coronary ostia results in coronary insufficiency. These complications in all cases are due to obliterative endarteritis of the vasa vasorum with resultant damage to the intima and media of the great vessels. This results in dilation of the ascending aorta and eventually in stretching of the ring of the aortic valve, producing aortic insufficiency. The valve cusps remain normal.

The disease usually begins within 5–10 years after initial infection, but may not become clinically manifest until 20 or 30 years after infection. Cardiovascular syphilis is thought to be more common in men than in women and possibly in blacks than in whites. The effects of genetic and nutritional factors on development of this and other complications of late syphilis are unclear. Approximately 10%–25% of patients with cardiovascular syphilis have coexistent neurosyphilis, and it is therefore mandatory to do a lumbar puncture in all patients with cardiovascular syphilis.

Neurosyphilis Neurosyphilis may be divided into four groups: asymptomatic, meningovascular, tabes dorsalis, and general paresis. Division is not absolute and there may be considerable overlap between syndromes.

Human Papillomavirus (HPV)/Condyloma Virus/Wart Virus

The widespread prevalence of condyloma virus infection (HPV, warts) of the female cervix is of great concern to us all because of its potential premalignant capabilities (Audio-Digest, 1989c, 1990a; American College of Obstetricians and Gynecologists Update, 1990a). Recent evidence has identified HIV infection as promoting more rapid progression of HPV infection to advanced stages of dysplasia and cancer (Maiman et al., 1991). In high-prevalence areas, women who develop cervical dysplasia are being encouraged to be tested for HIV. The HPV virus infects the epithelial cells of the cervix by integrating into the host genetic material. Early stages of HPV infection are not diagnosable on routine pap smear testing. Only viral-specific DNA analysis will identify presence of the virus at this stage. It is unclear what triggers dysplastic alterations or progressive disease. There are theories to support that certain cofactors such as cigarette smoking and possibly some vaginal infections may promote premalignant morphologic changes in the cells (American College of Obstetricians and Gynecologists Update, 1990b; Audio-Digest, 1989c).

There are now 66 recognized HPV viral types. HPV types 6 and 11 are very rarely malignant. HPV 16 is commonly found in premalignant lesions (CIN, cervical intraepithelial neoplasia) and is a high-risk virus. HPV 18 is the highest-risk virus. Commonly found in high-grade CIN, it is found in invasive cervical cancer, both squamous and endocervical. HPV is further classified into four additional groupings: 30s, 40s, 50s, and 60s. Types 31, 33, and 35 are intermediate-risk viruses. The important viruses in the 40s are types 42 and 45. Type 42 is associated with a significant number of penile diseases, and in the 40s group, only type 45 is found to be highly oncogenic. In the 50s group, type 51 has been found associated with malignant disease. Type 56 appears to be a significant oncogenic virus (Audio-Digest, 1989b). The 60s are newly discovered, and their behavior is not clearly defined.

A significant number of "normal" women carry HPV. In the absence of symptoms, in the absence of a colposcopic lesion, and with a negative pap smear, 10%–12% of women screened will be positive for HPV DNA. Men would have similar findings. Surprisingly large numbers of HPV types 16, 18, 31, 33, and 35 are found in totally asymptomatic people. Cervical adenocarcinomas are also HPV-induced and have principally HPV types 16 and 18, with type 18 predominating.

Management of condyloma virus infection without significant dysplastic alterations as documented by colposcopically directed biopsies is a highly controversial topic. Currently, treatments such as cryosurgery, trichloroacetic acid, laser, 5-FU, and, possibly, interferon are alternative approaches. For CIN, the need for specific treatments as outlined previously is obvious. In the absence of CIN, with evidence of HPV virus present only, the known data documenting spontaneous regression and resolution of visible viral lesions (20%–40%) makes treatment decisions difficult. Further studies are needed to clarify many of the above issues (Carmichael & Maskens, 1988; Syrjanen et al., 1985).

REFERENCES

American College of Obstetricians and Gynecologists Update. (1990a). *Advances in the treatment of cervical cancer, 16*(5). Port Washington, NY: Medical Information Systems, Inc.

American College of Obstetricians and Gynecologists Update. (1990b). *Genital herpes, 15*(8). Port Washington, NY: Medical Information Systems, Inc.

Aminoff, M.J. (Ed.). (1989). *Neurology and general medicine.* New York: Churchill Livingstone.

Audio-Digest Obstetrics/Gynecology Cassette Series. (1989a). *Advances in the management of genital infection, 36*(18). Glendale, CA: Audio-Digest Foundation.

Audio-Digest Obstetrics/Gynecology Cassette Series. (1989b). *Evaluation of pap smears, 36*(10). Glendale, CA: Audio-Digest Foundation.

Audio-Digest Obstetrics/Gynecology Cassette Series. (1989c). *Human papillomavirus (HPV) in the genital tract: Biology and management, 36*(21). Glendale, CA: Audio-Digest Foundation.

Audio-Digest Obstetrics/Gynecology Cassette Series. (1990a). *Geriatric gynecology, 37*(12). Glendale, CA: Audio-Digest Foundation.

Audio-Digest Obstetrics/Gynecology Cassette Series. (1990b). *New CDC guidelines for the treatment of PID, 37*(13). Glendale, CA: Audio-Digest Foundation.

Beeson, P.B., McDermott, W., & Wyngaarden, J.B. (Eds.). (1979). *Cecil textbook of medicine.* Philadelphia: W.B. Saunders.

Carmichael, J.A., & Maskens, P.D. (1988). Cervical dysplasia and human papillomavirus. *American Journal of Obstetrics and Gynecology, 160*(4), 916–918.

Centers for Disease Control. (1987). Frequency and distribution in the United States of strains of *Neisseria gonorrhoeae* with plasmid-mediated, high-level resistance to tetracycline. *Journal of Infectious Diseases, 155*(4), 819–822.

Centers for Disease Control. (1990a). National surveillance of antimicrobial resistance in *Neisseria gonorrhoeae. Journal of the American Medical Association, 264,* 1413–1417.

Centers for Disease Control. (1990b). Pelvic inflammatory disease: Review of treatment options. *Reviews of Infectious Diseases, 12*(6), 5656–5664.

Centers for Disease Control. (1990c). Sexually transmitted diseases. In *Healthy people 2000: National health promotion and disease prevention objectives* (pp. 19.1–19.15).

Centers for Disease Control. (1990d). Therapy for gonococcal infections: Options in 1989. *Reviews of Infectious Diseases, 12*(6), S633–S644.

Glass, R.H. (Ed.). (1988). *Office gynecology* (3rd ed.). Baltimore: Williams & Wilkins.

Heilman, K.M., Watson, R.T., & Greer, M. (1977). *Handbook for differential diagnosis of neurologic signs and symptoms.* New York: Appleton-Century-Crofts.

Jacobsen, L., & Westrom, L. (1969). Objective diagnosis of acute pelvic inflammatory disease. *American Journal of Obstetrics and Gynecology, 105,* 1088.

Maiman, M., Tarricone, N., Vieira, J., Suarez, J., Serur, E., & Boyce, J.G. (1991). Colposcopic evaluation of human immunodeficiency virus-seropositive women. *Obstetrics and Gynecology, 78*(1), 84–88.

Syrjanen, K., Vayrynen, M., Saarikoski, S., Mantyjarvi, R., Parkkinen, S., Hippelainen, M., & Castren, O. (1985). Natural history of cervical human papillomavirus (HPV) infections based on prospective follow-up. *British Journal of Obstetrics and Gynaecology, 92,* 1086–1092.

Vitale, J.J. (1976). *Vitamins.* Kalamazoo, MI: Upjohn Company.

Williams, C.L., & Strobino, B.A. (1990). Lyme disease transmission during pregnancy. *Contemporary Ob/Gyn, 35*(6), 48–64.

26

Pathophysiology of Sexual Dysfunction in Males with Physical Disabilities

Craig F. Donatucci and Tom F. Lue

Human sexuality plays an integral role in the well-being of the individual. Any process that interferes with the expression of normal human sexual function greatly affects the quality of life. Serious illness of any type is known to decrease sexual activity in most men. Dysfunction can be the direct result of the illness or a consequence of the psychosocial effects of the disease. Often the pathologic process causing the dysfunction does not specifically involve the genitourinary organs. Whatever the etiology, the net result is a decrease in the expression of normal human sexual function. With an understanding of the underlying problem, and familiarity with current modalities of therapy, the health care practitioner can positively improve quality of life for these patients.

ANATOMY OF THE PENIS AND PHYSIOLOGY OF ERECTION

The penis consists of three spongy cylinders, the paired corpora cavernosa, and a single corpus spongiosum, encased within Buck's fascia. The urethra and the third erectile cylinder, the corpus spongiosum, lie in the ventral groove formed by the paired corpora cavernosa. The glans penis is a distal expansion of the corpus spongiosum. The sinusoids, multiple blood-filled cavernous spaces separated by trabeculae of supporting connective tissues, are the main structural component of the three corpora and the glans penis. The sinusoids, contain smooth muscles cells, arterioles, venules, and terminal nerve endings and are lined with endothelial cells.

Arterial inflow originates from the paired internal pudendal arteries. After giving off the perineal artery, the internal pudendal artery becomes the common penile artery, which courses through the pelvis to terminate in three branches: the bulbourethral, the dorsal, and the cavernous arteries (Figure 1). The cavernous arteries, running longitudinally in the corpora near the septum, are the major source of blood to the erectile tissue. Blood supplied by these paired arteries fills the corpora cavernosa during tumescence (Tanagho & Lue, 1990).

The venous drainage of the penis regulates the outflow of blood during erection (Breza, Aboseif, Orvis, Lue, & Tanagho, 1989). The superficial dorsal veins, small venous channels in the subcutaneous layer, usually empty into the saphenous vein (Figure 2). Venous blood from the corporal sinusoids drains initially into tiny venules

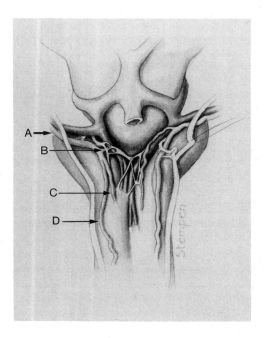

Figure 1.   The internal pudendal artery (A) gives origin to the urethral artery (B), the cavenous artery (C), and the dorsal artery (D) of the penis. (From Breza, J., Aboseif, S.R., Orvis, B.R., Lue, T.F., & Tanagho, E.A. [1989]. Detailed anatomy of penile neurovascular structures: Surgical significance. *Journal of Urology, 141*, 437–443. Copyright © 1989 by American Urological Society; reprinted by permission.)

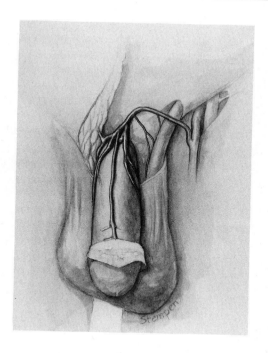

Figure 2. The superficial veins of the penis drain to the saphenous vein. (From Breza, J., Aboseif, S.R., Orvis, B.R., Lue, T.F., & Tanagho, E.A. [1989]. Detailed anatomy of penile neurovascular structures: Surgical significance. *Journal of Urology, 141,* 437–443. Copyright © 1989 by American Urological Society; reprinted by permission.)

under the tunica albuginea. These venules form subtunical venular plexuses that penetrate the tunica albuginea as the emissary veins. In the mid- and distal shaft, emissary veins course through the tunica albuginea before joining the deep dorsal vein (Figure 3). Emissary veins exiting laterally drain to the circumflex veins, which exit ventrally to the periurethral veins. The deep dorsal vein receives several circumflex veins, then penetrates the urogenital diaphragm behind the pubic bone to become the periprostatic plexus. Emissary veins in the proximal third of the penis join to form the cavernous veins, which drain directly into the internal pudendal vein.

REGULATION OF HEMODYNAMIC BALANCE

The hemodynamic balance between arterial inflow and venous outflow occurs at the microvascular level, under neurogenic control (Fournier, Juenemann, Lue, & Tanagho, 1987). In the flaccid state, the inflow vessels, the arterioles, are constricted. The sinusoids,

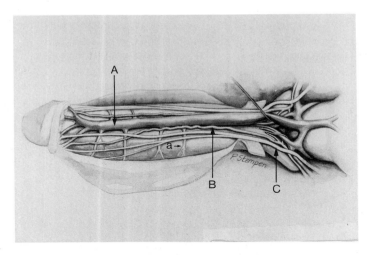

Figure 3. The emissary veins (a) drain to the deep dorsal vein (A), which then joins the periprostatic plexus. The dorsal arteries (B) and dorsal vein (C) lie adjacent to the deep dorsal vein. (From Breza, J., Aboseif, S.R., Orvis, B.R., Lue, T.F., & Tanagho, E.A. [1989]. Detailed anatomy of penile neurovascular structures: Surgical significance. *Journal of Urology, 141*, 437–443. Copyright © 1989 by American Urological Society; reprinted by permission.)

microscopic sinusoidal spaces whose walls are composed of endo-thelial cells and smooth muscles, are contracted. Together they exert a high resistance against arterial flow, allowing only a small amount of blood to flow to the tissue. At initiation of erection, the smooth muscles of the sinusoids and arterioles relax (control of this process is discussed below), increasing sinusoidal compliance and lowering the peripheral resistance to a minimum. Arterial inflow increases immediately, with dilation of the entire penile arterial tree and rapid filling of the sinusoidal spaces. The arteries and arterioles become straight and larger, leading to markedly distended smooth-appearing sinusoids.

The extensive network of subtunical venules join to form intermediary venules of about 100 microns in diameter. The larger of these subtunical venules join to form the emissary veins, which then exit through the tunica albuginea. Compression of the subtunical venules between the sinusoidal walls and the tunica albuginea restricts the venous outflow to a minimum during erection (Figure 4). Uneven stretching of the layers of the tunica albuginea also contributes to the close of the emissary veins.

Neurologic Control of Erection

Nervous system control of erection is both central and peripheral. The erection centers of the central nervous system include the sep-

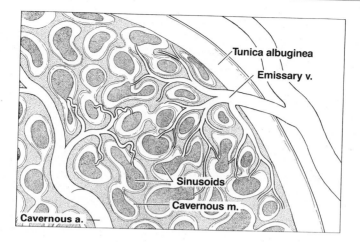

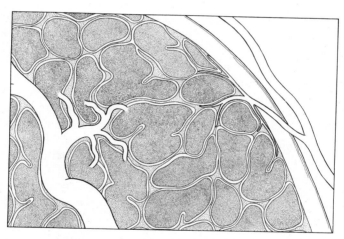

Figure 4. Mechanism of penile erection: In the flaccid state (A), the arteries, arterioles, and sinusoids are contracted. The intersinusoidal and subtunical venules are open with free flow to the emissary veins. During erection (B), the muscles of the sinusoidal wall and the arterioles relax, allowing maximal flow to fill the new compliant sinusoidal spaces. The small venules are compressed between sinusoids. The larger intermediary venules are sandwiched and compressed between the distended sinusoidal wall and the non-compliant tunica albuginea thus restrict the venous flow to a minimum. (From Lue, T.F. [1992]. Male sexual dysfunction. In E.A. Tanagho & J.W. McAninch [Eds.], *Smith's general urology* (13th ed., pp. 696–713). East Norwalk, CT: Appleton & Lange; reprinted by permission.)

tal portion of the hippocampus, the anterior cingulate gyrus, the anterior thalamic nuclei, the mammillothalamic tract, and the mammillary bodies. There are two spinal centers responsible for penile erection: the thoracolumbar and the sacral erection centers. From these nuclei, axons issue ventrally to join the inferior hypogastric and the pelvic plexuses. Nerve bundles from these plexuses innervate the bladder, prostate, rectum, and the penis (Lue, Zeineh, Schmid, & Tanagho, 1984; Walsh & Donker, 1982). The fibers innervating the penis (the cavernous nerves) travel along the posterolateral aspect of the seminal vesicle and the prostate, then penetrate the genitourinary diaphragm. These fibers are located near the lateral aspect of the membranous urethra and ascend gradually to the 1 and 11 o'clock positions to enter the corpora cavernosa with the cavernous arteries and veins. The autonomic nervous system is responsible for the vascular event of penile erection and detumescence.

The sensory component originates in the nerve endings of the glans and penile skin and possibly the corpora cavernosa. These nerves bundles join to form the paired dorsal nerve or the penis. After passing through the genitourinary diaphragm, the dorsal nerve of the penis joins the perineal nerve to form the pudendal nerve. The messages from the sensory receptors may pass to the sacral or thoracolumbar erection center to induce reflexogenic erection or travel through the ascending spinal tracts to the thalamus and the brain for sensory perception. This sensory input is also the afferent arm of the bulbocavernous reflex.

The somatic efferent pathway originates in the motor cortex. The impulses are carried via the corticospinal tract to the anterior horn of the second, third, and fourth sacral spinal cords. The messages are relayed via the anterior sacral roots to the pudendal nerve to innervate the ischiocavernosus and bulbocavernosus muscles. Contraction of the ischiocavernosus muscle after the corpora are filled with blood produces rigidity of the penis, with the pressure in the corpora cavernosa rising well above the systolic pressure (Lue & Tanagho, 1987). Rhythmic contraction of the bulbocavernosus muscle helps expel the semen from the urethra during ejaculation.

DIAGNOSTIC TESTS FOR ERECTILE DYSFUNCTION

Because impotence is a functional disease, diagnostic tests can be tailored according to the treatment the patient desires and his physical and mental conditions. This approach is based on: 1) the most recent advances of diagnostic techniques and therapy of impotence; and 2) the patient's physical and mental health, motivation, and goal and is termed the patient's goal-directed management of impotence.

Combined Intracavernous Injection and Stimulation Testing

After initial history, physical examination, and basic laboratory studies, selected groups of patients are asked to undergo a combined injection and stimulation test (CIS test, Lue, 1989). This test utilizes tactile input to improve the quality of erection obtained after intracavernous injection. In addition, self-stimulation can also give some indication of the integrity of the patient's reflexogenic erectile response and whether he is under psychologic inhibition at the time of testing.

Nocturnal Penile Tumescence Monitoring

The patient who has a full response to the CIS test suffers either from neurogenic or psychogenic impotence. It is difficult to differentiate between the two. However, since normal men experience erections during rapid eye movement sleep, monitoring these erections can document an intact neurovascular erectile mechanism (Karacan & Howell, 1988). A simple method is to place a ring of stamps around the base of the penis, and expansion during sleep may result in breakage of the perforations of the ring. A significant disadvantage of the above method is that it only records information about a single event during sleep. To overcome this disadvantage, several electronic monitors that can record the number and quality of nocturnal erections have been developed. Mercury strain gauges measure penile tumescence, length, and rigidity at predetermined intervals, the results are downloaded into a computer, and 8-hour recording sessions can be scanned for composite patterns of rigidity and tumescence.

Diagnostic Tests For Arterial Insufficiency

Penile Brachial Pressure Index Testing   Because of its low cost and wide availability, penile brachial index testing can also serve as a good office screen. Utilizing Doppler ultrasound, the pressure in the penile arteries is divided by the systolic pressure obtained in the brachial artery. Most authors consider a value above 0.7 as normal. Correlation between the Doppler penile brachial index testing and arteriographic findings have been fair. Because this test is based on Doppler wave forms, the information obtained is not specific for the cavernous arteries. The Doppler may pick up the dorsal artery of the penis, and perfusion of the dorsal artery may not be an accurate reflection of the integrity of the corporal arterial system.

Duplex Ultrasound Scanning   Duplex ultrasound testing combines real-time ultrasonography to visualize the cavernous arteries with pulsed Doppler scanning to measure the velocity of blood flow through those arteries (Lue, Hricak, Marich, & Tanagho, 1985). The echogenicity of the penile tissues is observed, and the diameters of the cavernous arteries are measured before and after intracavernous injection of a vasodilator as a functional test of the cavernous arterial function. The thickness of the cavernous artery wall can be measured and the artery observed for pulsation; healthy arteries will be noted to a have thin walls with strong pulsations. The peak flow velocity of blood within the cavernous arteries is measured after injection, and the values obtained are then compared with normal controls. Normal values are a post-injection diameter of more than 0.07 cm, peak flow velocity over 25 cm/sec, and a strong pulsation of the cavernous arteries.

The advantages of duplex ultrasound scanning are its noninvasiveness and sensitivity. Further, it can be combined with the CIS test in the office to arrive at a simple, minimally invasive differential diagnosis of erectile dysfunction. Duplex ultrasonography performed properly may be superior to pharmacologic arteriography (see below) for the diagnosis of arteriogenic impotence (Mueller, van Wallenberg-Pachaly, Voges, & Schild, 1990). The disadvantages of this procedure are the high cost of the equipment to perform the test and its operator-dependency of results.

Cavernous Arterial Occlusion Pressure   After reaching maximal tumescence during the filling phase of erection, the rigidity of the corpus cavernosum increases with further arterial inflow. Thus, by artificially increasing the intracorporal pressure beyond the systolic level and then allowing the pressure to fall until cavernous arterial flow resumes, the cavernous arterial occlusion pressure is obtained and the functional integrity of these vessels can be directly measured (Padma-Nathan, 1989).

Pharmacologic Arteriography   Long considered the "gold standard" in the evaluation of arterial function, pharmacologic arteriography has many potential pitfalls. Because of the low flow rate in the flaccid penis and the inhibition because of anxiety and apprehension during penile arteriography, the cavernous arteries may be poorly visualized and mistakenly judged to be diseased. With the introduction of intracavernous vasodilator injection, excellent visualization of the cavernous arteries with local anesthesia can be obtained and their true function properly evaluated. Yet, because of the potential for complications and its high cost, arteriography should be reserved for those patients who are to undergo reconstructive surgery of the penile arteries.

Diagnostic Tests for Venous Leakage

The CIS test can be used to gain an indirect assessment of the integrity of the penile veno-occlusive mechanism. The patient with a suspected venous leak would achieve a full erection, but would be unable to sustain the erection for at least 5 minutes.

At the University of California School of Medicine, San Francisco, pharmacologic cavernosometry is performed as a preoperative procedure to confirm the diagnosis of venous leak, and cavernosography is performed to identify the site of venous leakage (Lue Hricak, Schmidt, & Tanagho, 1986).

TREATMENT OPTIONS FOR IMPOTENCE

Psychosexual Therapy

In previous decades, 90% of cases of impotence were believed to be psychogenic (Masters & Johnson, 1970). Current thinking is that 50% of impotent patients have an underlying organic disorder, and in the older population, the percentage is probably higher. After appropriate history, physical examination, and diagnostic evaluation have established the probable diagnosis of psychogenic impotence, an attempt at psychosexual therapy is indicated. Among the goals of sex therapy intervention are the correction of misinformation and myths, establishment of mutual responsibility for satisfaction, and the elimination of interference in the form of performance demand or anxiety (Smith, 1988).

There are few controlled studies establishing the effectiveness of behavior therapy for functional impotence. Patients are often resistant to referral. Seagraves, Schoenberg, Goldman, and Ivanoff (1986) reported that 38% of patients referred to psychiatry never contacted the clinic, and of those who did, 83% refused therapy or terminated therapy early. The establishment of a satellite psychiatry service in the urology clinic may lead to an improved rate of success.

Oral Medication

Despite great patient desire for an effective oral therapy for impotence, yohimbine, an alpha-2 blocker, is the only agent available. It has had only moderate success (compared to placebo) in treating impotent patients in several clinical studies. The response rate seems higher in the patients with psychogenic impotence (31% complete and 31% partial) than organic impotence (18% complete and 27% partial) (Susset et al., 1989). It is often prescribed for patients seeking treatment for impotence because of its relatively mild side effects (i.e., anxiety, nervousness, slight increase of blood pressure).

Endocrine Therapy

After diabetes, the three most common endocrine conditions associated with impotence are:

1. Hypergonadotropic hypogonadism—the loss of end-organ androgen production may be the result of infection, trauma, surgery, or congenital abnormalities of sex chromosome or gonadal differentiation. Impotent men may present with depressed serum testosterone and elevated serum gonadotropins. The treatment is testosterone enanthate 200 mg intramuscularly every 2–3 weeks.

2. Hypogonadotropic hypogonadism—the loss of gonadotropin production with secondary decrease in end-organ androgen production, this condition is rare and often associated with prolactinomas or Kallmann syndrome. Treatment is directed at eliminating the primary cause and the institution of supplementary parenteral testosterone therapy.

3. Hyperprolactinemia—in most patients suffering from this condition, there is found to be an iatrogenic cause. Many medications are known to cause overproduction of prolactin (i.e., estrogens, reserpine, phenothiazine, or alpha-methyldopa), and secondary impotence may result. Only a small portion of patients with impotence due to hyperprolactinemia have pituitary tumors. In those patients with iatrogenic hyperprolactinemia, treatment consists of a change of medication. Patients with pituitary tumors may be treated with bromocriptine (Parlodel) or pituitary surgery.

Intracavernous Injection

Self-injection of papaverine or papaverine with phentolamine has become a popular treatment (Brindley, 1983; Virag, 1982; Zorgniotti & Lefleur, 1985). Sexual stimulation enhances the response (64% of impotent patients improve the quality of their erections with self-stimulation) (Donatucci & Lue, 1992) and lessens the amount of agent required to induce erection. Nearly all patients with neurogenic impotence, and about 60%–70% of patients with vasculogenic impotence, respond to intracavernous injections (Sidi & Chen, 1989). Intracavernous injection of prostaglandin E_1 was recently introduced with encouraging results (Ishii et al., 1989; Stackl, Hasun, & Marberger, 1988). Prostaglandin E_1 is metabolized during a single pass through the lungs and may be metabolized in the corpora to some degree. The major side effect is painful erection in about 20% of patients, which may be related to the concentration of the drug or penile neuropathy.

The major complications of self-injection therapy are priapism and fibrosis of the erectile tissues (Juenemann & Alken, 1989). Although incidence of priapism has been reported to range from 3% to 10%, with careful instruction and titration of doses, this complication can be avoided Other minor complications include hematoma, drop in blood pressure, vasovagal reflex, subcutaneous injection, and mild chemical hepatitis (Levine et al., 1989).

Vacuum Constriction Device

Several vacuum constriction devices (VCD) are now available commercially. The standard VCD consists of a suction cylinder and pump to induce erection and a constricting band placed at the base of the penis to maintain the erection-like state after the suction device is removed. To prevent ischemia of the penis, the patient is advised to remove the constriction band within 30 minutes.

Satisfactory use of these devices has been reported in a large number of patients. A retrospective study of 1,517 patients revealed that 92% achieved an erection or erection-like state sufficient for intercourse, and 77% were able to have intercourse at least every 2 weeks (Witherington, 1985). The reported complications (30, 50) include petechiae (27%), ecchymosis (10%), initial penile pain (41%), ejaculatory difficulty, usually from erectile pivoting (12%), dusky discoloration of the glans, penile numbness, and trapping of the ejaculate (Nadig, Ware, & Blumoff, 1986; Witherington, 1985).

Combined VCD and Intracavernous Injection

Simultaneous injection of intracavernous vasodilating drugs with use of a vacuum constriction device may be of help to patients who could not achieve adequate erection with either therapy alone. This is especially helpful for patients with severe vascular disease and for those with fibrosis of the erectile tissues secondary to priapism. An additional subgroup of patients who may benefit from the use of the VCD are those who have failed penile prosthesis insertion. The use of VCD in this group of patients markedly improves the erection obtained by intracavernous injection alone.

Vascular Reconstruction

Despite the high success rates of the new medical therapies described above, many patients are reticent to perform self-injection therapy and dislike the lack of spontaneity inherent in the use of the vacuum constriction device. However, many of these men still wish to avoid a penile prosthesis, thus stimulating the need to create and develop rational vascular reconstructive procedures to correct the varied forms of vasculogenic impotence.

Arterial Surgery   The common goal of all vascular reconstructive procedures is to improve cavernosal perfusion. This is achieved primarily through creation of an arterio-arterial anastomosis in an attempt to improve perfusion via the cavernous artery or through the arterialization of the deep dorsal vein, attempting to improve perfusion retrograde into the corpora cavernosa. The ideal arterial reconstructive method would provide rich arterial run-off in the flaccid state without concomitant increase in intracavernous pressure; avoid poor arterial run-off, which can lead to thrombotic obstruction of the anastomosis; and not result in high intracavernous pressure that may result in sinusoidal damage (Breza, Aboseif, Lue, & Tanagho, 1990).

Anastomosis of a donor artery to a cavernous artery would appear to be ideal, but the small size of the recipient artery and the poor run-off in the flaccid penis limit the success of this technique. Anastomosis of a donor artery to the dorsal artery of the penis would be adequate for those patients in whom large communicating branches can carry enough flow to the corpora cavernosa, but these are seen in less than 20% of cases. With the hypogastric and pudendal arteries, because of the size and greater flow rate of these vessels, balloon dilation or reconstructive surgery of an isolated lesion has a reasonable success rate. In patients with generalized atherosclerosis, however, impotence usually recurs with progression of their arterial disease.

Venous Surgery   As understanding of the importance of the integrity of the venous occlusive mechanism to the development of erection has been gained, a new era in penile vascular surgery has dawned. The ability to diagnose patients with severe arterial disease by duplex ultrasonography and to confirm the diagnosis in patients with venous leakage by cavernosometry and cavernosography allows patients with pure venogenic impotence to be selected for surgical correction. Early work involved ligation of the deep dorsal vein of the penis only, but many investigators found results unsatisfactory. Recent authors have described a variety of technical improvements, among them crural ligation to stop proximal drainage, or separation of the corpora cavernosa from the spongiosum to ligate the communicating branches. Success rates usually fall in the 50%–70% range (DePalma et al., 1989; Knoll, Furlow, & Benson, 1990). Complications include numbness of the penile skin, shortened penile length, penile curvature, and hematoma (Lewis, 1990; Wespes & Schulman, 1985).

Combined Arterial and Venous Surgery   In patients with mixed arterial-venous insufficiency, which is the most common cause of vasculogenic impotence, a reconstructive operation must increase arterial inflow as well as reduce venous leak. Virag introduced an operation utilizing an epigastric artery to deep dorsal vein anastomosis directed toward both the arteriogenic and venogenic components (Virag, Saltiel, Floresco, Shoukry, & Dufour, 1988). With dorsal vein arterialization, additional arterial blood would be supplied retrograde into the corpora cavernosa through the deep dorsal vein and emissary veins. A corporo-venous fistula may be added between the corpora cavernosa and the deep dorsal vein to improve the retrograde perfusion of the corpora cavernosa. Virag has reported return of normal erectile function in 49% of patients and improvement in an additional 20% (Virag, Bennett, & Shoukry, 1989). The reported complications include hypervascularization of glans, hematoma, and early thrombosis of the anastomosis. Theoretically, these procedures should achieve a higher success rate because they simultaneously correct problems of supply and drainage.

Prosthetic Surgery

Before the introduction of intracavernous vasodilator injection therapy, testosterone injections or placement of a penile prosthesis were the only effective treatment for erectile dysfunction besides psychological counseling. Today, the high success rate of less invasive therapies, such as intracavernous injection and vacuum constriction devices (VCD), has dramatically reduced prosthetic surgery.

There are two major categories of penile prostheses: 1) the semirigid prosthesis, and 2) the inflatable prosthesis. The semirigid prosthesis has the advantage of simple design and ease of insertion. Further, because of its simple design, it is resistant to mechanical failure. The disadvantage of the semirigid prosthesis is its permanently erect state and lack of concealability. The inflatable prosthesis has the advantage that it both elongates and expands in girth while inflated, which results in a more natural erection. However, the complexity of its design and the need for a fluid reservoir make placement more exacting and increase the chances for mechanical failure. Over the years, numerous modifications have been made to improve the concealment (semirigid) and durability (inflatable) of the penile prostheses and to reduce the complication rate of prosthetic surgery. The complications include device failure, perforation, infection, persistent pain, and aneurysmal dilation of the inflatable devices. With improved design and more durable material, the complication rate has been significantly reduced over the past few years, and the patient–partner satisfaction rate approaches 90% (Benson & Boileau, 1987).

SPECIFIC DISABILITY

Individual medical conditions may lead to sexual dysfunction by a variety of pathologic mechanisms, but all serious illness will affect sexual function adversely. Lack of communication about sexual concerns is common between physician and patient when both are concerned about the primary disease. Cultural traditions generally inhibit both patient and physician from speaking about sexual function (Wagner, 1981). There may be a direct relationship between the development of postsurgical sexual problems and the lack of discussion about sexuality prior to discharge from the hospital (Renshaw & Karstaedt, 1988). An important factor is the ability of the partner to cope with a mate's disease and the change in sexual behavior caused by the condition. The fear of death during intercourse may lead a couple to sleep apart.

Cardiovascular Disease

Despite recent advances, cardiovascular disease continues to be the leading cause of death in the U.S. Those patients who do not succumb to their initial myocardial event suffer significant sequelae, not the least of which is sexual dysfunction. Of patients who suffer a first myocardial infarction (MI), 25% never resume sexual activity, 50% resume sex but at a reduced frequency, and only 25% return to their normal, premyocardial infarction level of sexual activity (Gould, 1989). While some men post-MI suffer from ejaculatory problems, the greatest problems are impotence and decreased sexual drive. Impotence may be due to a progression of the generalized atherosclerotic process that now involves the penile vasculature or may be secondary to cardiac medications. Patients with primary vasculogenic impotence respond to a number of conventional therapeutic measures as mentioned above. Individualized therapy should be offered in accordance with the patient's goals.

Decreased sexual drive may be due to a variety of factors. A significant cause is the fear of death during coitus. However, the actual risk of such an event is small. In a study of nearly 6,000 patients with sudden death after myocardial infarction only 6 deaths were directly attributable to the stress of coitus (Ueno, 1969). Decreased self-esteem and preexisting sexual problems can also contribute to decreased sexual function after a cardiovascular event (Wolbroehl, 1984). Cerebrovascular accidents can also lead to a similar decrease in sexual function. Again, the dysfunction can be secondary to generalized atherosclerosis with vasculogenic impotence, or due to loss of motor control, inability to communicate, or diminished capacity for arousal (Sjogren & Fugl-Meyer, 1982).

Transplantation

The severe impact of end-stage heart disease and cardiac transplantation on patients' sexuality was documented by Tabler, Gunther, Kern, and Sanger (1990). Twenty-one of 45 patients who underwent heart transplantation responded to a written questionnaire concerning post-transplant sexual activity. Sexual dysfunction was present to some degree in the majority of patients, with impotence, ejaculatory problems, and altered libido most common. Many patients avoided sexual opportunities out of fear of death during coitus. The health care practitioner needs to discuss sexuality and sexual practice post-transplant before surgery to minimize sexual difficulty postoperatively. Specific therapy can be individualized to the patient's goals. Several transplant patients have utilized intracavernous injection therapy with excellent results at the University of San Francisco.

Ostomy

Patients' perceptions of sexuality after ostomy surgery were explored by Gloeckner (1991) using a questionnaire to examine sexual adjustment and attitudes in patients who had undergone ostomy surgery. Seventy-eight patients with permanent ostomies, at least 1 year after surgery, were asked to participate and 40 chose to do so. The majority of patients had undergone bowel diversion, the rest had undergone urinary diversion. Physical changes were evaluated, with the majority of men suffering impotence after surgery, and many women reporting dyspareunia. Intrapsychic changes were investigated by questioning changes in body image and conception of sexual attractiveness. Most patients suffered some loss in perception of sexual attractiveness in the postoperative period, with improvement in two thirds of them with time. Patients who had undergone bowel diversion had a higher sense of sexual attractiveness than those with continent diversion or urinary conduits, but the reason for this surprising finding was not explored. Finally, the author noted that the majority of respondents report growing closer to their partners after the experience of major surgery. This study again reinforces the need for the urologist to discuss the sexual consequences of surgery with both patient and partner.

Male patients who have undergone creation of an ostomy after major pelvic surgery often develop secondary erectile dysfunction.

The neurovascular supply to the penis is particularly prone to injury during these procedures. Utilizing one of the therapeutic regimens mentioned previously, normal sexual function can be restored in these patients.

Spinal Cord Injury

Sexual concerns are often of significant importance to the patient with a spinal lesion. Three factors are important when considering the effect of the spinal injury on sexual function: the sex of the patient, the neurologic level of the lesion, and the degree of completion of the lesion (Bennet, Seager, Vasher, & McGuire, 1988). In both sexes, the level of the lesion affects the adequacy of sexual function. Men with partial upper motor neuron lesions may retain reflexogenic erectile and psychogenic erectile capability. If the upper motor lesion is complete, psychogenic erection is lost. The reflexogenic erection that remains may be unsatisfactory for sexual intercourse because the onset of tumescence and detumescence bear no relation to sexual arousal. A lower motor neuron lesion below or at the S-2, S-3, and S-4 levels will cause erectile function to be lost.

The majority of the data concerning sexual function in spinal cord injury patients is dated, but several series have been well studied. Munroe and associates studied 84 male patients ranging in age from 21 to 40 (Munroe, Horne, & Paull, 1948). Erectile function was noted in 74% of the patients overall, but injury to the sacral cord or caudal equina precluded erectile function. Bors and Comarr (1960) investigated 529 patients with spinal injury, 63.5%–94% retained erectile function. They noted that erectile function was greatest in patients with incomplete upper motor lesions, those with complete upper motor lesions had less, and those with complete lower motor lesions had least of all. Sexual intercourse was possible for only 23%–33% of these patients and ejaculation for 3%–19%. In another large series of 638 patients, Tsuji and associates found an overall potency rate of 54%, with 67% of the patients with incomplete lesions maintaining erectile function, and 50% of the patients with complete lesions retaining potency (Tsuji, Nakajima, Morimoto, & Nounaka, 1961).

Spinal cord injury patients are most sensitive to small doses of intracavernous vasoactive agents, and normal, natural erections can be restored by a self-injection regimen. In the future, these patients may benefit from electrostimulation of the cavernous nerves. Chronic electrostimulation of the cavernous nerves with resultant erection has been well documented in an animal model (Lue & Tanagho, 1988). Further, in a recent report, intraoperative stimulation of the cavernous nerves in patients undergoing radical prostatectomy was described (Lue, Gleason, Carroll, & Tanagho, 1991). Five of the seven patients who were potent preoperatively had erections, while none of the five who were impotent before surgery responded. Because most spinal cord injury patients are young and have an intact neurovascular bundle and normal cavernous nerves, they may be well suited to electrostimulation.

Women with spinal injuries may have insufficient vaginal secretions at the time of intercourse, a problem easily remedied with standard surgical lubricant. Psychogenic vaginal lubrication may persist in women with lower motor neuron lesions. Menstruation, ovulation, and fertility continue unimpaired, and deliveries are not uncommon in the patient with a spinal cord injury. These patients are at high obstetrical risk and require close prenatal supervision and care (Rieve, 1989).

SUMMARY

New, minimally invasive diagnostic tests can be utilized to clarify the underlying cause of the sexual dysfunction in individuals with disabilities. Recently developed therapeutic measures offer the patient a range of options to treat sexual dysfunction, from psychological counseling to intracavernous injection programs, vacuum constriction devices, and various reconstructive and prosthetic surgical procedures. Armed with a thorough understanding of the cause of sexual dysfunction in an individual with a disability, knowledge of the patient's goals can allow the health care practioner to provide direct therapy and positively affect the patient's quality of life.

REFERENCES

Bennet, C.J., Seager, S.W., Vasher, E.A., & McGuire, E.J. (1988). Sexual dysfunction and electroejaculation in men with spinal cord injury: Review. Journal of Urology, 139, 453–457.

Benson, G.S., & Boileau, M.A. (1987). The penis: Sexual function and dysfunction. In J.Y. Gillenwater, J.T. Grayhack, S.S. Howards, & J.W. Duckett (Eds.), Adult & pediatric urology (pp. 1407–1447). Chicago: Yearbook Medical Publishers.

Bors, E., & Comarr, A.E. (1960). Neurological disturbances of sexual function with special reference to 529 patients with spinal cord injury. Urologic Survey, 10, 191–222.

Breza, J., Aboseif, S.R., Lue, T.F., & Tanagho, E.A. (1990). Cavernous vein arterialization for the treatment of vasculogenic impotence: An animal model. Journal of Urology, 139, 298A.

Breza, J., Aboseif, S.R., Orvis, B.R., Lue, T.F., & Tanagho, E.A. (1989). Detailed anatomy of penile neurovascular structures: Surgical significance. *Journal of Urology, 141,* 437–443.

Brindley, G.S. (1983). Cavernosal alpha-blockade: A new technique for investigating and treating erectile impotence. *British Journal of Psychiatry, 143,* 332–337.

DePalma, R.G., Schwab, F., Druy, E.M., Miller, H.C., Emsellem, H.A., Edwards, C.M., & Bergrud, D. (1989). Experience in diagnosis and treatment of impotence caused by cavernosal leak syndrome. *Journal of Vascular Surgery, 9,* 117–121.

Donatucci, C.F., & Lue, T.F. (1992). The combined intracavernous injection and stimulation test. *Journal of Urology, 148,* 61–62.

Fournier, G., Jr., Juenemann, K.-P., Lue, T.F., & Tanagho, E.A. (1987). Mechanism of venous occlusion during canine penile erection: An anatomic demonstration. *Journal of Urology, 137,* 163–167.

Gloeckner, M.J. (1991). Perceptions of sexuality after ostomy surgery. *Journal of Enterostomal Therapy, 18*(1), 36–38.

Gould, L.A. (1989). Impact of cardiovascular disease on male sexual function. *Medical Aspects of Human Sexuality, 23,* 24–27.

Ishii, N., Watanabe, H., Irisawa, Y., Kubota, Y., Kubota, Y., Kawamura, S., Suzuki, K., Chiba, R., Tokiwa, M., & Shirai, M. (1989). Intracavernous injection of prostaglandin E_1 for the treatment of erectile impotence. *Journal of Urology, 141,* 323–325.

Juenemann, K.-P., & Alken, P. (1989). Pharmacotherapy of erectile dysfunction: A review. *International Journal of Impotence Research, 1,* 71–93.

Karacan, I., & Howell, J. (1988). Use of nocturnal penile tumescence in diagnosis of male erectile dysfunction. In E.A. Tanagho, T.F. Lue, & R.D. McLure (Eds.), *Contemporary management of impotence and infertility* (pp. 95–103). Baltimore: Williams & Wilkins.

Knoll, L.K., Furlow, W.L., & Benson, R.C. (1990). Penile venous surgery for the management of cavernosal venous leakage. *International Journal of Impotence Research, 2,* 21–27.

Levine, S.B., Althof, S.E., Turner, L.A., Risen, C.B., Bodner, D.R., Kursh, E.D., & Resnick, M.I. (1989). Side effects of self-administration of intracavernous papaverine and phentolamine for the treatment of impotence. *Journal of Urology, 141,* 54–57.

Lewis, R.W. (1990). Venous ligation surgery for venous leakage. *International Journal of Impotence Research, 2*(1), 1–19.

Lue, T.F. (1989). Impotence: A patient's goal-directed approach to treatment. *World Journal of Urology, 8,* 67–74.

Lue, T.F., Gleason, C., Carroll, P., & Tanagho, E.A. (1991). Intraoperative stimulation of the cavernous nerves in men. *Journal of Urology, 145*(4), 344A.

Lue, T.F., Hricak, H., Marich, K.W., & Tanagho, E.A. (1985). Vasculogenic impotence evaluated by high resolution ultrasonography and pulsed Doppler spectrum analysis. *Radiology, 155,* 777–781.

Lue, T.F., Hricak, H., Schmidt, R.A., & Tanagho, E.A. (1986). Functional evaluation of penile veins by cavernosography in papaverine-induced erection. *Journal of Urology, 135,* 479–482.

Lue, T.F., & Tanagho, E.A. (1987). Physiology of erection and pharmacologic management of impotence. *Journal of Urology, 137,* 829–836.

Lue, T.F., & Tanagho, E.A. (1988). Erection pacemaker. In E.A. Tanagho, T.F. Lue, & R.D. McClure (Eds.), *Contemporary management of impotence and infertility* (pp. 157–159). Baltimore: Williams & Wilkins.

Lue, T.F., Zeineh, S.J., Schmid, R.A., & Tanagho, E.A. (1984). Neuroanatomy of penile erection: Its relevance to iatrogenic impotence. *Journal of Urology, 131*, 273–280.

Masters, W.H., & Johnson, V.E. (1970). *Human sexual inadequacy.* Boston: Little, Brown.

Mueller, S.C., van Wallenberg-Pachaly, H., Voges, G.E., & Schild, H.H. (1990). Comparison of selective internal iliac pharmacoangiography, penile brachial index and duplex sonography with pulsed Doppler analysis for the evaluation of vasculogenic (arteriogenic) impotence. *Journal of Urology, 143*, 928–932.

Munroe, D., Horne, H.W., & Paull, D.P. (1948). The effect of injury to the spinal cord and cauda equina on the sexual potency of men. *New England Journal of Medicine, 239*, 903–911.

Nadig, P.W., Ware, J.C., & Blumoff, R. (1986). Noninvasive device to produce and maintain an erection-like state. *Urology, 27*, 126–131.

Padma-Nathan, H. (1989). Evaluation of the corporal veno-occlusive mechanism: Dynamic infusion cavernosometry. *Seminars in Interventional Radiology, 6*, 205–211.

Renshaw, D.C., & Karstaedt, A. (1988). Is there (sex) life after coronary bypass? *Comprehensive Therapy, 14*(4), 61–66.

Rieve, J.E. (1989). Sexuality and the adult with acquired physical disability. *Nursing Clinics of North America, 24*(1), 265–276.

Seagraves, R.T., Schoenberg, H.W., Goldman, L., & Ivanoff, J. (1986). Psychiatric treatment of erectile dysfunction in urology outpatient clinic. *Urology, 27*(4), 322–327.

Sidi, A.A., & Chen, K.K. (1989). Clinical experience with vasoactive intracavernous pharmacotherapy for treatment of impotence. *World Journal of Urology, 5*, 156–159.

Sjogren, K., & Fugl-Meyer, A.R. (1982). Adjustment to life after stroke with special reference to sexual intercourse and leisure. *Journal of Psychosomatic Research, 26*, 409–417.

Smith, A.D. (1988). Psychologic factors in the multidisciplinary evaluation and treatment of erectile dysfunction. *Urology Clinics of North America, 15*(1), 41–51.

Stackl, W., Hasun, R., & Marberger, M. (1988). Intracavernous injection of prostaglandin E$_1$ in impotent men. *Journal of Urology, 140*, 66–68.

Susset, J.G., Tessier, C.D., Wincze, J., Bansal, S., Mallhotra, C., & Schwacha, M.G. (1989). Effect of yohimbine hydrochloride on erectile impotence: a double-blind study. *Journal of Urology, 141*, 1360–1363.

Tabler, M., Gunther, I., Kern, R., & Sanger, H.L. (1990). Sexual concerns after heart transplantation. *Journal of Heart Transplantation, 9*(4), 397–403.

Tanagho, E.A., & Lue, T.F. (1990). Physiology of penile erection. In F.W. Chisholm (Ed.), *Scientific foundations in urology* (pp. 420). Chicago: Mosby-Year Book.

Tsuji, I., Nakajima, F., Morimoto, J., & Nounaka, Y. (1961). The sexual function in patients with spinal cord injury. *Urologia Internationalis, 12*, 270–280.

Ueno, M. (1969). The so-called coition death. *Japanese Journal of Legal Medicine, 17*, 333–340.

Virag, R. (1982). Intracavernous injection of papaverine for erectile failure. *Lancet, 2*, 938.

Virag, R., Bennett, A.H., & Shoukry, K. (1989). Arterial and venous surgery for vasculogenic impotence: A combined French and American experience. *Journal of Urology, 141*, 289A.

Virag, R., Saltiel, H., Floresco, J., Shoukry, K., & Dufour, B. (1988). Surgical treatment of vasculogenic impotence by deep dorsal vein arterialization. A study of 292 cases followed up for 1 to 8 years. *Chirurgie, 114*, 703–714.

Wagner, G. (1981). Erection physiology and endocrinology. In G. Wagner & R. Green (Eds.), *Impotence: Physiological, psychological, surgical diagnosis and treatment* (p. 37). New York: Plenum Press.

Walsh, P.C., & Donker, P.J. (1982). Impotence following radical prostatectomy: Insight into etiology and prevention. *Journal of Urology, 130*, 492–497.

Wespes, E., & Schulman, C.C. (1985). Venous leakage: Surgical treatment of a curable cause of impotence. *Journal of Urology, 133*, 796–798.

Witherington, R. (1985). The Osbon Erecaid System in the management of erectile impotence. *Journal of Urology, 133A*, 306.

Witherington, R. (1989). Vacuum constriction device for management of erectile impotence. *Journal of Urology, 141*, 320–322.

Wolbroehl, G.S. (1984). Sexual activity and the post coronary patient. *American Family Practitioner, 29*(3), 175–177.

Zorgniotti, A.W., & Lefleur, R.S. (1985). Auto-injection of corpus cavernosum with a vasoactive drug combination for vasculogenic impotence. *Journal of Urology, 133*, 39–41.

27

Electroejaculation and its Techniques in Males with Neurologic Impairments

Lauro S. Halstead and S.W.J. Seager

Ejaculatory failure is a major reproductive issue for many men with neurologic disorders. In the absence of a reliable technique to obtain semen by artificial ejaculation or some other method, biologic fertility is essentially impossible, although spermatogenesis may be normal. Over the years, this problem has led investigators to explore numerous approaches to retrieving sperm by artificial techniques, including vibratory stimulation (VS) (Brindley, 1981a; Comarr, 1970; Francois, Lichtenberger, Jouannet, Desert, & Maury, 1980; Tarabulcy, 1979), intrathecal (Chapelle, Jondet, Durand, & Grossiad, 1976; Guttman, 1949; Guttman & Walsh, 1970; Otani, Kondo, & Takita, 1985; Spira, 1956) and subcutaneous (Chapelle, Blanquart, Puech, & Held, 1983) chemical ejaculation (CE), electroejaculation (EE), and vas deferens aspiration (Bustillo, 1986).

The purpose of this chapter is to focus on one of these techniques (EE), which in our view provides the safest and most reliable method at the present time of obtaining semen from men with neurologic impairments. In addition to describing the technique and equipment currently used at our center and in an increasing number of facilities around the world, we present an historical review of the development of EE equipment and techniques as applied to humans since 1948.

HISTORY OF THE DEVELOPMENT OF
ELECTROEJACULATION EQUIPMENT AND TECHNIQUE

The first report of electroejaculation in men with neurologic impairments was by Horne, Paull, and Munro (1948). They described their experience with 18 men with spinal cord injuries with lesions from C5 through the cauda equina. They consistently obtained specimens containing spermatozoa in 11 of the 18, or in 61%. Electrical stimulation, using both sinusoidal and faradic currents, was delivered via a no. 28 curved urethral sound. The stimulation was applied in the region of each seminal vesicle and the prostate for approximately 4 seconds in each position. Following stimulation, the prostate and seminal vesicles were massaged and semen was milked from the urethra. Although no pregnancies were reported in spouses of subjects who underwent electrostimulation, two pregnancies occurred in spouses of men who could masturbate and have coitus.

Of special interest in this first report was the relatively low level of current used (45–60 milliamperes), the short duration of stimulation (approximately 4 seconds at each stimulation site), and the ability to obtain spermatozoa in one of three subjects with cauda equina injuries. In addition, the quality and quantity of the semen were generally quite good, especially considering the status of spinal cord injury care in the 1940s. The technique was apparently reproducible, although it did not induce antegrade ejaculation. What is particularly surprising, however, is that, despite this very positive and successful initial report, these authors apparently did not follow up this work with other studies and no one else, to our knowledge, has ever described using their technique successfully.

Between the first description of successful electroejaculation in 1948 and 1962 there were at least three additional reports in the U.S. and Australia that described efforts to stimulate the prostate using electrical stimulation in men without spinal cord injuries and men with spinal cord injuries (Bors, Engle, Rosenquist, & Holliger, 1950; Potts, 1957; Rowan, Howley, & Nova, 1962). None of the efforts, however, were successful in producing ejaculation.

In 1966, Bensman and Kottke reported their experience with five men with spinal injuries, four with cervical injuries, and one with a cauda equina injury. Electrostimulation was applied for 5–10 minutes using a continuous 2- to 10-cycle-per-second sinusoidal current of 20–30 milliamperes. Stimulation was delivered with a metal rectal diathermy electrode placed in proximity to the seminal vesicles. Three of the five subjects experienced retrograde ejaculation with variable sperm counts, but all of the sperm were nonmotile.

None of the subjects had antegrade ejaculation despite milking the urethra throughout the procedure. All five subjects had evidence of bladder contractions during the stimulation.

As in the report by Horne and colleagues, Bensman and Kottke were also able to obtain sperm using electrical stimulation from a man with a cauda equina lesion suggesting that this form of ejaculation does not require an intact spinal reflex arc. In addition, the level of current used was low (20–30 milliamperes) while the duration of stimulation was fairly long (5–10 minutes). Of particular interest was the observation that one subject noted a slight increase in muscle spasticity of the lower extremities during stimulation, and one experienced a headache and elevation of blood pressure. No mention is made of any treatment given the subject to reduce his blood pressure, and there is no record of the number of times each subject underwent stimulation. Again, despite this reasonably successful report, there were no follow-up published reports by these authors or others using their technique.

The first known pregnancy using EE was reported by Thomas and colleagues in 1975 (Thomas, McLeish, & McDonald, 1975). The father had a partially incomplete spinal injury at T12 and underwent repeated stimulations with a battery-operated rectal probe that had been developed for use in rams (Nichols & Edgar, 1964). The stimulation was a train of flat-topped pulses with an amplitude of 15 volts, a duration of $1/500$ second, and a frequency of 60 cycles per second. It was applied in a rhythmic fashion with a gradual increase until a maximum was achieved that was sustained for 6 seconds with a 6-second interval between each stimulus.

Although this was the first pregnancy using electroejaculation, the child, unfortunately, died shortly after birth from transposition of the great vessels. However, this report was noteworthy for several other reasons: 1) the use of a portable, battery-operated probe; 2) the acknowledged adaptation of experience gained in veterinary medicine; 3) the observation that repeated stimulations produced an improvement in ejaculate volume and sperm motility (sperm counts were not reported); 4) the use of rhythmic and gradually crescendoing applications of electrical stimulations; and 5) the use of prostatic massage and a Valsalva maneuver to compensate for an absent antegrade ejaculation.

Between 1975 and 1979, Francois, David, and their colleagues reported their experiences with electrostimulation techniques, first in monkeys (Francois, Maury, Vacant, Cukier, & David, 1975) and later in humans (David, Ohry, & Rozin, 1977–78; Francois, Maury, Jovannet, David, & Vacant, 1978). The study by David and colleagues described their experience with 16 men with SCI (6 with cervical injuries and 10 with thoracic). Rectal probe stimulation was delivered using 15–30 volts for 4–8 seconds at 170 Hz. The electrode was moved from side to side in the area of each seminal vesicle, and voltage was increased if no ejaculate was observed. Antegrade ejaculations with motile sperm were obtained in four subjects and one pregnancy occurred following homologous (artificial) insemination (AIH). There is no mention of post-stimulation bladder irrigation to evaluate for retrograde ejaculation, and there is no description of any complications.

A pregnancy that resulted in the delivery of a healthy child was described in a case report at about the same time by Francois and colleagues (Francois et al., 1978) using the same technique. It is unclear whether this represented a second, separate pregnancy or the same one alluded to by David et al. (1977–1978). In any event, it represented the successful culmination of 3 decades of work by many investigators from many different countries to achieve a live birth by using electrical stimulation in a man with a spinal injury. One factor that may have contributed to their success was the experience that they had obtained from working with nonhuman primates before applying the technique to men with spinal injuries.

Practical experience with animal models may also help explain Brindley's achievements in this field. Between 1980–1984, Brindley published a series of landmark articles dealing with various aspects of EE in over 100 men with SCI (Brindley, 1980; Brindley, 1981a, 1981b; Brindley, 1984). His experience as reported in these articles was noteworthy for several reasons: 1) the use of an electrode mounted on a fingerstall instead of a probe, which presumably gave him more flexibility and control over the precise location of the stimulating electrode; 2) previous experience with EE in nonhuman primates (rhesus monkeys and baboons); 3) the fullest description yet of various aspects of the technique, equipment, and safety issues involved in EE; 4) a detailed effort to correlate anatomic and physiologic factors with successful stimulations; and 5) because of the large number of subjects studied, the first attempt to correlate level of injury and successful ejaculation (none was noted). Pregnancies were reported in three separate papers, although the exact number is difficult to determine because of apparent overlap in the populations described.

Despite these enormous contributions by Brindley, however, the field of EE did not advance as far as might have been expected. Investigators who studied his papers were not able to duplicate his results, and researchers who were trained by him, as far as we know,

were unsuccessful in applying his techniques on a routine and re-
peatable basis to their own patients in their home institutions.
Thus, it was a successful technique that, for whatever reason, was
never successfully transferred to others.

Over the years, as EE techniques became more sophisticated
and successful, there was increasing interest and concern with the
safety parameters of repeated electrical stimulation to the rectal
mucosa. In 1983, Martin and colleagues described efforts to calcu-
late safe electrical parameters for electrostimulation (ES) and to
evaluate the effects of ES on both ejaculation and penile tumescence
in men without SCI ($N = 8$) and men with SCI ($N = 12$) (Martin et
al., 1983). The current density used in their subjects never exceeded
0.37 mA per mm^2, which they estimated is less than 50% of the
threshold for causing tissue damage of the local rectal mucosa. Pain
was too aversive in all but one of the subjects without SCI to achieve
erection, much less ejaculation. Discomfort in the subjects with
SCI, by contrast, was minimal, and tumescence was directly propor-
tional to the area of the electrode surface and applied current density. Rectoscopic exams post-stimulation showed mild erythema due
to the heating of the rectal mucosa. The number of subjects who
demonstrated this finding was not mentioned, nor was there any
description of the length of each stimulation session or of any attempt to measure directly the temperature of the local rectal mucosa or temperature of the rectal probe.

The first attempt to evaluate the effects of chronic EE in an SCI
animal model was reported by Seager, Savastano, Street, Halstead,
and McGuire (1984). In a group of 10 *Macacus fasculicularis* monkeys, complete cord transections were made above T6 in three animals and at L3 in three animals. Three others had complete sacral
rhizotomies and one was left intact as a control. Electrical stimulation per rectum was applied on a monthly basis for a period of 18
months. Evaluations of the ejaculates showed a decrease in the quality and quantity of the semen in the monkeys with high thoracic
lesions but preservation of pre-injury parameters in those with lower level lesions. Autopsy studies failed to reveal any abnormalities
associated with the chronic EE, and tissue samples from the rectum,
seminal vesicles, prostate, testes, and epididymis were normal.

Based on the success of this experience in SCI monkeys, we
established a Fertility Clinic for SCI Men at the Institute for Rehabilitation and Research (TIRR) in Houston, Texas, in late 1983. The
initial efforts involved a direct application of knowledge and experience gained in the laboratory experiment with SCI monkeys, as well
as experience accumulated in the wild and in zoos over the course of

almost 20 years by Seager with over 100 species of animals (Seager, 1983; Seager, Wildt, & Platz, 1980). In 1984, the first training session for colleagues in human medicine who were interested in applying this technique to patients in their home institutions was held. Although the initial training period was fairly extensive, it has now been shortened to approximately 2 days as the technique has become more refined and the trainers more experienced.

The EE technique developed at TIRR has evolved and is based on our collective experience of using EE in nonhuman primates and working with men with SCI in a clinical rehabilitation setting. A brief description of this technique has been published previously (Bennett, 1988; Halstead, 1989). However, because of the widespread interest, use, and success of this equipment and technique in more than 20 countries, it is timely to provide a more detailed description of the many changes and improvements incorporated in the equipment and methods over the years, along with observations and experience concerning advantages and limitations.

ELECTROEJACULATION EQUIPMENT

A recent model of the stimulator box (1990) and a set of probes are shown in Figures 1 and 2. Although the basic elements have remained essentially unchanged since 1980, modifications and im-

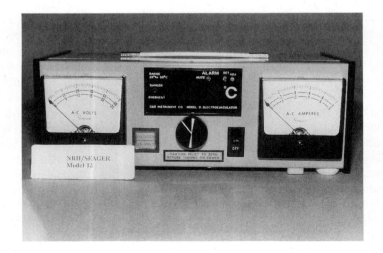

Figure 1. Photograph of the electroejaculation equipment (NRH/SEAGER Model 12) distributed by the National Rehabilitation Hospital, Washington, D.C.

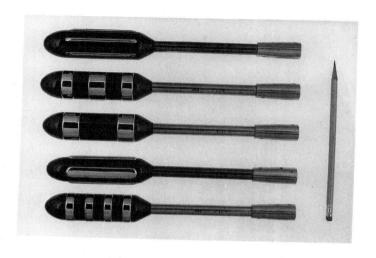

Figure 2. Photograph of electroejaculation probes with a variety of electrode configurations. (Note pencil for comparison of size.)

provements have been introduced in an attempt to develop equipment that is easier to use and more effective while maintaining rigorous standards of safety.

The stimulator operates from a standard 120-volt receptacle and delivers a sine wave current of 60 Hz. Voltage pulses are controlled by manipulating a comfortably sized knob, which is used as a voltage rheostat. A range switch provides optimum known sensitivity at low as well as high power levels. Accuracy over a wide range of power levels is made possible by dual level range meters for both voltage and milliamperes. The unit is protected by circuit breakers, which have visual trip indicators. Isolation transformers and current-limiting devices prevent even accidental delivery of excessive current to the subject (Figure 3). This is an essential design feature for use with anyone but especially for people with neurologic impairments, where sensation may be modified or absent in the rectal and genital areas.

The probes are precision-machined from solid bars of polyvinyl chloride with a thermosensor countersunk in the central electrode. This sensor is connected via the probe to a separate thermometer, which provides a direct and continuous digital readout of the temperature of the probe at the site of stimulation. Probes range in size from ½ inch to 1⁵/₁₆ inches and electrode size and placement are

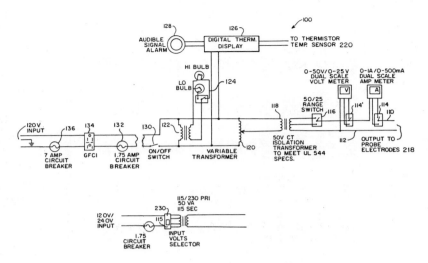

Figure 3. Diagram of electroejaculation equipment showing isolation transformers and current-limiting devices.

varied (Figure 2) to provide options in an effort to achieve the best possible stimulus with the least amount of current.

ELECTROEJACULATION TECHNIQUE

Initial Evaluation

Men presenting to the Male SCI Fertility Clinic for the first time undergo a standardized evaluation. This assessment includes a history and physical examination performed by a physician, with particular attention to the occurrence of urological problems—especially urinary tract infections and epididymitis—both pre- and post-injury, and to the level and completeness of the neurologic impairment. Persons with good-to-normal pain sensation in the groin and rectum are usually referred for EE under anesthesia, while patients with significant medical problems (e.g., chronic decubitus ulcer) are not seen until their medical problems are resolved or stabilized.

Following the history and physical, the patient is shown a video that demonstrates the procedure and outlines the precautions taken to make the procedure as comfortable and safe as possible. When a couple presents to a clinic for the purpose of having a child, the initial visit also includes a psychosocial evaluation by a social worker. The purpose of this evaluation is to help the couple consider emotional issues that are associated with the procedure and its outcome and to alert the Fertility Team to any psychological problems that might arise in the course of the couples' efforts to conceive.

When these initial assessments are completed, the patient gives informed consent and laboratory tests are obtained. These include a complete blood count (CBC), urinalysis, urine culture and sensitivity, and blood tests for FSH, LH, testosterone, and HIV. An intravenous pyelogram (IVP) or renal sonogram is obtained if one has not been performed in the previous year. Finally, other laboratory tests are ordered as indicated by the history and physical exam.

Preparation for EE

Prior to each EE procedure, patients are asked to limit their fluids for 8 hours, except for liquid needed to take medications. This is to reduce urinary output at the time of the procedure and help minimize the risk of urine contamination of either antegrade or retrograde ejaculations. To further limit this possibility, the bladder is emptied by catheterization within 10 minutes of EE. In addition, patients are requested to have their bowel programs either the night before or the morning of the procedure. This helps ensure a clear rectal vault and reduces the likelihood of fecal contamination of the rectal mucosa, which can significantly interfere with establishing satisfactory electrical contact.

The Procedure

Electroejaculation is performed by a three-person team that usually consists of a nurse who monitors and records vital signs and administers any required medications, a "catcher" who massages the urethra and collects the semen, and the "stimulator" who inserts the probe and controls the electrical stimulus. Over the years we have performed EE with patients in a variety of positions and have found the right or left lateral decubitus with the hips flexed and a small pillow between the knees is the most comfortable for the patient and the most convenient for the team members. We intentionally do not remove the patient's pants and underclothes but leave them below the knees where they help restrain excessive movements of the legs that often accompany electrical stimulation.

With the patient properly positioned, the first step of the procedure is to perform a careful digital exam of the rectum to ascertain the size and direction of the rectal vault and to determine if any residual stool is present. This is followed by visual inspection of the rectal mucosa using an illuminated anoscope. Based on this evaluation, a probe is selected that is suitable to the size of the rectal vault and will provide the best possible electrical contact with the prostate and seminal vesicles. For most patients, we have found a standard probe of 1$1/8$ or 1$1/4$ inches in diameter with three longitudinal electrodes is usually very effective. However, over the years we have developed a number of variations on this standard model and now have probes that range in diameter from $3/4$ inch to 1$5/16$ inches with a variety of electrode configurations, as shown in Figure 2.

For SCI men with lesions at T6 or above or for anyone who experiences hyperreflexia, nifedipine (Procardia) 10–20 mg is given, using the "chew and swallow" method (Stephen & Avila, 1991) approximately 10 minutes before starting electrostimulation. This method of administration provides rapid absorption from the gastric mucosa and is now felt to be superior to sublingual nifedipine for hypertensive crises (McAllister, 1986). In our experience, the chew and swallow method, which permits subjects to crush the capsule with their teeth and then swallow the liquid contents, is easier for the patient and provides more effective and predictable blood pressure control. In patients whose blood pressure is particularly sensitive to noxious stimuli (especially incomplete high quadriplegics), we supplement the initial dose of nifedipine as needed with an additional 10–20 mg or with sublingual nitroglycerine $1/150$ gr. Using this regimen, our objective during each EE procedure is to limit systolic pressure to under 180 mmHg and diastolic pressure to under 120 mmHg. When blood pressure cannot be readily controlled at these levels, it often means there is some other source of noxious stimuli present (e.g., infection in the GU tract or elsewhere, a large amount of retained feces high in the intestinal tract, skin irritation or ulceration. When blood pressure suddenly drops (20–25 mmHg) in the middle of a procedure, it generally indicates that the person has ejaculated.

There are six basic principles for delivering safe and effective levels of electrical stimulation: 1) maintain gentle but firm pressure on the ventral surface of the probe against the tissues being stimulated; 2) use a standard, systematic pattern of probe placement and movement for each patient so that all structures are adequately stimulated each time. Although our technique is modified depending on individual response, in general we begin at midline directly over the prostate and then, after 10–12 stimulations, rotate the probe to the left to stimulate the vicinity of the left seminal vesicle 3–5 times followed by rotation of the probe to the right to stimulate the contralateral seminal vesicle 3–5 times and finally return to midline for an additional 5–10 stimulations; 3) starting at 0 volts, use a rhythmic, turning movement of the hand on the knob of the volt meter to create a slowly crescendoing series of peaks and valleys, with each peak held for 1–2 seconds and 3–5 volts higher than the last, while each valley returns to 5 volts or lower (on a 0–25 volt scale) and to 10 volts or lower (on a 25–50 volt scale); 4) monitor the milliamp scale with each stimulation. The needle should reflect a parallel rise and fall of miliamperes with the changes visible on the volt meter if adequate surface contact is being maintained with the rectal mucosa; 5) never exceed 35 volts; and 6) never allow the temperature to exceed 37°C. Each stimulation is noted on a hand-held or automatic counter and the total number should not exceed 35–45.

In the majority of men, ejaculation begins after 10–15 stimulations at 10–15 volts while drawing 300–400 milliamperes of current. Once a subject has started to ejaculate, it usually takes 10–12 additional stimulations in order to obtain the entire ejaculate volume. When 20–25 stimulations have been given and no antegrade ejaculate has been detected, it usually means the person has ejaculated retrograde or the stimulation was given too rapidly and the ejaculation/emission is occurring at a lower rate than the stimulation. For this reason, it is usually advisable to stop stimulating at this point, leave the probe in the rectum, and allow the patient to rest quietly for 3 or 4 minutes. When stimulation is resumed, the semen catcher should be alert to the possibility of a rapid and possibly forceful ejaculate within several stimulations.

If no ejaculate or sperm are obtained after 3 or 4 EE sessions (either antegrade or retrograde), then a vasogram is usually indicated to rule out ductal blockage and, if that is negative, then a testicular biopsy is performed to assess spermatogenesis.

Throughout the procedure, careful note is made of the presence of goose flesh on the hip and/or leg, the degree of tumescence, the presence of spasms, and the moment of the first appearance of an emission or ejaculate. Goose flesh usually occurs at 3–5 volts and indicates good electrical contact has been made with the rectal mucosa, resulting in stimulation of sympathetic nerves. The degree of tumescence also appears to reflect, in a general way, the amount of electrical stimulation that is occurring. However, the degree of tumescence and the presence and amount of ejaculate is not strongly correlated. We have observed good ejaculates with a flaccid penis as well as one that is fully erect, but more typically ejaculation occurs between 20%–80% of full erection. In patients who have increased tone, spasms of striated muscle almost always accompany EE. These usually begin in the abdominal wall and then spread to the hips and legs. Sometimes the spasms are so forceful that they require a leg restraint or an additional person to hold the ankles.

When a particularly viscous antegrade ejaculation occurs, 1–2 mL of a semen enrichment medium such as Hamm's F-10 is used to wash the ejaculate into the bottom of the collection cup to enhance liquefaction. Regardless of the presence or absence of antegrade ejaculation, each procedure should be followed by a vigorous digital massage of the prostate and posterior urethra. This frequently produces several milliliters of ejaculate.

Following each procedure, the rectal mucosa is reexamined with the anoscope and any changes noted. In over 3,000 procedures, we have observed minor changes—principally hyperemia—on fewer than a dozen occasions. However, since changes that cannot be appreciated by the human eye may occur after multiple stimulations, we are undertaking a biopsy study of potential rectal mucosa pathology in patients who have undergone repeated stimulations.

After the rectal exam, a bladder wash-out is performed using 10–20 mL of sperm enrichment medium. The resulting wash is centrifuged and examined for sperm count and motility. If an adequate antegrade sample has been obtained with a sperm count and motility percentage sufficient for artificial insemination, then repeated bladder catheterization to check for a retrograde ejaculate is not necessary. Whether the emission actually is ejaculated completely back into the bladder is a question that requires further study. It may simply be deposited in the posterior urethra and then pushed into the bladder during catheterization. Our experience with posterior urethral massage suggests that retrograde ejaculation is deposited both in the posterior urethra as well as back into the bladder. Hence, the term "retrograde bladder ejaculation" is probably a misnomer.

Post-procedure the probes are cleansed using a soft brush and mild soap and then rinsed. They are immersed, with the electric connections maintained above fluid levels, in an approved, cold sterilization agent for 20 minutes or more. After sterilization, the probes are rinsed, dried, and stored for subsequent use. With proper care and maintenance, probes have been used for more than 500 procedures and still provide reliable, consistent results.

Fresh semen is evaluated in the laboratory for color, volume, pH, viscosity, motility percentage, progressive motility (movement across the microscope stage based on a scale of 0–4, with 4 being optimal movement), total sperm count, total live sperm count, and abnormal morphology. If the ejaculate contains many abnormal forms, it is sent to the histopathology laboratory for staining and further examination.

Most men and their significant others want to see the ejaculate, especially if there are live sperm. To make this practical, it is useful to have a TV monitor or direct screen attached to the microscope.

Altogether, a typical EE procedure takes 30–40 minutes from the time of transfer to the examination table to the transfer back to the wheelchair. The major side effects are related either to hyper-reflexia (headache, sweating, temporary increase in spasticity) or to the nifedipine or nitroglycerine given to control hypertension (headache, fatigue, light-headedness). One or more of the symptoms of hyperreflexia occur in approximately 80% of men with high paraplegia and quadriplegia, and one or more symptoms in approximately 25% of those given medications. Usually, the side effects are less pronounced after undergoing several procedures. Another unexpected side effect is the significant reduction in spasticity for 6–8 hours, which occurs in 70%–80% of those patients who experience moderate to severe spasticity. This phenomenon is currently being investigated in both men and women with spinal cord injuries.

ELECTROEJACULATION UNDER GENERAL ANESTHESIA (GA)

General anesthesia is used for patients who have fair-to-normal pain sensation in the rectal area. This usually includes men with SCI who are Frankel E and D and occasionally those who are Frankel C and B. Many of these latter patients have pain–touch dissociation. That is, they report good sensation in the perineal area on history only to find on exam that they do, indeed, have good preservation of light and deep touch but poor to absent preservation of pain sensation, which makes it practical to perform EE without anesthesia.

Even if pain sensation is poorly preserved or absent in the patient with an incomplete lesion, great care must be taken, especially during the first EE procedure, to increase the electrical input extremely slowly and to very closely monitor the patient's level of discomfort. The tension and anxiety of the unknown often make the first procedure more uncomfortable than subsequent ones, in which case the patient often elects to proceed without GA and finds that he can tolerate it quite satisfactorily. If the discomfort persists at a minimal to moderate level, however, there are still other options short of general anesthesia (GA). These include pre-medication with meperadine or diazepam given by mouth or intramuscularly or midazolam given intravenously. None of these medications given in moderate doses appear to interfere with ejaculatory function. We have also tried lining the rectal wall with a local anesthetic agent such as 2% lidocaine jelly, which has been successful on several occasions.

When GA is used, the overall procedure is performed in a manner similar to that described for unanesthetized patients. Intubation is performed at the discretion of the anesthesiologist, and the patient is placed in the lateral decubitus position. The anesthetic agents commonly used are intravenous barbiturates and/or a combination of inhalation gasses. Nitrous oxide is felt by some to be deleterious to sperm quality and, therefore, is not recommended. As a general rule, anesthesia needs to be deep enough to perform rectal surgery.

Another important guideline is to plan general anesthesia around the partner's ovulatory cycle. Ordinarily, this is not necessary for regular EE, but considering the costs associated with GA, it is advisable to be prepared to perform artificial insemination in case an ejaculate suitable for fertilization is obtained.

Finally, for all patients who do not have SCI, general anesthesia is required to perform EE. These include psychogenic and anejaculatory men and those with a diagnosis of multiple sclerosis (MS), diabetes, spina bifida, and retroperitoneal lymph node dissection (RPLND).

SELECTED RESULTS

Between 1984 and June 1991, we have performed approximately 3,000 EE procedures in over 330 men with SCI. Ejaculations were obtained from patients whose ages ranged from 17 to 52 years and in whom length of injury ranged from 2.5 months to 39 years. Causes of spinal cord damage have included most conceivable forms of traumatic injury and many forms of nontraumatic injury, such as tumors, disk surgery, and neural tube defects. Of these 331 men, 201 (61%) had thoracic injuries, 118 (36%) had cervical lesions, and only 12 (4%) had lumbar injuries. Clinical assessment revealed that the majority (220, or 66%) had complete injuries (Frankel A) while the remainder (111, or 34%) had incomplete lesions (Frankel B–D).

Over the years, it has been assumed by clinicians and researchers alike that spermatogenesis would most likely decline over time following spinal injury. While this may be true for some men, it is clearly not true for all. Table 1 summarizes EE data on six patients who had been injured 17 years or longer at the time of their first EE. The number of years post-injury ranged from 17 to 37 years and ages at injury from 7 to 19 years. Ages at time of first EE ranged from 28 to 52 years and year of injury from 1950 to 1973. In these patients,

Table 1. Electroejaculation patients with spinal cord injury of 17 or more years of duration

Age	Patient subject	Years injured (year of first EE)	Age at injury (year)	Injury level	Complete or incomplete	Number of EE procedures	Antegrade or retrograde ejaculation	Total sperm count	Semen results	
									% Motility	Progressive motility[a]
35	1	17 (1987)	18 (1970)	T5	C	42	A	116×10⁶	50	4
28	2	17 (1990)	11 (1973)	T2	C	11	R	775×10⁶	50	3
38	3	20 (1987)	18 (1967)	C5	I	9	A	125×10⁶	50	4
36	4	29 (1989)	7 (1960)	T5	C	1	R	—	0	0
49	5	30 (1988)	19 (1958)	C5	I	2	A	203×10⁶	0	0
52	6	37 (1987)	15 (1950)	T8	C	5	A	210×10⁶	40	4

[a]Ranked on a 4-point scale, with 0 = least motility, and 4 = optimal motility.

five of six had good ejaculates and four of six had sperm counts and quality suitable for insemination. The two men with the poorest results (patients 4 and 5) were ejaculated only one and two times, respectively.

Another concern has been how often and how many times a man with SCI can undergo artificial ejaculation. Table 2 provides an anecdotal answer for a 40-year-old man who underwent 42 EE procedures over a 57-month period, or almost one ejaculation per month for 5 years. He was injured in a motor vehicle accident in 1970 at 18 years of age and has a T5 complete injury (Frankel A). His first ejaculate since injury was obtained on 10/2/86 using EE and was suitable for insemination. The quality of semen improved with subsequent ejaculations and "peaked" in early 1990 when he had 1.4 billion total sperm and 700 million live sperm with 4+ forward motility. There have been several occasions when repeat EE procedures performed at short intervals (less than 14 days) have resulted in much lower numbers and, in one instance, no ejaculate at all.

A third issue concerns how SCI changes semen compared to pre-injury levels. Table 3 summarizes data on a 24-year-old man who had routine laboratory semen analysis as part of a fertility evaluation 4 months before sustaining a complete T9 SCI (Frankel A) in July, 1990. Approximately 4 months following his injury, he underwent EE and produced an ejaculate with a semen analysis essentially identical to that obtained pre-injury.

In addition to the 331 men with SCI reported here, we have also performed EE on 52 patients with other neurologic impairments, including retroperitoneal lymph node dissection (RPLND), multiple sclerosis (MS), spina bifida (SB), diabetic neuropathy, and idiopathic anejaculation. These procedures have been performed at the National Rehabilitation Hospital and at other fertility clinics in the U.S.

Table 2. Multiple antegrade ejaculates in 40-year-old with complete T5 SCI sustained at age 18 (1970)

Procedure #	Date	Volume (mLs)	% Motility	Progressive motility[a]	Total sperm count
1	10/3/86	2.0	20	3	264×10^6
2	11/7/86	2.5	35	4	544×10^6
36	1/6/90	7.0	50	4	1.4×10^9
41	6/3/91	5.5	50	4	748×10^6
42	7/2/91	5.6	50	4	822×10^6

[a]Ranked on a 4-point scale, with 0 = least motility and 4 = optimal motility.

Table 3. Semen analysis pre- and post-SCI in a 24-year-old with complete T9 SCI

Procedure	Date	Volume (mLs)	Total sperm count	% Motility	Progressive motility
Semen analysis	3/30/90	2.0	400×10^6	50	3
T-9 complete SCI	7/22/90	—	—	—	—
Electroejaculation (antegrade)	11/15/90	2.5	993×10^6	50	4

and abroad, using the equipment and techniques described in this chapter.

THE FUTURE

The success of the equipment and techniques outlined here have not occurred in a vacuum. In reviewing the historical development of EE, it is clear that many aspects of our technique are not new. The major difference has not been in any dramatic breakthrough of knowledge or a quantum improvement in equipment, but rather in the ability to teach others the skills and knowledge of using this technique and equipment successfully. The fact that many clinicians and researchers can now perform EE safely and reliably has, at the same time, been enormously abetted by the spectacular advances in the area of human reproduction. These combined elements have made it possible for colleagues around the world to participate in a revolution in the fertility management of men with neurologic impairments. This revolution is attested to by the many reports of pregnancies obtained for the first time in various populations using this technique and equipment (Bennett, Seager, & McGuire, 1987; Bennett, Seager, Vasher, & McGuire, 1988; Hirsch, Seager, Sedor, King, & Staas, 1990; Ohl, Grainger, Bennett, Randolph, Seager, & McCabe, 1989). It is also reflected in the results of an informal survey of 40 centers using NRH/Seager equipment, which showed that there have been more than 65 pregnancies in wives of men with SCI between 1988 and mid-1991.

While progress in this area of SCI management has been impressive, the gains have not been achieved without a certain price. Troubling issues have been raised that need to be addressed. Expanded reproductive rights for persons with disabilities have been achieved at the expense of individual privacy and discretion. At this stage in our knowledge, technology depersonalizes what should be a personal, spontaneous, and intimate activity. What is more, it imposes a financial burden that excludes some altogether and limits availability for others. In response to these drawbacks, a major challenge to the fields of rehabilitation and reproductive technology at the turn of this century is to develop equipment and techniques that are affordable to all who want them and that can be used safely and routinely in the comfort and privacy of one's home.

REFERENCES

Bennett, C.J., Seager, S.W.J., & McGuire, E.J. (1987). Electroejaculation for recovery of semen after retroperitoneal lymph node dissection: Case report. *Journal of Urology, 137,* 513–515.

Bennett, C.J., Seager, S.W., Vasher, E.A., & McGuire, E.J. (1988). Sexual dysfunction and electroejaculation in men with spinal cord injury: Review. *Journal of Urology, 139,* 453–457.

Bensman, A., & Kottke, F.J. (1966). Induced emission of sperm utilizing electrical stimulation of the seminal vesicles and vas deferens. *Archives of Physical Medicine and Rehabilitation, 47,* 436.

Bors, E., Engle, E.T., Rosenquist, R.C., & Holliger, V.H. (1950). Fertility in paraplegic males: A preliminary report of endocrine studies. *Journal of Clinical Endocrinology, 10,* 381.

Brindley, G.S. (1980). Electroejaculation and the fertility of paraplegic men. *Sexuality and Disability, 3*(3), 223–229.

Brindley, G.S. (1981a). Electroejaculation: Its technique, neurological implications and uses. *Journal of Neurology, Neurosurgery, & Psychiatry, 44,* 9.

Brindley, G.S. (1981b). Reflex ejaculation under vibratory stimulation in paraplegic men. *Paraplegia, 19,* 299–302.

Brindley, G.S. (1984). The fertility of men with spinal injuries. *Paraplegia, 22,* 337.

Bustillo, M., & Rajfer, J. (1986). Pregnancy following insemination with sperm aspirated directly from vas deferens. *Fertility and Sterility, 46*(1), 144–146.

Chapelle, P.A., Blanquart, F., Puech, A.J., & Held, J.P. (1983). Treatment of anejaculation in the total paraplegic by subcutaneous injection of physostigmine. *Paraplegia, 21,* 30.

Chapelle, P.A., Jondet, M., Durand, J., & Grossiad, A. (1976). Pregnancy of the wife of a complete paraplegic by homologeous insemination after an intrathecal injection of neostigmine. *Paraplegia, 14,* 173.

Comarr, A.E. (1970). Sexual function among patients with spinal cord injury. *Urology International, 25,* 134.

David, A., Ohry, A., & Rozin, R. (1977–1978). Spinal cord injuries: Male infertility aspects. *Paraplegia, 15,* 11.

Francois, N., Maury, M., Jovannet, D., David, G., & Vacant, J. (1978). Electroejaculation of a complete paraplegic followed by pregnancy. *Paraplegia, 16,* 248.

Francois, N., Maury, M., Vacant, J., Cukier, J., & David, G. (1975). Etude experimental de l'electro-ejaculation chez la babouin [Experimental study of electroejaculation of African monkeys]. *Journal of Urology and Nephrology, 81*, 533.

Francois, N., Lichtenberger, J.M., Jouannet, P., Desert, J.F., & Maury, M. (1980). L'ejaculation per le vibromassage chez le paraplegique a propos de 50 cas avec 7 grossesses [Ejaculation by vibratory stimulation of paraplegics with reference to 50 cases with 7 pregnancies]. *Annales de Med. Phys., 23*, 24.

Guttman, L. (1949). The effect of prostigmin on the reproductive functions of the spinal man. *International Neurological Congress, 2*, 69.

Guttman, L., & Walsh, J.J. (1970). Prostigmin assessment test of fertility in spinal man. *Paraplegia, 9*, 39–51.

Halstead, L.S., VerVoort, S., & Seager, S.W.J. (1989). Rectal probe electrostimulation in the treatment of anejaculatory SCI men, *Paraplegia, 25*, 120–129.

Hirsch, I.H., Seager, S.W.J., Sedor, J., King, L., & Staas, W.E., Jr. (1990). Electroejaculatory stimulation of a quadriplegic man resulting in pregnancy. *Archives of Physical Medicine and Rehabilitation, 71*, 54–57.

Horne, M.W., Paull, D.P., & Munro, D. (1948). Fertility studies in the human male with traumatic injuries of the spinal cord and cauda equina. *New England Journal of Medicine, 239*, 959.

Martin, D.E., Warner, H., Crenshaw, T.L., Crenshaw, R.T., Shapiro, C.E., & Perkash, I. (1983). Initiation of erection and semen release by rectal probe electrostimulation (RPE). *Journal of Urology, 129*, 637–642.

McAllister, R.G., Jr. (1986). Kinetics and dynamics of nifedipine after oral and sublingual doses. *American Journal of Medicine, 81*(6A), 2–5.

Nichols, G. De La M., & Edgar, D.G. (1964). A transistorized rectal probe for ejaculating rams, *New Zealand Veterinary Journal, 12*, 145.

Ohl, D.A., Grainger, R., Bennett, C.A., Randolph, J.F., Seager, S.W.J., & McCabe, M. (1989). Successful use of electoejaculation in two multiple sclerosis patients including report of a pregnancy utilizing intrauterine insemination. *Neurology and Urodynamics, 8*, 195–198.

Otani, T., Kondo, A., & Takita, T. (1985). A paraplegic fathering a child after an intrathecal injection of neostigmine: Case report. *Paraplegia 23*, 32–37.

Potts, I.F. (1957). The mechanisms of ejaculation. *Medical Journal of Australia, 1*, 495.

Rowan, R.L., Howley, T.F., & Nova, H.R. (1962). Electrojaculation. *Journal of Urology, 87*, 726.

Seager, S.W.J. (1983). The breeding of captive wild species by artificial methods. *Zoological Biology, 2*, 235.

Seager, S.W.J., Savastano, J.A., Street, J.W., Halstead, L., & McGuire, E.J. (1984). Electroejaculation, semen quality, and penile erection in normal and chronic spinal non-human primates. *Journal of Urology, 131*, 234A.

Seager, S.W., Wildt, D.E., & Platz, C. (1980). Semen collection by electroejaculation and artificial vagina in over 100 species of animals. *Proceedings of the Ninth International Congress on Animal Reproduction and Artificial Insemination*, p. 571.

Spira, R. (1956). Artificial insemination after intrathecal injection of neostigmine in a paraplegic. *Lancet, 1*, 670.

Stephen, J.M., & Avila, J.A. (1991). Letter to the editor. *New England Journal of Medicine, 324*(14), 993.

Tarabulcy, E. (1979). Sexual function in the normal and in paraplegia. *Paraplegia, 10,* 201–208.

Thomas, R.J.S., McLeish, G., & McDonald, I.A. (1975). Electroejaculation of the paraplegic male followed by pregnancy. *Medical Journal of Australia, 2,* 798.

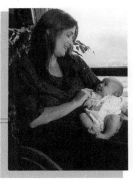

IV

POLICY
AND THE FUTURE

28

Future Directions in Research and Training in Reproductive Issues for Persons with Physical Disabilities

William H. Graves

This topic, future directions in reproductive issues for persons with physical disabilities, carries with it a great risk of errors of ignoring the obvious or of being oblivious to those factors in the environment that make a difference in the outcome of predictions. These errors are more likely to occur because it is not clear what is obvious, and since we have few facts or relatively little research to guide us in the first place, it is easy to be oblivious to environmental factors outside the rehabilitation research and training arena affecting the accuracy of predictions of future directions.

Reproductive issues for people with physical disabilities as a research topic has a brief history. The earliest sponsored project of the National Institute on Disability and Rehabilitation Research (NIDRR) or its predecessors, such as the Rehabilitation Services Administration and the National Institute on Handicapped Research, in the related area of sexuality of people with disabilities was reported in 1968. This first study was "Sex Education for Handicapped Adolescents," by J.L. Bloom of the University of Pittsburgh Vocational Rehabilitation Research and Training Center. The paper describes the results of a study that presented a sex education course to a group of adolescents with physical disabilities and to a group of

adolescents with emotional disturbances to determine the level of
sex knowledge of the youth, their ability to learn, and if sex education caused anxiety. I know all of you share with me pride in the
considerable progress that has been achieved since that early paper
was written.

   I would like to share with you a brief review of research reports
on sexual aspects of disability collected by the National Rehabilitation Information Center, or NARIC. This information was a response to a query from my office for a bibliography of NIDRR-
sponsored research on sexual and reproductive issues affecting individuals having disabilities. From 1968 to 1990, 62 project reports or
other types of materials that focus on sexual functioning of people
with disabilities have been deposited at NARIC. Of these materials,
39% address spinal cord injury and 31% address severe disability.
The other impairments on which there was more than one report
included hearing impairments (3, or 5%), end stage renal disease (3,
or 5%), and mental illness (2, or 3%). Other impairments for which
there were single references or entries included chronic obstructive
pulmonary disease, genitourinary diseases, visual impairments, cerebral palsy, traumatic brain injury, and multiple sclerosis. There
was also a single entry under families. The information contained
in these materials by and large is not current. Sixty percent, or 37,
were reported between 1979 and 1984. Fifteen, or 24%, of the entries
were published between 1973 and 1978. Fully 84% of the references were published between 1973 and 1984. Only six entries, or
10%, had been received between 1985 and 1990. Most of you would
probably agree that NARIC's holdings do not represent the universe
of literature in the area. Moreover, even when the universe has been
identified, it will be small, and the number of reports addressing
sexuality issues for people other than those with spinal cord injuries
is woefully limited. Some might agree with me that the holdings
in sexual functioning and spinal cord injury are also limited.

   NARIC was able to locate few citations in rehabilitation research in the area of reproduction. The need for research literature
in this important area reflects the evolution of understanding of the
needs of people with physical disabilities by the rehabilitation research community and, more importantly, an increased understanding of people with disabilities of what some would call the inevita-
ble relationship between sexual functioning and reproduction. The
topics addressed in this volume are the obvious, as well as natural
and logical, consequences of the earlier work of such researchers as
Ted and Sandra Cole on sexual functioning. For example, their earlier work on sexual functioning laid the foundation for the current

intersystem collaborative research project conducted under the leadership of the University of Alabama–Birmingham Model Spinal Cord Injury Center on gynecologic and obstetric complications in females with spinal cord injury (SCI). For the period 1990–1995, the study will:

Describe gynecologic and obstetric conditions in females with acute and chronic spinal cord injuries.

Determine if females with SCI experience increased gynecologic and obstetric complications after injury.

Determine if females with SCI experience unique gynecologic and obstetric complications after injury.

Determine the effects of menses on bodily responses that occur following injury such as spasticity, bladder function, and autonomic hyperreflexia.

Determine if females with SCI experience unique hormonal and/or physiologic responses following SCI.

This research is a natural, perhaps obvious, consequence of earlier work on males with spinal cord injury. It also reflects the societal pressure on medical research to address issues affecting women. NIDRR, like National Institutes of Health (NIH), responds to these kinds of societal and congressional interests.

If one had read the research in sexuality and disability carefully and had asked the question, "What is the next research frontier?", the obvious, natural, and logical answer would have been reproduction.

One, however, would not have had to read the literature to come to this conclusion if one had been observing events within the disability and rehabilitation communities. Only a person oblivious to the interests of people with physical disabilities for integration and independence could have missed predicting that reproduction would come to the forefront as a research topic for disability and rehabilitation research. With advances in medical technology and rehabilitation practices, individuals with physical disabilities are living longer and wish to engage in the full range of community activities, including marriage and procreation.

People with disabilities are not isolated from factors affecting the rest of society; factors such as aging and becoming a parent. The zeitgeist surrounding the baby boom of the late 1980s also affected people with physical disabilities. Should we as rehabilitation researchers not expect people with disabilities to want babies, to be parents, and to participate in all aspects of community living in the same ways that people without disabilities participate? The answer is, of course we should. As rehabilitation researchers, we have a responsibility to respond to the needs of people with physical disabilities for integration, independence, and increased personal freedom and choice by conducting a research program that enables a person with a disability to become empowered in all aspects of community living, including those that are the most personal and intimate. Studying reproductive issues and developing techniques and strategies that enable people with physical disabilities to become parents is a powerful affirmation of the commitment of the rehabilitation research and training community to the empowerment of individuals with physical disabilities.

The next step is to put forth a vision of the future direction of rehabilitation research and training in this significant area affecting the lives of people with disabilities.

Research in this area may be conceptualized as having three major strands. The first, where there is some research but not a great deal, is sexuality. The second, and the major focus of this volume, is in the area of reproduction. The third, and where NIDRR is placing its emphasis, is parenting and schooling. Let me take each of these topic areas separately.

The first is sexuality. Rehabilitation researchers will be examining sexual functioning as it relates to wider ranges of disabilities. The listing of disabilities in which there is ample research is staggeringly short with little depth of coverage. More research is needed, for example, on individuals with multiple disabilities, such as arthritis and diabetes or deaf-blindness. Additional research is needed that examines issues that may also be related to the aging process, such as post-polio syndrome and sexual functioning. There is a need for gender and role identification research among children with such disabilities as cerebral palsy, muscular dystrophy, and Down syndrome.

The second area of research is the area of reproduction. The topics of the chapters in this book certainly can serve as a listing of future directions, given the limited knowledge that we currently have. We need to know more about genetic factors related to reproductive failure. We need to know how trauma affects sexual and reproductive functioning. We need to know more about fertility and contraceptive choices for people with physical disabilities and how these choices are affected by medications and lifestyles of people with disabilities. We need to know more about the gynecologic and obstetric conditions of a number of disabilities and how they might be managed by the woman with the disability and her physician so that she can make choices about childbearing and sexual functioning.

The third area, an obvious consequence of reproduction, is parenting and education of the child. As society progresses to complete inclusion and integration of individuals with disabilities, more persons with disabilities have and will become parents. Parents with mental retardation, who have learning disabilities, who are blind, who have cognitive impairments due to a traumatic brain injury, who are deaf, who have mobility impairments, or who have other disabilities are like all other parents. They are their child's first teacher. Their newborn is theirs to love, to nurture, to assist in being all that that newborn might be, and to prepare for his or her role in society. However, parents with disabilities must frequently deal with the inexperience, lack of training, and, sometimes, skepticism of education, health, and childcare professionals; they must overcome self-doubts and adapt conventional parenting knowledge and resources to meet their individual circumstances. Often the needs of individual parents are recognized when it is too late, for example, when a parent with multiple sclerosis is losing custody of a child because he or she lacked the skills or support to provide basic childcare. In the area of school readiness, parents may need help with their own organizational or communication skills, as well as to learn techniques or assistive technologies to help their children to be ready for school.

Rehabilitation and disability research needs to provide research-based information and training materials that respond to the needs of parents with physical disabilities to be their child's first teacher. The research literature in this area is nonexistent. There is almost no information that is research based, for example, that provides guidance to parents who are congenitally blind on how to assist their sighted child in reading or to dunk a basketball. Similarly, for parents who are congenitally deaf, there is not information that is research based that enables them to provide their hearing child with the oral language and syntax and grammatical structure of the hearing community. For parents who use personal attendants, there is little research-based information on the best way for the child to learn mobility-related tasks, or for the parent with the mobility impairment to teach tasks such as toileting, dressing, and bathing or the role of the personal attendant.

Now back to the concern that the obvious not be ignored—the obvious is that people with disabilities are marrying and wishing to become parents. The rehabilitation and medical communities are dedicated to assisting them to achieve their goals. As more and more people with disabilities are successful in achieving their goals of marriage and procreation, the obvious becomes the birth, care, feeding, and teaching of the newborn. Rehabilitation research and training agendas must respond to this next step in the evolution of inclusion, independence, and integration of people with disabilities. Not to respond to this need would be a descriptor of a rehabilitation research and training community that is oblivious to changes in the disability community and oblivious to advances not only in medical sciences, but also to advances in the empowerment of people with disabilities.

I can assure you that NIDRR will not ignore the obvious and will not be oblivious to these changes in the disability community. It will continue to join with the disability and rehabilitation community in promoting a rehabilitation research and training agenda at NIDRR that promotes the independence, integration, and freedom of choice of people with disabilities. These factors will determine the future direction of rehabilitation research and training at NIDRR, especially as it relates to sexuality, reproduction, and parenting.

29

Future Directions for Research on Reproductive Issues for People with Physical Disabilities

David B. Gray and Aimée B. Schimmel

No body of scientific evidence has been accumulated that addresses fundamental questions facing people with disabilities who wish to form intimate friendships, have children, and be good parents. Indeed, the traditional approach to research on sexual behavior, reproduction, and parenting has focused on improving the understanding of normal development and on developing treatments for the health problems of people without physical disabilities. Such reductionistic, theoretical, and mechanistic research is frequently developed and conducted by a single discipline. These studies often explicitly exclude people with disabilities as subjects because they are at the extremes of the distributions in some, but not all, dimensions of physical structure, function, and behavior. The rationale for this approach to research study design is that inclusion of people with disabilities would limit the generality of the research findings. Sexual identity, sexuality, sexual behaviors, pregnancy, labor, delivery, and parenting are activities that have a great amount of variability within the "normal" population, much of it unexplained. Knowing what to expect when the entire body is functioning without impairment may be the first step in understanding how to cope with and treat individual differences that are associated with disability. Many of the findings discussed in this book were based on this approach and form the basis for some of the research directions contained in this chapter. Such an approach to designing research programs would prompt the question: What does the study of normal sexual, reproductive, and parenting behaviors have to contribute to people with disabilities? Does having a physical impairment in one organ or organ system necessarily mean that other body systems do not respond in a physiologically normal way? What are the comorbidities (co-occurrences) of different physical disabilities with sexual behaviors and reproductive capacity? Are these problems qualitatively different from those that confront people without disabilities?

The section of this book, "Personal Issues," provided chapters that described how individuals with disabilities adapt to reproduce and be good parents. The variations on "normal" solutions to functional limitations in these examples of adaptive behaviors illustrate the basis of a newly developing approach to scientifically studying problems. The paradigm shift in the direction of research is from a focus on topics of theoretical interest to the application of the scientific method to discover, develop, and implement the most effective and efficient solutions to problems. Problem-oriented research is characterized by client involvement, multidisciplinary cooperation, empirically derived hypotheses, functional analyses conditional on physical impairment, and environmentally (context) relevant study designs. This approach has a goal of constructing a scientifically valid and reliable database that provides a context for the determination of structures and functions that are adaptive ("normal" for successful problem resolution) for a specific physical impairment. For example, the range of successful adaptive behaviors (i.e., positive self-image), body structure modifications (i.e., internal or external prostheses), or environmental alterations (i.e., accessible bed) that people with spina bifida adopt will determine their low, moderate, or high quality of sexual and family life.

The paradigms and methods used by the research community interested in the reproductive issues for people with physical disabilities differ. The chapters of this book illustrate that all approaches are needed to bring better understanding of basic mechanistic issues and to develop improved functional solutions to pragmatic problems of everyday living and loving of people with physical disabilities. The following discussion provides a glimpse into possible directions that research may take in developing both new questions and answers to some of the challenges and opportunities described by the authors of this book.

CHILDHOOD

There is a lack of scientifically valid and reliable information on the development of sexual identities and sexual relationships of people with disabilities. Frequently, children with disabilities are not provided the education and access to socialization that would allow them to build healthy interpersonal relationships. This stage of maturation is essential to developing individual sexual identity as well as future associations with others of the same or opposite sex. Misconceptions of the potential growth and limits of the functional abilities of children with physical disabilities prevent parents, teachers, and health professionals from teaching children with disabilities about sex, birth control, sexually transmitted diseases, pregnancy, reproduction, and parenting or exposing them to basic experiences that help children develop gender identity. Research needs to be conducted that will develop a sound basis for implementing training by parents and educators that sensitively incorporates issues of sex education, health maintenance, and disease prevention.

Often, lack of access to buildings and recreational settings prevents children with disabilities from attending social functions where they would be able to make friends and acquire needed social skills. Studies of ways to make neighborhoods, schools, community centers, playgrounds, and transportation accessible to all people need to be encouraged. Effective methods should be developed to remove all physical, psychological, or financial barriers that hamper the abilities of any child or adult. Studies such as these and those listed below must take into consideration all issues that affect the people studied (e.g., socioeconomic background, level and type of disability, cultural background).

Research Issues

How do individuals born with a disability develop or acquire sexual identities and learn socially acceptable sexual behaviors?
What are the intersections of gender and disability?
How can scientific methods be used to improve the options for accessible homes, recreational facilities, and educational settings?

Research Directions

Develop effective, vigorous, explicit, and factual training tools for educating caregivers of children with disabilities.
Conduct longitudinal studies that assess development of individuals with and without disabilities.

Conduct comparative studies of the maturation of individuals with
disabilities in an accessible, inclusive environment with the
maturation of individuals with disabilities in an environment
that lacks specific aspects of accessibility.

SEXUALITY

The complex and controversial issues involved in the study of human sexuality are compounded when scientifically examining behavioral and physiologic measures of the sexual experience for people with physical disabilities is considered. Sexual pleasure may be
qualitatively and quantitatively different for people with physical
disabilities, but with the current level of research activity, little
hope can be held for developing answers for people with disabilities
who want to know if sexual experiences are possible, what can be
expected, and if interventions are available to improve their sexual
experiences.

Thirty years after Dr. Money's report on phantom orgasms of
males with spinal cord injuries, several researchers have begun to
address some fundamental issues involved in understanding the sexual experience of men and women with spinal cord injuries (SCI).
Drs. Whipple and Komisaruk challenge the commonly held view
that orgasm is not possible for people with spinal cord injury. They
use physiologic measures found to correlate with the cognitive aspects of orgasm in women without injury to serve as markers for
sexual arousal and orgasm in individuals with SCI. They postulate
that orgasm may not be an all-or-none phenomenon and that orgasm
may not be dependent totally upon tactile genital stimulation. The
differences and similarities of sexual response were compared for
women without disabilities and for those with spinal cord injury by
Dr. Marca Sipski. She provided a scientific framework for studying
sexual arousal in specific types of spinal cord injury in women that
includes both physiologic changes and self-reports of levels of sexual
pleasure.

A nearly neglected area of clinical services and research is the
sexuality of persons who have experienced traumatic brain injury.
Dr. Zasler described portions of the neural anatomy that if damaged
have serious consequences on both sexual relations (formation or
continuation of intimate relationships) and sexual performance
(masturbation to intercourse). He has suggested several important
clinical considerations for treatment and counseling that need verification through scientific study.

Research Issues

What are the sexual experiences of people with disabilities and their partners?

How does the sexual experience of people with disabilities compare pre- and post-injury? What are the differences and similarities?

Compared to others with similar or different impairments, what sexual behaviors provide maximum pleasure?

What are the sexual arousal stages of people with disabilities in relation to people without disabilities?

What are the mechanisms responsible for vaginal changes (e.g., lubrication), pain sensation alterations, and pleasurable touch sensitivities during sexual arousal in women with physical disabilities?

Can areas of the body other than the genital be conditioned to induce orgasm?

What is the relationship between the perception of muscular exertion and CNS-induced (generated) orgasm?

How does methylprednisolone treatment immediately post-injury affect sexual responsiveness?

How frequently are people with disabilities sexually exploited?

What can be done to prevent abuse and exploitation to persons with disabilities?

Research Directions

Encourage studies of people with different disabilities such as the assessment of the frequency and preferences of sexual activities of women and men with physical disabilities with the variables: age of onset of disability, level and type of physical impairment, gender preference, opportunity to date, marital status, spousal relationship, sexual position preferences, need for personal assistant care (e.g., bowel and bladder control, mobility, assistance in and out of bed), level of independence, self-image, culture, employment, and economic resources.

Develop a research program that will provide a basis for diagnosis and therapeutic interventions for people with disabilities and for those who counsel them.

Examine the effects of traumatic physical impairment on secretions of gonadal hormones, development of secondary sex characteristics, relay of sensory afferents from reproductive/sexual organs, brain function alterations in frontal involvement or hemispheric laterality, relationships between mood and sexuality,

increase or decrease in sexual intercourse post-injury, and non-
injured partner's sexual responsiveness.
Build a research program for the restoration of sexual functioning
based upon the recent animal studies that show promise
through grafting of fetal neurons, disinhibition of regeneration
of neurons by pharmacologic agents, and stimulation or enhanced sensitivity of touch sensation by pharmacologic agents.

CONTRACEPTION

Having a choice in controlling conception is important for all men
and women. Methods of contraception available to people without
disabilities have not been explored for use by people with physical
disabilities. Dr. Haseltine described a number of contraceptive devices and techniques available to people without physical disabilities. As she points out, the risks and benefits of these approaches to
contraception have not been described or evaluated for people with
physical disabilities. The following are some research issues that
need to be addressed, and directions for building future research
programs are suggested.

Research Issues

What forms of contraception can be used by people with different
physical impairments and functional abilities?
How effective are various contraceptives in preventing pregnancy in
women with disabilities?
What forms of contraception can be put in place independently by
men and women with disabilities?
Do different types of contraception carry special risks for infection,
skin ulcers, or induce hyperreflexia? Which types allow some
degree of privacy? Which types enhance or diminish sexual
arousal? Which types have detrimental long-term effects?
Can birth control pills be packaged in a manner that makes them
accessible to women with little finger dexterity?
How do women without finger dexterity check the intactness of an
IUD?
Does the lack of pain sensation prohibit use of common contraceptive devices or necessitate special precautions by people with
disabilities?
Is it safe to leave an external condom catheter (to control urine
output) on during intercourse?
What is the relationship between bladder infection and types of
contraception in both men and women?

Research Directions

Initiate a research program that develops contraceptive devices modified or redesigned for use by individuals with limited functional abilities, limited fine motor control, poor planning abilities, or limited mobility.

Study the frequency of common complications that have not been determined for people with disabilities, such as toxic shock syndrome and complications from the contraceptive sponge and birth control pills.

SEXUALLY TRANSMITTED DISEASES

The spread of AIDS has sensitized American society to the need for effective prevention of sexually transmitted diseases and the need for the development of treatments for all types of sexually transmitted diseases. Little attention has been paid to the risks of people with physical disabilities of contracting AIDS or any other disease that is transmitted through intimate human contact.

Research Issues

What are the causes and treatment of pelvic inflammatory disease (PID) in women with physical disabilities?

Can home use of temperature sensitive devices replace the traditional diagnostic indicator of pain to detect STD infection?

Are the base rates for STDs different for men and for women with neurogenic disorders?

What effects do drugs for the treatment of sexually transmitted diseases have on the fertility of men and women with physical disabilities?

Research Directions

Develop effective methods of assessing and treating sexually transmitted diseases in people with disabilities.

Assess the frequency and type of sexually transmitted diseases in people with different disabilities.

FERTILITY

Being able to have children is a life goal of many people with or without disability. Unfortunately, for many couples, having children is not possible. The reasons for infertility in people without disabilities are not well understood. With the added complexity of a physical impairment, diagnosing the cause of infertility is even more difficult. Common treatments for urinary tract infections, hyper-reflexia, and other conditions secondary to primary physical impairments may reduce fertility. The methods for the production of sperm reduce their viability. The effects of these methods on the genes contained in sperm may need study. The comorbidity of unknown infertility and physical disability challenges the research and clinical communities to consider idiopathic infertility when designing studies or prescribing treatments. The base rates for co-occurrence need to be determined.

Research Issues

What effects do different bladder emptying routines have on spermatogenesis and the viability of sperm?

For individuals with frequent urinary tract infections, does the repeated use of certain drugs reduce fertility?

What are the pharmacokinetics of drugs on sperm viability in men who are immobile? Does immobility preclude the use of some drugs or merely mean the dose, rate, or site of administration need to be considered?

Are treatments used for repair or protection of sperm in men without physical disability useful for treatment of sperm in men with physical disabilities?

Does spinal or head injury incite antibody formation that affects sperm formation and viability?

Are testosterone or gonadal replacement therapies appropriate for men with physical disabilities?

What is the differential effectiveness of sexual counseling, implants, or surgical changes on sexual activity?

Given that electrostimulation of the cavernous nerves works in animals, is this technique appropriate for human trials?

Why do men with bowel diversion have a sense of sexual attractiveness greater than those with bladder diversion?

What is the frequency and nature of the complications of penile prostheses in terms of device failure, perforation, infection, or pain?

What are the advantages, disadvantages, and acceptance rates of inflatable versus semirigid penile implants?

What complications arise from the self-injection of papaverine or prostaglandin?

What are the long-term effects of the use of electroejaculation?

How can the major negative side effects (autonomic hyperreflexia and reactions to drugs to control hypertension) of electroejaculation be controlled?

Can the positive side effects of electroejaculation (reduced spasticity) be utilized to improve therapeutic options for controlling spasticity?

Research Directions

Develop methods to improve and simplify electroejaculation so that it can be used in settings more private than clinics.

Investigate the impact that medications and antibiotics have on fertility.

Evaluate the effects of common medications for disability conditions on sexual response.

Develop devices that allow for spontaneity and that are attractive and manageable.

Continue to refine techniques to achieve erection in males with SCI.

Focus on infertility in males with disabilities (e.g., difficulties that males with SCI have in achieving enough viable sperm for insemination).

MARRIAGE

The possibility of marriage for individuals growing up with a disability was often discouraged. Several chapters describe the responses of parents and friends to people with disabilities who announced their intentions to marry. Increasingly, people with disabilities have chosen to marry and are now role models for the next generation. The description of the decision to marry and the nature of the spousal relationships in a marriage where one or both of the partners has a disability provides a good base for developing research projects to provide guidance to people with disabilities who choose to get married and to those who counsel them.

The problems of adjustment to new lifestyles and new spousal roles in people who were injured after marriage have rarely been the focus of scientific studies. The transition from a mutually interdependent relationship to a relationship with a high dependency factor can strain even the best of marriages. Developing strategies for spousal adjustment, reducing personal assistance requirements, and rebuilding interdependent relationships will help marriages withstand the effects of a traumatic injury.

Research Issues

Does some type of counseling help individuals with disabilities prepare for the possibility of marriage?

What types of counseling are needed and when? Are they effective?
Does peer counseling provide sufficient information for marriage
 decisions?
What compensatory skills does the spouse of the person with a
 disability need to acquire or bring to a relationship?
What steps can be taken to effectively prepare and sustain the
 spouse of a traumatically injured partner for a substantially
 different lifestyle and altered marital role?

Research Directions

Conduct studies of the effectiveness of different types of counseling
 preparatory to marriage, after a traumatic injury to a spouse,
 and during periods of stress induced by functional needs of the
 spouse with a disability.

PREGNANCY, LABOR, AND DELIVERY

The need for research on the special concerns of women with disabilities who have children is becoming increasingly important as
more women with disabilities choose to have children. This decision to have a child could be made significantly easier if the problems specific to the pregnancies of women with disabilities were
better understood, new treatments developed, and knowledge of existing treatments more widely disseminated. Pregnant women with
disabilities encounter changes that force them to modify their daily
living activities. Their bodily sensations may change, their endurance and respiratory capacity may decrease, and their bodies'
abilities to regulate temperature may fluctuate. These discomforts
are common during the pregnancy of all women, but may be exacerbated by a disability. As the fetus grows, the mother is increasingly
impaired. She may outgrow her wheelchair or find it difficult to
utilize her assistive devices. She may also experience autonomic
hyperreflexia, which may physically and psychologically impair her
ability to function.

It is essential for physicians and other members of the woman's
medical team to communicate regularly with each other and the
patient. These health professionals should acquire training related
to the special needs of their patients as well as listen to their patients. Physicians should publish the results of their experiences,
making them available to other health care professionals who may
have patients with disabilities. Women with disabilities should also
communicate with other women with disabilities who have given

birth. These mothers are excellent sources of guidance, reassurance, and educational tips on methods to overcome traditional barriers.

Research Issues

What medications are often taken during pregnancy and what are the possible effects on the fetus?

Must bladder management regimes necessary during pregnancy be continued after a woman has given birth?

What are the complication rates in the pregnancies of women with disabilities and how do they compare with those in women without disabilities?

Which complications are universal to pregnancy and which are specific to disabilities?

When does hyperreflexia occur during pregnancy? How severe is it?

When and how can intervention safely be performed for the mother and the child?

What is the frequency of bladder infections? What are safe treatments for bladder infections during pregnancy?

How can transfers to and from wheelchairs be safely made without increasing the risk of skin abrasions and breakdown?

Is carpal tunnel syndrome due to overuse of wrists during pregnancy frequent and how is it prevented?

What changes develop in spasticity during pregnancy and do pharmaceutical interventions carry significant risk?

What exercise is possible during pregnancy for women with disabilities?

Do sensory changes during pregnancy contribute to better understanding of pain inhibition (i.e., decreased pain during intercourse while pregnant accompanied by more pleasurable sensation)?

How can community physicians, nurses, and therapists be better informed about effective clinical treatments for pregnant women with disabilities?

What are the early indicators of the onset of labor?

Can Lamaze courses be adjusted for disability?

What constitutes an accessible office and hospital in terms of examination tables (bed versus table) and positions for examination or delivery?

What are the attitudes of staff at hospitals toward pregnant women with disabilities? Can training programs include information on treatment of pregnant women with disabilities?

Do adjustments need to be made in the type and dosage of the anesthesia typically used in delivery?

When is a c-section justified? What are the indications for its use?
How and why is arthritic pain reduced during pregnancy?
When should delivery be induced?
What are safe delivery techniques?

Research Directions

Assess the needs and procedures to alleviate the discomfort of women with disabilities during pregnancy regarding medication, care, assistive devices, and physiologic changes.

Focus on infertility in women with disabilities.

Develop practical and scientifically based training programs for birthing, controlling autonomic hyperreflexia, dispensing medications, monitoring during pregnancy, and the need for cesarean sections.

Evaluate methods of delivery for women with all types of disabilities.

Research the anesthesia and delivery needs of women with disabilities.

Encourage the development of devices and materials that reduce the problems of women with disabilities who are pregnant.

PARENTING

Studies of individuals with disabilities who have successfully developed sexual identities and married and raised children are missing from the research literature. The attitudes of family, neighbors, and professionals toward parenting by individuals with disabilities has often been negative. Clearly, individuals with disabilities can be effective parents. There is a need for studies that explore the strengths and weaknesses of parenting by people with disabilities and of research on when, where, and how much, if any, social support is needed. The type of support that best fits the needs of the individual should be explored in terms of informal and formal sources. Carol Ann Roberson's account of prejudice and negative expectations cries out for effective strategies for educating all Americans on the rights and ability of people with disabilities to have families.

The primary care providers in traditional and single-parent families are women. Yet, few studies of mothers with SCI, head injury, spina bifida, cerebral palsy, or other common disabilities have appeared in the scientific literature. Based on the assumption of poor parenting by women with disabilities, social service agencies continue to remove children from women with disabilities. The mothering skills described in this volume illustrate that while the basic functions of mothering do not change with disability the manner in which they are performed does. Most of the solutions described by the authors in this book were developed through trial and error. Books on parenting for mothers without physical disabilities do not prepare the mothers with disabilities for the special challenges they face. Most of the scientific literature on mothering explicitly excludes women with disabilities. Can a research effort be made to provide a basis for best solutions to the problems faced by mothers with disabilities?

Some of the questions raised by chapters in this book that should be addressed by research are described in the following lists.

DECISION TO BECOME A PARENT

Research Issues

What are the attitudes of people without disabilities toward the parenting rights and abilities of people with disabilities?
How do people with disabilities develop the skills for family management?

Research Directions

Conduct demographic studies that provide descriptions of populations of parents with disabilities.
Examine the variables influencing the decision of an individual with a disability to adopt or to give birth.

PARENTING ABILITIES

Research Issues

How does the factor of disability compare to personality, education, finances, employment, culture, or other variables that may predict success in parenting?
Is severity of impairment a significant factor in limiting or eliminating some aspects of parenting?
What early mothering skills (i.e., diapering, holding, bonding, nursing, communicating) need to be studied to determine effective methods for the acquisition of these important behaviors?
For each type of physical impairment, what aspects of parenting require personal assistance or technical devices?
What are the characteristics of successful fathers and mothers with disabilities?

Does disability predict poor or dangerous parenting?

How do the theoretical models used in studies of normal parenting apply to parenting with a disability?

What relationships are difficult, different, or similar in parents and children with and without disabilities?

Research Directions

Begin longitudinal comparative studies of families, where one or both parents has a disability, that examine the decision to become parents; the types of parenting skills that develop; and the form, level, and source of assistance needed to parent.

INFLUENCES ON CHILDREN

Research Issues

Does mother–child bonding occur, and is it different for mothers with disabilities?

What skills do children with parents with a disability need to develop that are different from children with parents without disabilities?

Is it possible that children of women with disabilities are better equipped to face life challenges?

What communicative, disciplinary, reinforcing, intellectual, motivational, or emotional differences exist in children with a mother or father who has a disability?

Research Directions

Develop longitudinal approaches to the study of children of parents with disabilities to clarify the importance of having a parent with a disability in relation to other factors including personality, education, finances, employment, and culture.

Encourage the field of health economics to study the costs of adopting children, including health care insurance issues.

CONCLUSION

The extent of problems associated with reproduction by people with physical disabilities are clearly described in the personal perspectives presented in this book. The personal accounts illustrate the importance of continued support for research and training to enhance sexuality, reproduction, adoption, and parenting for people with physical disabilities. Advances in understanding normal gender identity, sexuality, marriage, reproduction, and parenting can provide scientists with an excellent knowledge base for developing studies of these topics in populations of persons with disabilities. The research issues and directions listed in this chapter point to a rich area of inquiry for scientific attention.

EPILOGUE

Six months after the conference on which this book was based, Congress passed and the President signed into law P.L. 101-613. This bill, The National Institutes of Health Amendment of 1990, contained the legislation authorizing the creation of a National Center for Medical Rehabilitation Research (NCMRR) within the National Institute of Child Health and Human Development at the National Institutes of Health. The mission of the NCMRR is to support research and research training, disseminate health information, and coordinate other programs with respect to the rehabilitation of individuals with physical disabilities resulting from diseases or disorders of the neurologic, musculoskeletal, cardiovascular, pulmonary, or other physiologic systems.

One of NCMRR's first initiatives was to set aside approximately $1 million for research on issues related to reproduction by individuals with physical disabilities. The aim of this initiative is to encourage scientists to conduct research that reestablishes, improves, or assists the reproductive function in people with physical disabilities. Many of the research directions outlined in this chapter are part of the effort to stimulate new research in this field. One outcome of this effort is the funding of six research studies that include: a comparative study of testicular-epididymal dysfunction in men and animals, a standardized protocol for the study of electro-ejaculation of men with spinal cord injury, the impact of disability on the sexuality of women with disabilities, the female sexual response using physiologic measures, the control of spasticity and attenuation of pain through the elicitation of sexual responses in women with spinal cord injury, and basic research on autonomic innervation of the reproductive tract.

The chapters of this book contain many more issues that need the attention of the scientific and broader social community. Numerous changes are needed in our society to allow each person with a disability to develop a sexual identity, to express sexuality, to decide to marry, to choose to have children, and to become a parent. This agenda requires significant alterations in attitudes and approaches to people with disabilities. It is the responsibility of the social, applied, clinical, and basic research scientists to provide effective alternatives to unsatisfactory treatment practices. This book is, to paraphrase Winston Churchill, not the beginning but the end of the beginning of dialogues between people with disabilities and scientists who have the interest, skill, and dedication to resolve some of the reproductive issues faced by people with disabilities.

Index

Page numbers followed by "t" or "f" indicate tables or figures, respectively.